"Knowing is not enough; we must apply.
Willing is not enough; we must do."

—Goethe

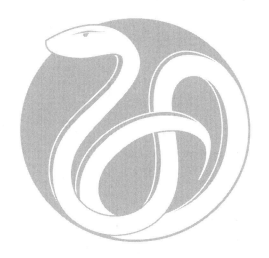

INSTITUTE OF MEDICINE
OF THE NATIONAL ACADEMIES

Advising the Nation. Improving Health.

THE NATIONAL ACADEMIES
Advisers to the Nation on Science, Engineering, and Medicine

The **National Academy of Sciences** is a private, nonprofit, self-perpetuating society of distinguished scholars engaged in scientific and engineering research, dedicated to the furtherance of science and technology and to their use for the general welfare. Upon the authority of the charter granted to it by the Congress in 1863, the Academy has a mandate that requires it to advise the federal government on scientific and technical matters. Dr. Ralph J. Cicerone is president of the National Academy of Sciences.

The **National Academy of Engineering** was established in 1964, under the charter of the National Academy of Sciences, as a parallel organization of outstanding engineers. It is autonomous in its administration and in the selection of its members, sharing with the National Academy of Sciences the responsibility for advising the federal government. The National Academy of Engineering also sponsors engineering programs aimed at meeting national needs, encourages education and research, and recognizes the superior achievements of engineers. Dr. Wm. A. Wulf is president of the National Academy of Engineering.

The **Institute of Medicine** was established in 1970 by the National Academy of Sciences to secure the services of eminent members of appropriate professions in the examination of policy matters pertaining to the health of the public. The Institute acts under the responsibility given to the National Academy of Sciences by its congressional charter to be an adviser to the federal government and, upon its own initiative, to identify issues of medical care, research, and education. Dr. Harvey V. Fineberg is president of the Institute of Medicine.

The **National Research Council** was organized by the National Academy of Sciences in 1916 to associate the broad community of science and technology with the Academy's purposes of furthering knowledge and advising the federal government. Functioning in accordance with general policies determined by the Academy, the Council has become the principal operating agency of both the National Academy of Sciences and the National Academy of Engineering in providing services to the government, the public, and the scientific and engineering communities. The Council is administered jointly by both Academies and the Institute of Medicine. Dr. Ralph J. Cicerone and Dr. Wm. A. Wulf are chair and vice chair, respectively, of the National Research Council.

www.national-academies.org

COMMITTEE ON FOOD MARKETING AND
THE DIETS OF CHILDREN AND YOUTH

J. MICHAEL MCGINNIS *(Chair)*, Institute of Medicine, Washington, DC

DANIEL R. ANDERSON, Department of Psychology, University of
Massachusetts, Amherst

J. HOWARD BEALES III, School of Business, George Washington
University, Washington, DC

DAVID V. B. BRITT, Sesame Workshop *(emeritus)*, Amelia Island, FL

SANDRA L. CALVERT, Children's Digital Media Center, Georgetown
University, Washington, DC

KEITH T. DARCY, Ethics Officer Association, Waltham, MA

AIMÉE DORR, Graduate School of Education and Information Studies,
University of California, Los Angeles

LLOYD J. KOLBE, Department of Applied Health Science, Indiana
University, Bloomington

DALE L. KUNKEL, Department of Communication, University of
Arizona, Tucson

PAUL KURNIT, KidShop, Kurnit Communications, and Lubin School of
Business at Pace University, Chappaqua, New York

ROBERT C. POST, Yale Law School, New Haven, CT

RICHARD SCHEINES, Department of Philosophy, Carnegie Mellon
University, Pittsburgh, PA

FRANCES H. SELIGSON, Nutrition Consultant, Hershey, PA

MARY STORY, Division of Epidemiology, School of Public Health,
University of Minnesota, Minneapolis

ELLEN A. WARTELLA, Office of the Executive Vice Chancellor and
Provost, University of California, Riverside

JEROME D. WILLIAMS, Department of Advertising, University of
Texas, Austin

Liaison from the Food and Nutrition Board

NANCY F. KREBS, Department of Pediatrics, University of Colorado
Health Sciences Center, Denver

Staff

JENNIFER APPLETON GOOTMAN, Study Director
VIVICA I. KRAAK, Study Director
LESLIE J. SIM, Research Associate
SHANNON L. WISHAM, Research Associate
AMIEE M. ADASCZIK, Health Science Intern (January 2005 through May 2005)
KELLY D. HORTON, Christine Mirzyan Science and Technology Policy Fellow (June 2005 through August 2005)

Staff
LINDA D. MEYERS, Director
GERALDINE KENNEDO, Administrative Assistant
ANTON BANDY, Financial Associate
ELISABETH RIMAUD, Financial Associate (through May 2005)

IOM boards do not review or approve individual reports and are not asked to endorse conclusions and recommendations. The responsibility for the content of the reports rests with the authoring committee and the institution.

Staff
ROSEMARY CHALK, Director
WENDY KEENAN, Senior Program Assistant (through April 2005)
DEBORAH JOHNSON, Senior Program Assistant

Reviewers

This report has been reviewed in draft form by individuals chosen for their diverse perspectives and technical expertise, in accordance with procedures approved by the National Research Council's Report Review Committee. The purpose of this independent review is to provide candid and critical comments that will assist the institution in making its published report as sound as possible and to ensure that the report meets institutional standards for objectivity, evidence, and responsiveness to the study charge. The review comments and draft manuscript remain confidential to protect the integrity of the deliberative process. We wish to thank the following individuals for their review of this report:

MARK P. BECKER, Office of the Executive Vice President and Provost, University of South Carolina, Columbia

ODILIA BERMUDEZ, Friedman School of Nutrition Science and Policy, Tufts University, Boston, MA

RONETTE BRIEFEL, Mathematica Policy Research, Inc., Washington, DC

KATE CLANCY, Union of Concerned Scientists, Washington, DC

JANICE DODDS, School of Public Health, University of North Carolina, Chapel Hill

ADAM DREWNOWSKI, Department of Epidemiology, University of Washington, Seattle

RACHEL GELLER, The Geppetto Group, New York, NY

JAMES O. HILL, Center for Human Nutrition, University of
    Colorado, Denver
DONNA JOHNSON, Center for Public Health Nutrition, University
    of Washington, Seattle
MILTON KOTELCHUCK, Department of Maternal and Child
    Health, Boston University School of Public Health, MA
SHIRIKI K. KUMANYIKA, Center for Clinical Epidemiology and
    Biostatistics, University of Pennsylvania School of Medicine,
    Philadelphia
MICHAEL MUDD, Kraft Foods *(emeritus)*, Chicago, IL
JOHN C. PETERS, Food and Beverage Technology, Procter &
    Gamble Company, Cincinnati, OH
BARRY M. POPKIN, School of Public Health, University of North
    Carolina, Chapel Hill
JULIET SCHOR, Department of Sociology, Boston College, MA
STEPHEN D. SUGARMAN, School of Law, University of California,
    Berkeley
JANET TENNEY, Alexandria, VA
LARRY WALLACK, School of Community Health, College of Urban
    and Public Affairs, Portland State University, OR

Although the reviewers listed above have provided many constructive
comments and suggestions, they were not asked to endorse the conclusions
or recommendations nor did they see the final draft of the report before its
release. The review of this report was overseen by JOHANNA DWYER,
Office of Disease Prevention, National Institutes of Health, and ELENA
NIGHTINGALE, Institute of Medicine, the National Academies.

Appointed by the National Research Council, they were responsible for
making certain that an independent examination of this report was carried
out in accordance with institutional procedures and that all review comments were carefully considered. Responsibility for the final content of this
report rests entirely with the authoring committee and the institution.

Preface

Marketing works. It is a primary engine of our economy and its content can sometimes give us a glimpse of the forces shaping our futures. How marketing affects the perspectives and behaviors of our children and youth, including their diets, has been a subject of active discussion and debate for more than three decades, beginning in a time when marketing could generally be characterized in terms of the advertising done through the traditional media—television, radio, print. Times have changed markedly. Marketing is now a regular feature of virtually all the venues and communication vehicles we encounter in our daily lives. Television advertising remains the dominant form of marketing reaching children and youth that is formally tracked, but the expansion of alternative advertising and marketing strategies is evolving rapidly.

Against the backdrop of pressing public concern over the rapid and widespread increase in the prevalence of childhood obesity, Congress, through the FY2004 Health, Labor, and Education Committee appropriation, directed the Centers for Disease Control and Prevention (CDC) to undertake a study of the role that marketing of food and beverages may play as a determinant of the nutritional status of children and youth, and how marketing approaches might be marshaled as a remedy. The CDC turned to the Institute of Medicine (IOM) of the National Academies to conduct this study, a natural corollary to the IOM report released in 2004, *Preventing Childhood Obesity: Health in the Balance.*

The IOM Committee on Food Marketing and the Diets of Children and Youth is pleased to present this report, *Food Marketing to Children and*

Youth: Threat or Opportunity? The report represents the most comprehensive review to date of the scientific studies designed to assess the influence of marketing on the nutritional beliefs, choices, practices, and outcomes for children and youth. In conducting our study, the committee not only developed and applied a rigorous analytic framework to the assessment of the relevant scientific literature but also undertook an extensive review of the nutritional status and trends for children and youth, what is known about the full range of factors that influence their dietary patterns, the broad and evolving food and beverage marketing environment, and the relevant policy levers that might be brought to bear to improve our children's nutritional status. Important and relevant findings from our committee's review are distributed throughout the body of the text. A summary list of the findings is provided in the final chapter, along with the committee's overall conclusions and recommendations.

This report notes that the prevailing pattern of food and beverage products marketed to children and youth has been high in total calories, sugar, salt, fat, and low in nutrients. A dietary profile that mirrors the products marketed would put our children and youth at risk for the types of nutritional problems that we see occurring today—increasing rates of obesity, and inadequacies of certain important micronutrients—and for the development of various serious chronic diseases later in life. Dietary choices are made in the midst of myriad social, cultural, and economic environmental influences. The focus of the committee was on the role of food and beverage marketing as one of these intersecting influences.

In our review, the committee faced certain challenges related to the nature of the available research material. First, virtually all of the published scientific research has focused on advertising—and television advertising in particular. While television maintains an important place in food and beverage marketing, industry strategies have moved far beyond television advertising. Second, much of the research underpinning the development and implementation of food and beverage marketing activities is proprietary and unpublished, and, given the National Academies' requirement that information used be in the public domain, a large amount of marketing research was unavailable for the committee's use.

Nonetheless, ample information and studies were available for the committee to draw certain key conclusions, including that television advertising influences the food preferences, purchase requests, and diets, at least of children under the age of 12 years, and is associated with the increased rates of obesity among children and youth. The committee could not state the relationship in quantitative terms, but it is clear that even a small effect across the entire population would represent an important impact. Although we could not draw conclusions about the impact of the broader marketing environment, it is highly likely that the influences reinforce those seen from advertising. Moreover, the committee found that, for an issue of this potential magnitude, there was both a need and an opportunity for substantially more industry and government attention and action—and cooperation—on an agenda to turn food and beverage marketing forces toward better diets for American children and youth. These recommendations are detailed in Chapter 7.

A word is indicated about the members of the IOM Committee on Food Marketing and the Diets of Children and Youth. Befitting the breadth of the topic, this was a committee of unusually varied expertise, experience, and perspective. It was, in addition, a committee that engaged the task with extraordinary energy, commitment, and resolve—both to undertake a rigorous assessment and to do it cooperatively. Shared leadership has been a central feature of the work, as members worked both individually and in groups to ensure that each dimension of the task was skillfully executed. The process has been thorough, the discussions vigorous, and the report represents a consensus document in the best sense of the word. We believe readers will find the documentation to be extensive, the evidence analyses to be seminal, and the findings to be carefully considered.

As is so often the case with these studies, vital guidance and tireless energy were contributed to the work by the co-study directors, Jennifer Gootman and Vivica Kraak, who received highly skilled support from research associates Leslie Sim and Shannon Wisham. We are also grateful for the careful shepherding of the study by the directors of the two sponsoring boards: Linda Meyers of the Food and Nutrition Board and Rosemary Chalk of the Board on Children, Youth, and Families.

There can be few matters of such compelling importance as the health of America's children and youth. The committee is grateful for the opportunity to contribute this report as a resource for insight and action, and we are hopeful that its recommendations will help turn the threat of the current trends into an opportunity for change.

> J. Michael McGinnis, *Chair*
> Committee on Food Marketing
> and the Diets of Children and Youth

Acknowledgments

Beyond the hard work of the committee and IOM project staff, this report reflects contributions from various other individuals and groups that we want to acknowledge.

The committee greatly benefited from the opportunity for discussion with the individuals who made presentations and attended the committee's workshops and meetings including: Leann Birch, Brady Darvin, Mary Engle, Lance Friedmann, Marvin Goldberg, Bob McKinnon, Elizabeth Moore, Alisa Morris, Marlena Peleo-Lazar, Ken Powell, Morris Reid, Victoria Rideout, Marva Smalls, Ellen Taaffe, as well as all those who spoke during the open forum (Appendix H).

This study was sponsored by the U.S. Department of Health and Human Services' Centers for Disease Control and Prevention. We wish to thank William Dietz, Casey Hannan, Barbara Polhamus, and their colleagues for their support and guidance on the committee's task.

We appreciate the extensive contribution of Courtney Carpenter, Kunter Gunasti, Alan Mathios, Marvin Goldberg, and Edward Palmer for authoring commissioned papers that were used as background in the report. University students Amiee Adasczik, Frederick Eberhardt, Emily Evans, Shimada Hall, Kelly Horton, Glynnis Johnson, Linda Kao, Heather Kirkorian, and Meghan Malloy all provided outstanding assistance in reviewing literature and organizing data for the committee. We also thank the University of Texas at Austin students for their contribution to the product proliferation analysis working paper cited in the report.

The committee acknowledges the contribution of Collier Shannon Scott and Georgetown Economic Services that shared three brief and relevant summaries of analyses—two of which had been prepared for the Grocery Manufacturers Association (GMA) and the Association of National Advertising, and the third was a collaborative endeavor between four GMA food and beverage company members—General Mills, Inc., Kellogg Company, Kraft Foods, Inc., and PepsiCo—which collectively responded to specific questions about advertising and marketing trends and company activities that were requested by the committee. We also thank Nielsen Media Research and Nielsen//Net Ratings, The Geppetto Group, KidShop, Strottman International, and Yankelovich for sharing relevant data. There were other colleagues who provided useful international data and reports to the committee: Martin Caraher in the United Kingdom, Corinna Hawkes, Filippa von Haartman in Sweden, Gitte Laub Hansen in Denmark, and Anne-Marie Hamelin in Quebec.

There are others at the IOM who provided support to this project: Wendy Keenan for logistical support; Anton Bandy, Elisabeth Rimaud, and Gary Walker for financial oversight; and guidance from Clyde Behney, Jennifer Bitticks, Mark Chesnek, Jim Jensen, Jennifer Otten, and Christine Stencel. The report has been greatly enhanced by the public relations and creative work of Spectrum Science Communications staff including Erika Borodinsky, Susannah Budington, Rosalba Cano, Victoria Kirker, Pamela Lippincott, Leslie Priest, Susie Tappouni, Mark Trinkaus, Clarissa Vandersteen, and Jane Woo. We thank them for their creative efforts.

J. Michael McGinnis, *Chair*
Committee on Food Marketing
and the Diets of Children and Youth

Contents

Executive Summary

Creating an environment in which children and youth can grow up healthy should be a very high priority for the nation. Yet the prevailing pattern of food and beverage marketing to children in America represents, at best, a missed opportunity, and, at worst, a direct threat to the health of the next generation. Dietary patterns that begin in childhood give shape to the health profiles of Americans at all ages. Because these patterns reflect the intersecting influences of our cultural, social, and economic environments, ensuring that these environments support good health is a fundamental responsibility, requiring leadership and action from all sectors.

The dramatic rise in the number of U.S. children and youth who are obese, have type 2 diabetes, and are at increased risk for developing obesity and related chronic diseases in adulthood, is a matter of national concern. Obesity among children and youth has more than tripled over the past four decades—from about 5 percent in 6- to 19-year-olds in the 1960s to 16 percent in 1999–2002. More than 9 million U.S. children and youth are obese and another 15 percent are at risk for becoming obese. The prevalence of type 2 diabetes among children and youth—previously known as "adult-onset" diabetes—has more than doubled in the past decade.

As a society, we have moved well beyond the era when our dietary focus was on ensuring caloric sufficiency to meet basic metabolic needs. We are now confronted with nutritional inadequacy of a different sort. Diets that are high in calories and other constituents such as saturated fats, and low in certain nutrients are putting our children and youth at risk for diseases later in life, such as heart disease, stroke, circulatory problems, some cancers, diabetes, and osteoporosis. Parents, communities, the government, public health sector, health care systems, and private enterprise all face significant challenges to create an environment for our children and youth that turns the course and enhances their prospects for healthy lives.

DIETARY PATTERNS FOR CHILDREN AND YOUTH

Health-related behaviors such as eating habits and physical activity patterns develop early in life and often extend into adulthood. A healthful and balanced diet provides recommended amounts of nutrients and other food components to promote normal growth and development, reduce chronic disease risk, and foster appropriate energy balance and a healthy weight trajectory. Yet the diets of America's children and adolescents depart substantially from recommended patterns that puts their health at risk. Although there have been some improvements with respect to the intake of certain micronutrients, overall our children and youth are not achieving basic nutritional goals. They are consuming excess calories and added sugars and have higher than recommended intakes of sodium, total fat, and saturated fats. Moreover, dietary intakes of whole grains, fiber, calcium, potassium, magnesium, and vitamin E are well below recommendations and are sufficiently low to warrant concern. Adolescent girls and low-income toddlers are especially at risk for inadequate intakes of iron.

The result is that the health of children and adolescents is not as good as it should or could be. Because of improvements in immunization levels, injury rates, and the availability of and access to children's services, death and disease rates for children are generally low. But more sedentary lifestyles and diets that are too high in calories, fat, sugars, and sodium, are putting children's futures at risk. Those who are poor face the greatest risk, as a result of their already greater health, social, and nutrition disparities.

If children and youth of all income and ethnic groups are to develop dietary patterns that will provide lifelong health promotion and disease prevention benefits, their diets will need to change significantly. They need to increase their intakes of fruits, vegetables, legumes, whole grains, and low-fat dairy products, and reduce their intakes of high-calorie and low-nutrient foods and beverages, including snack foods and sweetened beverages.

The dietary and related health patterns of children and youth result from the interplay of many factors (Figure ES-1)—genetics and biology, culture and values, economic status, physical and social environments, and commercial and media environments—all of which, apart from genetic predispositions, have undergone significant transformation over the past three decades. Among the various environmental influences, none has more rapidly assumed a central socializing role for young people than the media,

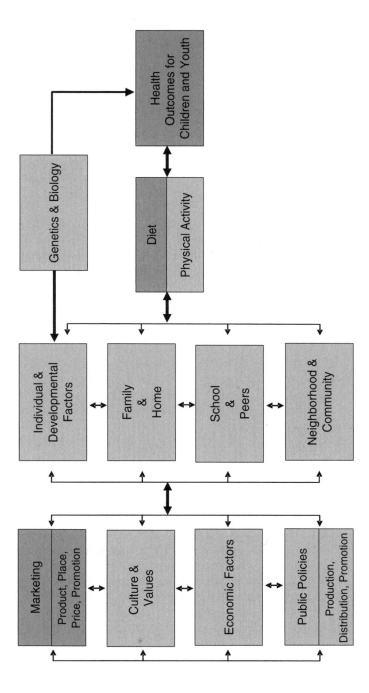

FIGURE ES-1 Influences on the diets and related health outcomes of children and youth.

in its multiple forms. With its growth in variety and penetration has come a concomitant growth in the promotion of branded food and beverage products in the marketplace, and the influence addressed in this report on the diet and related health patterns of children and youth.

FOOD AND BEVERAGE MARKETING

The commercial advertising and marketing of foods and beverages influences the diets and health of children and youth. With annual sales now approaching $900 billion, the food, beverage, and restaurant industries take a central place in the American marketplace. Total marketing investments by these industries have not been clearly identified, although advertising alone accounted for more than $11 billion in industry expenditures in 2004, including $5 billion for television advertising. Television remains the primary promotional vehicle for measured media marketing, but a shift is occurring toward unmeasured sales promotion, such as marketing through product placement, character licensing, special events, in-school activities, and advergames. In fact, only approximately 20 percent of all food and beverage marketing in 2004 was devoted to advertising on television, radio, print, billboards, or the Internet.

Children and youth represent a primary focus of food and beverage marketing initiatives. Between 1994 and 2004, the rate of increase in the introduction of new food and beverage products targeted to children and youth substantially outpaced the rate for those targeting the total market. An estimated more than $10 billion per year is spent for all types of food and beverage marketing to children and youth in America. Moreover, although some very recent public announcements by some in the industry suggest an interest in change, the preponderance of the products introduced and marketed to children and youth have been high in total calories, sugars, salt, and fat, and low in nutrients.

How this marketing affects children and youth is the focus of this report. The process begins early in life. Children develop consumer socialization skills as they physically and cognitively mature. Over the span of ages 2–11 years, they develop consumption motives and values as they are exposed to commercial activities; they develop knowledge about advertising, products, brands, pricing, and shopping; and they begin to develop strategies for purchase requests and negotiation. The family is the first socializing agent, as parents and older siblings act as sources of information and provide social support and pressure that affect children's behaviors.

Media now have a more central role in socializing today's children and youth than ever before. Advertising and marketing messages reach young consumers through a variety of vehicles—broadcast and cable television, radio, magazines, computers through the Internet, music, cell phones—and in many different venues—homes, schools, child-care settings, grocery stores, shopping malls, theaters, sporting events, and even airports. Virtually all children ages 2–18 years now live in households with a television, and more than half of today's children and youth report that their families have no rules for television viewing. Children and youth under the age of 18 years comprise 20 percent of those using the Internet. Myriad marketing approaches are now available, and targeted and integrated marketing has become more prevalent.

With new outlets, attractions, and tools, children and youth represent a powerful demographic force. Collectively, children and youth spend more than $200 billion annually, and they influence many food and beverage purchases beyond those they make directly. Although children's choices are strongly influenced by their parents and siblings, they are increasingly making decisions at younger ages in the marketplace, either in ways that are independent of parental guidance, or as agents influencing the choices and purchasing decisions of their parents and caregivers. Of the various items that children and youth purchase and influence, food and beverages— particularly candy, carbonated soft drinks, and salty snacks—consistently represent the leading categories.

An important issue in discussions about the influence of food and beverage advertising and marketing reaching children and youth relates to the stages of discernment. Before a certain age, children lack the defenses, or skills, to discriminate commercial from noncommercial content, or to attribute persuasive intent to advertising. Children generally develop these skills at about age 8 years, but children as old as 11 years may not activate their defenses unless explicitly cued to do so. Concern about young children's limited ability to comprehend the nature and purpose of advertising, and about the appropriateness or impact of food marketing to which younger children might be exposed, led to a Federal Trade Commission (FTC) rulemaking process in the late 1970s on the question of whether advertising to young children should be restricted or banned as a protective measure. Congress eventually intervened, and the FTC terminated the rulemaking in 1981.

The question persists, however, about the effects of advertising exposure on children, and it has been deepened and broadened by a developing appreciation of the influence of environmental signals on personal behaviors, regardless of age; by the expansion and the nature of youth and child-oriented food and beverage products in the marketplace; by the dramatic augmentation of strategic tools and vehicles for marketing activities; and, in particular, by concern about the relation of the marketing environment, among the multiple influences, to the rapid growth of childhood obesity in the United States.

This concern is not unique to the United States. In addition to the discussions in this country, several related activities have been initiated in other countries and through international organizations. Certain countries have instituted formal bans or restrictions on televised food and beverage advertising to children. Others have undertaken reviews of the issue. Prior to this study, the most recent systematic evidence review of the scientific literature was the report of Hastings and colleagues in 2003, sponsored by the Food Standards Agency in the United Kingdom. That study found that food advertising to children affected children's preferences, purchase behaviors, and consumption, not just for different brands but also for different food and beverage categories. In 2004, the World Health Assembly, drawing on a number of key documents, endorsed marketing practices and policies that acknowledged the vulnerability of children and encouraged marketing practices that promote healthful foods and beverages. Our review has been undertaken in a context of global interest in the issue.

COMMITTEE APPROACH AND EVIDENCE REVIEW

The Committee on Food Marketing and the Diets of Children and Youth was established in 2004. Its charge was to explore what is known about current food and beverage marketing practices, the influence of these practices on the diets and health of U.S. children and youth, and public and private strategies that have been used or could be used to promote healthful food and beverage choices among children and youth. The committee recognizes that a variety of interacting factors affect the health and weight of children and youth, including societal norms, culture, socioeconomic factors, race/ethnicity, education, and physical activity. Although important, these are not the subject of this report, which specifically examines the role of food and beverage marketing in the diets of children and youth.

The committee drew on multiple sources of evidence in its review, including peer-reviewed literature, as well as industry and marketing sources. Particular attention and emphasis was given to the development and implementation of a disciplined process of gathering, classifying, and considering the available scientific literature relevant to the committee's charge. Articles identified in an initial search of the literature were scanned for relevance and methodologic rigor. Approximately 200 of the strongest and most pertinent articles were further reviewed and, of these, 123 were subjected to a systematic evidence review using a protocol established by the committee. Each study was coded on several dimensions, including the relationship of marketing to diet, the cause and effect variables studied, the methods used, and the comparative relevance of the evidence. The results drawn from this assessment provide much of the foundation for the recommendations of this report and are discussed in Chapter 5.

It is important to underscore several points about the literature. First, the importance of this issue commands much more study. Although thousands of papers touch on the topic, the number of carefully designed studies is far too limited for a problem that may so substantially affect the nation's health and that is so intrinsically complicated. Second, the available peer-reviewed literature focuses predominantly on television advertising, but food and beverage marketing extends far beyond television and is changing rapidly to include integrated marketing campaigns that extend to new media platforms that target multiple venues simultaneously. Virtually no scientific studies are available to assess these other techniques. Third, the great bulk of the available research that deals with health outcomes involves direct measures only of overall television viewing, not exposure to television advertising. Because the overall amount of television viewing is highly correlated with the amount of exposure to television advertising, this measurement strategy is informative, but interpretation requires adjusting for other factors, such as sedentary behavior, snacking frequency, or the types of foods consumed. Finally, the committee acknowledges that there are certain constraints that apply to any literature of this sort. It concludes that although publication bias is possible in such research, if it exists it is small and would not influence the conclusions of the report.

On the matter of characterizing commercial marketing practices and trends, the committee faced several notable challenges. Substantial proprietary market research data were either not publicly accessible, or available only for purchase at considerable cost and with prohibitive constraints on public use of the data. Public use provisions were required because the National Academies are subject to section 15 of the Federal Advisory Committee Act of 1997, which requires that the National Academies make available to the public all written materials presented to an expert committee in order for its recommendations to be used by a sponsoring government agency. The result was highly limited availability to the committee of potentially relevant proprietary information that could be considered for the review.

The committee was also asked, if feasible, to estimate costs and provide benchmarks to evaluate progress. Because of the complexity of the issues, the multiplicity of stakeholders, and the unavailability of data necessary on which to establish estimates and baselines, the committee lacked the evidence and resources to address these dimensions with confidence. As noted below, it did, however, include in its recommendations the designation of a public agency responsible for tracking progress, and the establishment of a mechanism for commercial marketing data to be made available as a publicly accessible resource, so that such estimates and benchmarks could be developed and tracked in the future.

KEY FINDINGS

The committee's review indicates that, among many factors, food and beverage marketing influences the preferences and purchase requests of children, influences consumption at least in the short term, is a likely contributor to less healthful diets, and may contribute to negative diet-related health outcomes and risks among children and youth. The literature indicates relationships among marketing, dietary precursors, diets, diet-related health, and, in particular, adiposity (body fatness).

Specifically, the committee's systematic evidence review found that:

With respect to *dietary precursors*, food and beverage advertising on television has some influence on the preferences and purchase requests of children and youth:

• There is strong evidence that television advertising influences the food and beverage preferences of children ages 2–11 years. There is insufficient evidence about its influence on the preferences of teens ages 12–18 years.

• There is strong evidence that television advertising influences the food and beverage purchase requests of children ages 2–11 years. There is insufficient evidence about its influence on the purchase requests of teens ages 12–18 years.

• There is moderate evidence that television advertising influences the food and beverage beliefs of children ages 2–11 years. There is insufficient evidence about its influence on the beliefs of teens ages 12–18 years.

• Given the findings from the systematic evidence review of the influence of marketing on the precursors of diet, and given the evidence from content analyses that the preponderance of television food and beverage advertising relevant to children and youth promotes high-calorie and low-nutrient products, it can be concluded that television advertising influences children to prefer and request high-calorie and low-nutrient foods and beverages.

With respect to *diets*, food and beverage advertising on television has some influence on the dietary intake of children and youth:

• There is strong evidence that television advertising influences the short-term consumption of children ages 2–11 years. There is insufficient evidence about its influence on the short-term consumption of teens ages 12–18 years.

• There is moderate evidence that television advertising influences the usual dietary intake of younger children ages 2–5 years and weak evidence that it influences the usual dietary intake of older children ages 6–

11 years. There is also weak evidence that it does *not* influence the usual dietary intake of teens ages 12–18 years.

With respect to *diet-related health*, food and beverage advertising on television is associated with the adiposity (body fatness) of children and youth:

- Statistically, there is strong evidence that exposure to television advertising is associated with adiposity in children ages 2–11 years and teens ages 12–18 years.
- The association between adiposity and exposure to television advertising remains after taking alternative explanations into account, but the research does not convincingly rule out other possible explanations for the association; therefore, the current evidence is not sufficient to arrive at any finding about a causal relationship from television advertising to adiposity. It is important to note that even a small influence, aggregated over the entire population of American children and youth, would be consequential in impact.

Most children ages 8 years and under do not effectively comprehend the persuasive intent of marketing messages, and most children ages 4 years and under cannot consistently discriminate between television advertising and programming. The evidence is currently insufficient to determine whether or not this meaningfully alters the ways in which food and beverage marketing messages influence children.

CONCLUSIONS AND RECOMMENDATIONS

The prevalence of obesity in children and youth has occurred in parallel with significant changes in the U.S. media and marketing environments. This relationship has lead to the committee's primary inquiry about what the available data indicate as to the influence of food and beverage marketing on the diets and health of American children and youth. This issue was the focus of the committee's systematic evidence review which is described in Chapter 5 and Appendix F.

Embedded in relevant sections throughout the text of the report, the committee presents findings in these key dimensions: health, diet, and eating patterns of children and youth; food and beverage marketing to children and youth; the influence of food and beverage marketing on the diets and diet-related health of children and youth; and the policy environment. These findings are listed again in Chapter 7. Based on these findings, the committee has identified five broad conclusions that serve as the basis for its recommendations (Box ES-1).

Reflective of the responsibilities of multiple sectors, the committee's recommendations address actions related to food and beverage production, processing, packaging, and sales; marketing practice standards; media and

---

BOX ES-1
Broad Conclusions

- Along with many other intersecting factors, food and beverage marketing influences the diets and health prospects of children and youth.

- Food and beverage marketing practices geared to children and youth are out of balance with healthful diets and contribute to an environment that puts their health at risk.

- Food and beverage companies, restaurants, and marketers have underutilized potential to devote creativity and resources to develop and promote food, beverages, and meals that support healthful diets for children and youth.

- Achieving healthful diets for children and youth will require sustained, multisectoral, and integrated efforts that include industry leadership and initiative.

- Public policy programs and incentives do not currently have the support or authority to address many of the current and emerging marketing practices that influence the diets of children and youth.

---

entertainment initiatives; parents, caregivers, and families; school environments; and public policy. Recommendations are also offered for research activities necessary to chart the path of future improvements, and the monitoring capacity to track improvements in marketing practices and their influence on children's and youths' diets and health. These recommendations reflect the current context and information in a rapidly changing environment, and should be implemented together as a package to support and complement one another.

Food and Beverage Production and Promotion

Central to making progress toward more healthful diets for children and youth will be carefully designed and sustained commitments by the food, beverage, and quick serve restaurant industries to promote the availability, accessibility, affordability, and appeal of nutritious foods and beverages.

Recommendation 1: *Food and beverage companies should use their creativity, resources, and full range of marketing practices to promote and support more healthful diets for children and youth.*

To implement this recommendation, companies should
- Shift their product portfolios in a direction that promotes new and

reformulated child- and youth-oriented foods and beverages that are substantially lower in total calories, lower in fats, salt, and added sugars, and higher in nutrient content.

- Shift their advertising and marketing emphasis to child- and youth-oriented foods and beverages that are substantially lower in total calories, lower in fats, salt, and added sugars, and higher in nutrient content (see later recommendations on public policy and monitoring).
- Work with government, scientific, public health, and consumer groups to develop and implement labels and advertising for an empirically validated industrywide rating system and graphic representation that is appealing to children and youth to convey the nutritional quality of foods and beverages marketed to them and their families.
- Engage the full range of their marketing vehicles and venues to develop and promote healthier appealing and affordable foods and beverages for children and youth.

Recommendation 2: *Full serve restaurant chains, family restaurants, and quick serve restaurants should use their creativity, resources, and full range of marketing practices to promote healthful meals for children and youth.*

To implement this recommendation, restaurants should
- Expand and actively promote healthier food, beverage, and meal options for children and youth.
- Provide calorie content and other key nutrition information, as possible, on menus and packaging that is prominently visible at the point of choice and use.

Recommendation 3: *Food, beverage, restaurant, retail, and marketing industry trade associations should assume transforming leadership roles in harnessing industry creativity, resources, and marketing on behalf of healthful diets for children and youth.*

To implement this recommendation, trade associations should
- Encourage member initiatives and compliance to develop, apply, and enforce industry-wide food and beverage marketing practice standards that support healthful diets for children and youth.
- Provide technical assistance, encouragement, and support for members' efforts to emphasize the development and marketing of healthier foods, beverages, and meals for children and youth.
- Exercise leadership in working with their members to improve the availability and selection of healthful foods and beverages accessible at

eye level and reach for children, youth, and their parents in grocery stores and other food retail environments.

- Work to foster collaboration and support with public-sector initiatives promoting healthful diets for children and youth.

Marketing Practice Standards

A reliable barometer of the commitment of the members of the food, beverage, and restaurant industries to promote the nutritional health of children and youth will be the rigor of the standards they set and enforce for their own marketing practices.

Recommendation 4: *The food, beverage, restaurant, and marketing industries should work with government, scientific, public health, and consumer groups to establish and enforce the highest standards for the marketing of foods, beverages, and meals to children and youth.*

To implement this recommendation, the cooperative efforts should
- Work through the Children's Advertising Review Unit (CARU) to revise, expand, apply, enforce, and evaluate explicit industry self-regulatory guidelines beyond traditional advertising to include evolving vehicles and venues for marketing communication (e.g., the Internet, advergames, branded product placement across multiple media).
- Assure that licensed characters are used only for the promotion of foods and beverages that support healthful diets for children and youth.
- Foster cooperation between CARU and the Federal Trade Commission in evaluating and enforcing the effectiveness of the expanded self-regulatory guidelines.

Media and Entertainment Initiatives

Because no element of the lives of Americans has a broader reach than the media and entertainment industry, their opportunities and responsibilities are great to depict and promote healthful diets and eating habits among children and youth.

Recommendation 5: *The media and entertainment industry should direct its extensive power to promote healthful foods and beverages for children and youth.*

To implement this recommendation, media, and the entertainment industry should

- Incorporate into multiple media platforms (e.g., print, broadcast, cable, Internet, and wireless-based programming) foods, beverages, and storylines that promote healthful diets.
- Strengthen their capacity to serve as accurate interpreters and reporters to the public on findings, claims, and practices related to the diets of children and youth.

Parents, Caregivers, and Families

Parents and families remain the central influence on children's attitudes and behaviors, and social marketing efforts that aim to improve children's and youths' diets therefore must be tied directly to that influence.

Recommendation 6: *Government, in partnership with the private sector, should create a long-term, multifaceted, and financially sustained social marketing program supporting parents, caregivers, and families in promoting healthful diets for children and youth.*

To implement this recommendation

- Elements should include the full range of evolving and integrated marketing tools and widespread educational and community-based efforts, including use of children and youth as change agents.
- Special emphasis should be directed to parents of children ages birth to 4 years and other caregivers (e.g., child-care settings, schools, afterschool programs) to build skills to wisely select and prepare healthful and affordable foods and beverages for children and youth.
- The social marketing program should have a reliable and sustained support stream, through public-appropriated funds and counterpart cooperative support from businesses marketing foods, beverages, and meals to children and youth.

School Environments

If schools and parents are to remain the strongest allies working to promote and advance the interests of American children and youth, the school environment must be fully devoted to preparing students for healthful lifelong dietary patterns.

Recommendation 7: *State and local educational authorities, with support from parents, health authorities, and other stakeholders, should educate about and promote healthful diets for children and youth in all aspects of the school environment (e.g., commercial sponsorships, meals and snacks, curriculum).*

To implement this recommendation, companies should

- Develop and implement nutrition standards for competitive foods and beverages sold or served in the school environment.
- Adopt policies and best practices that promote the availability and marketing of foods and beverages that support healthful diets.
- Provide visible leadership in this effort by public and civic leaders at all levels such as the National Governors Association, the state and local Boards of Education, and the National Parent Teacher Association, as well as trade associations representing private-sector businesses such as distributors, bottlers, and vending machine companies that directly interface with the school administration.

Public Policy

A first obligation of public policy is to protect the vulnerable and a second is to create the conditions for a desirable future. Both call for the careful use of policy initiatives to foster healthy prospects for children and youth.

Recommendation 8: *Government at all levels should marshal the full range of public policy levers to foster the development and promotion of healthful diets for children and youth.*

To implement this recommendation

- Government should consider incentives (e.g., recognition, performance awards, tax incentives) that encourage and reward food, beverage, and restaurant companies that develop, provide, and promote healthier foods and beverages for children and youth in settings where they typically consume them (e.g., restaurants, schools, amusement parks, sports venues, movie theaters, malls, and airports).
- Government should explore combining the full range of possible approaches (e.g., agricultural subsidies, taxes, legislation, regulation, federal nutrition programs) for making fruits and vegetables readily available and accessible to all children, youth, and families.
- The U.S. Department of Agriculture should develop and test new strategies for promoting healthier, appealing school meals provided through the School Breakfast Program and the National School Lunch Program as well as other federal programs designed for after-school settings (Special Milk Program) and child-care settings (Child and Adult Care Food Program).
- If voluntary efforts related to advertising during children's television programming are unsuccessful in shifting the emphasis away from high-calorie and low-nutrient foods and beverages to the advertising of

healthful foods and beverages, Congress should enact legislation mandating the shift on both broadcast and cable television.*

Research

Knowledge is the bedrock of effective action and progress, yet current resources are scant to expand the knowledge base, from all sources, on the changing ways in which marketing influences the diets and health of children and youth.

Recommendation 9: *The nation's formidable research capacity should be substantially better directed to sustained, multidisciplinary work on how marketing influences the food and beverage choices of children and youth.*

To implement this recommendation
- The federal research capacity, in particular supported by the agencies of the U.S. Department of Health and Human Services (e.g., National Institutes of Health, Centers for Disease Control and Prevention, Food and Drug Administration), the U.S. Department of Agriculture, the National Science Foundation, and the Federal Trade Commission should be expanded to illuminate the ways in which marketing influences children's attitudes and behaviors. Of particular importance are studies related to newer promotion techniques and venues, healthier foods and beverages and portion sizes, product availability, the impact of television advertising on diet and diet-related health, diverse research methods that systematically control for alternative explanations, stronger measurement, and methods with high relevance to every day life.
- A means should be developed for commercial marketing data to be made available, if possible as a publicly accessible resource, for better understanding the dynamics that shape the health and nutrition attitudes and behaviors of children and youth at different ages and in different circumstances, and for informing the multifaceted social marketing program targeting parents, caregivers, and families to promote healthful diets for children and youth.

Monitoring Progress

The saying goes that "what gets measured gets done." Yet no single public body exists with responsibility or authority to track the influences of

---

*See text at pages 349 and 362.

marketing on the dietary practices and health status of children and youth in the United States.

Recommendation 10: *The Secretary of the U.S. Department of Health and Human Services (DHHS) should designate a responsible agency, with adequate and appropriate resources, to formally monitor and report regularly on the progress of the various entities and activities related to the recommendations included in this report.*

To implement this recommendation
* The Secretary should consult with other relevant cabinet officers and agency heads (e.g., U.S. Department of Agriculture, U.S. Department of Education, Federal Trade Commission, Federal Communications Commission) in developing and implementing the required monitoring and reporting.
* Within 2 years, the Secretary should report to Congress on the progress and additional actions necessary to accelerate progress.

The review and recommendations presented in this report are anchored in the presentation and interpretation of the evidence. This was the central charge to the committee, and the effort represents the most comprehensive and rigorous review of existing scientific literature done to date. It is important to point out that the committee was not charged with, nor did it engage in, addressing some of the broader philosophical, social, and political issues related to food and beverage marketing to children and youth. Perspectives about basic responsibilities to shepherd the welfare of those most vulnerable or impressionable, conjecture about insights from studies not yet done or information not available on the strength of relationships between marketing and behavior of children and youth, and social urgency prompted by the rapidly increasing prevalence of childhood obesity, all are legitimate and important matters for public discussion. But they were not central features of the committee's charge or work. Neither was the related, but vital, matter of physical activity, which is so inextricably a part of the challenge of childhood obesity. What the committee can contribute to the ongoing and imperative public policy questions raised by this challenge is to conclude, based upon a thorough and impartial review of existing scientific data, that the dietary patterns of our children and youth put their health at risk, that the patterns have been encouraged and reinforced by prevailing marketing practices, and that the turnaround required will depend upon aggressive and sustained leadership from all sectors, including the food and beverage industries. This is a public health priority of the highest order.

1

Setting the Stage

What influence has food and beverage marketing had on the dietary patterns and health status of American children and youth? The answer to this question has the potential to shape the health of generations and is the focus of this report. The dramatic rise in the number of U.S. children and adolescents who are obese, have type 2 diabetes,[1] have the metabolic syndrome,[2] and are at increased risk for developing other chronic diseases in adulthood has been a complex and troubling trend over the past 40 years. There is growing evidence that the early life environment is an important determinant of obesity later in life (Reilly et al., 2005).

The term obesity is used in this report to refer to children and youth who have a body mass index (BMI) equal to or greater than the 95th percentile of the age- and gender-specific BMI charts developed by the Centers for Disease Control and Prevention (CDC) in 2000 (Kuczmarski et al., 2000). In most children, such BMI values are associated with elevated body fat and reflect the presence or risk of related chronic diseases (IOM, 2005). CDC uses the term overweight to refer to children and youth with

---

[1]Previously known as adult-onset diabetes, in the 1990s, cases of type 2 diabetes in children accounted for 8 to 45 percent of all newly diagnosed childhood cases of diabetes when compared to less than 4 percent before the 1990s (Fagot-Compagna et al., 2000).

[2]The metabolic syndrome is diagnosed when an individual has at least three of five metabolic abnormalities: glucose intolerance, abdominal obesity, elevated triglyceride level, low high-density lipoprotein (HDL) level, and high blood pressure.

the same BMI values. Obese children have a greater chance of becoming obese adults than children of normal weight. Children of obese parents have an even greater likelihood of becoming obese. An obese preschooler with normal weight parents has approximately a 25 percent chance of becoming an obese adult; however, the same child with an obese parent has greater than a 60 percent chance of becoming an obese adult (Whitaker et al., 1997). Moreover, an obese 2- to 5-year-old is more than four times as likely to become an obese adult when compared to a child who is below the 50th percentile of the CDC BMI charts[3] (Freedman et al., 2005).

Although childhood-onset obesity accounts for only a quarter of adult obesity cases, obesity that is present before a child is 8 years of age, and persists into adulthood, is associated with severe obesity—a BMI greater than 40 kg/m² —in adulthood as compared with a BMI of 35 kg/m² for adult-onset obesity (Freedman et al., 2001). Between 1990 and 2000, severe obesity, which is associated with more serious health complications, more than doubled, increasing from 0.78 percent to 2.2 percent in U.S. adults (Freedman et al., 2002). Additionally, concerns about childhood-onset obesity are supported by documented associations between childhood obesity and increased cardiovascular disease risk and mortality in adulthood (Li et al., 2004; Srinivasan et al., 2002). The most promising way to prevent future adult obesity is to promote an environment conducive to healthy eating among children and youth (Taylor et al., 2005).

Obesity is not the only diet-related problem children and youth face. In addition to the consumption of excess calories and added sugars, the consumption of sodium, saturated fats, and *trans* fats are well above recommended levels and the consumption of vegetables, fruits, whole grains, and calcium are well below recommended levels. American children and youth are therefore at increased risk for developing conditions such as heart disease, stroke, certain cancers, type 2 diabetes, and osteoporosis later in life. As discussed in Chapter 2, the most current data indicate that the overall nutrient intakes of children and adolescents[4] depart substantially from recommended patterns and reflect a pattern that puts young people's health at risk (Box 1-1).

---

[3]The CDC BMI charts are mathematically smoothed curves of the pooled growth parameters of children and adolescents sampled in cross-sectional national health surveys conducted from 1963 to 1994. The current CDC guidelines for healthy weight in children and youth are in the range of the 5th to the 85th percentiles.

[4]See discussion later in this chapter for age categories and related terms used throughout this report.

BOX 1-1
Trends in U.S. Children's and Adolescents' Nutrient Intakes and Eating Patterns, 1970s to 2004

- Children and youth are in energy imbalance as reflected by an aggregate calorie intake that has increased significantly for both younger children and adolescents, with modest increases also experienced among older children ages 6–11 years.

- Calorie intake by infants and toddlers substantially exceeds their estimated requirements.

- Carbohydrate intake has increased over the past 25 years among children and youth.

- Infants and toddlers are consuming diets disproportionately high in sweetened foods and beverages and fried potatoes, and disproportionately low in green leafy vegetables.

- Added sugars consumed by younger children are well above recommended levels, and older children and adolescents are consuming about double the recommended amounts of added sugars in their diets.

- Sweetened beverage consumption by children and youth has steadily increased over the past 35 years, and now represents a major source of calories and added sugars.

- Consumption of milk by children and youth, a major source of dietary calcium, has declined over the past 35 years, and most have lower calcium intakes than recommended.

- Total fat and saturated fats consumed by children and youth remain at levels that exceed dietary recommendations.

- Mean sodium intake of children and youth has increased over the past 35 years, and the majority of children and adolescents are consuming sodium in greater amounts than recommended levels.

- Consumption of vegetables, fruits, and whole grains falls short of the daily recommended servings for most children and youth.

- Snacking by children and youth has increased steadily over the past 25 years.

- Children and youth consume a large proportion of their total calories from foods and beverages that are of high-calorie and low-nutrient content.

- Foods consumed outside of the home have steadily increased and now represent about a third of the daily calories consumed by children and youth.

Creating an environment in which children and youth can grow up healthy should be a high priority for the nation. Health is more than the absence of physical or mental illness—it also is the extent to which children and youth have the capacity to reach their full potential (NRC and IOM, 2004). Many factors affect children's and youths' dietary patterns and overall health. The Institute of Medicine's (IOM's) recent report, *Preventing Childhood Obesity: Health in the Balance* (IOM, 2005), recognizes that children, youth, and their parents are immersed in a modern milieu where the physical, social, commercial, and media environments have all undergone significant transformations over the past several decades. These broader environments now contribute to the rising prevalence of obesity in children and youth, thereby impacting their diets and health through a chain of events that can have profound effects extending far into adulthood (IOM, 2005; NRC and IOM, 2004). On the other hand, there exists unrealized potential to shift the broader environmental signals to encourage healthy lifestyles in which eating habits and physical activity behaviors promote healthy energy balance and nutritional status, and therefore work to prevent obesity and related chronic diseases (IOM, 2005; Peters et al., 2002).

Like adults, children and adolescents acquire new information and knowledge through both explicit and implicit learning—that is, through the processes of dedicated, didactic, and educational experiences, as well as through passive, automatic, and unconscious acquisition of abstract knowledge that remains robust over time (Cleeremans et al., 1998). In addition, they acquire information through the socialization process that helps them to develop their roles and behaviors as consumers and as members of society. The family is the first socializing agent because parents and older siblings act as sources of information and provide social support and pressure that affect children's behaviors (Moore et al., 2002). There are also diverse social and cultural norms and values that influence eating and physical activity. Whether influenced by their parents and siblings, or by other signals in their environments, children buy food and other goods and influence the purchasing decisions of their parents and caregivers (McNeal, 1999).

Children acquire consumer socialization skills early in life, developing consumption motives and values as they are exposed to commercial activities. They develop knowledge about advertising, products, brands, pricing and shopping, and they adopt purchase requests and negotiation strategies that may be the result of marketing activities (John, 1999). Children must have certain basic information-processing skills to fully understand advertising messages (Gunter et al., 2005; Kunkel, 2001). They must be able to discriminate, at a perceptual level, commercial from noncommercial content, and they must be able to attribute persuasive intent to advertising and to adjust their interpretation of commercial messages based on that knowledge. Each of these capabilities develops over time, largely as a function of cognitive growth and development rather than the accumulation of any particular amount of experience with media content (John, 1999; Young, 1990), including the acquisition of media literacy skills. Although cognitive defenses are critical, actual activation of these defenses must be assessed, as children as old as 11 years of age may not activate their defenses unless explicitly cued (Brucks et al., 1988; Moore and Lutz, 2000).

FOOD AND BEVERAGE MARKETING TO
CHILDREN AND YOUTH

Choices are influenced by the way options are presented to individuals. Food and beverages are now marketed to children, youth, and their families in ways that are dramatically different from 40 years ago, and this marketing today strongly influences their preferences and choices. Advertising does not exist or operate in isolation from other aspects of marketing activities. In most advertising, the commercial is an element of a larger marketing design that includes competition for securing market share of branded products, attention to retailers, point-of-purchase displays, attractive packaging, strategic placement of items on store shelves, and the use of coupons, premiums, and price incentives to promote consumer purchases (Schudson, 1986). Children and youth are subsequently exposed to influences from an array of marketing venues and vehicles including school-based marketing, promotions, television and movie product placement, and marketing through the Internet, digital television, and mobile phones.

Moreover, integrated marketing communications have begun to permeate the lives of children and youth. They are now being exposed to a changing landscape of media and promotional activities (Moore, 2005). It is not simply a proliferation of existing media, but the advent of newer media that are interactive and that blend entertainment with advertising and other forms of promotion. Thus, children and youth are now exposed to media and marketing influences to a much greater extent, and through many more diverse and integrated venues embedded in their daily lives, when compared to previous generations.

With new outlets, attractions, and tools, children and youth collectively represent a powerful demographic segment. They are a primary market, spending discretionary income on a variety of products that they acquire by spending their own money; an influence market, determining a large proportion of what is spent by parents and households; and a future market, representing tomorrow's adult customers for branded products and services (McNeal, 1999; MPA, 2004). Children and youth collectively spend more than $200 billion annually (MPA, 2004; Teenage Research Unlimited, 2004), and also determine a large proportion of what is spent by parents and households (Chapter 4).

Parents and their children report that young people have the largest purchase influence on food when compared to other nonfood spending categories such as music, electronics, and home decor. Of the various spending categories, one-third of children's direct purchases are for sweets, snacks, and beverages, followed by toys and apparel (Schor, 2004). Of the top 10 items that children ages 8–12 years report they can select without parental permission, the leading four are food or beverage categories: candy or snacks, soft drinks, fast food from quick serve restaurants, and breakfast cereals (Chaplin, 1999). Similarly, food or beverages—particularly candy, sweetened soft drinks, and salty snacks—represent the top items that teens ages 13–17 years buy with their own money (MPA, 2004; Chapter 4).

Approximately half of all commercials during children's television programming consists of branded foods and beverages that are disproportionately high in salt and calories (e.g., high fat, high sugar), and low in essential nutrients (IOM, 2005)—primarily sweetened cereals, candies and snacks, carbonated soft drinks and sweetened beverages, and fast food (Gamble and Cotugna, 1999). Additionally, companies use advertising and other marketing techniques that associate these specific foods with fun and pleasurable experiences (Hawkes, 2002; Schlosser, 2001).

When high-calorie and low-nutrient foods and beverages are marketed to infants, toddlers, and young children who have an innate biological preference for high-calorie foods that are sweet and salty (Benton, 2004; Mennella and Beauchamp, 1998), or when these types of products are marketed to parents, schools, or child-care settings and made easily available and accessible in their environments, there is a much greater opportunity and likelihood that children will develop sustained preferences for these products. Indeed, young children typically reject new foods and may need to be introduced to a new food as many as 5 to 10 times before they will accept it (Birch, 1999). Children's preferences for foods that lack sweet and salty tastes are learned and require repeated positive experiences, especially to accept fruits, vegetables, and other nutrient-rich foods later in life (Birch 1999; Skinner et al., 2002; Chapter 3). When accompanied by physical inactivity, preferences for and consumption of high-calorie foods and beverages over time set in motion the circumstances that contribute to weight gain and obesity, especially for children and youth who are genetically predisposed to gaining weight in an obesogenic environment (IOM, 2005).

Moreover, the contemporary media landscape offers many more options to market messages about foods and beverages to children and youth than just a decade ago, encompassing broadcast, satellite, and cable television; the video cassette recorder and digital video disk (DVD) recorder; portable audio media (e.g., radio, tapes, CDs, DVDs, MP3 players); print media (e.g., magazines, newspapers, books); computers and the online activities they provide with Internet access (e.g., e-mail, instant messaging, advergaming); and cell phones that can connect to the Internet and provide text messaging and digital screens (Roberts et al., 2005; Chapter 4). The entertainment industry focuses more time and resources than ever before on trying to understand the desires of children and youth (Schor, 2004), and there are cable television networks exclusively devoted to reaching young audiences (Nickelodeon, 2005).

STUDY BACKGROUND AND RATIONALE

In FY 2004, Congress directed the CDC to support a comprehensive, evidence-based review of the effects of food marketing on children's and youths' diet and health. With this congressional directive, the CDC turned to the IOM in July 2004 to assess the effects of food marketing on children's and youths' diet and health. It had been nearly 25 years since a similar review of the available evidence was undertaken in the United States for this topic (Elliott et al., 1981). Several notable changes and innovations have occurred with food and beverage marketing and the media environments that directly affect the lives of U.S. children and youth during this time frame.

Committee Charge and Approach

The IOM appointed a 16-member committee on Food Marketing and the Diets of Children and Youth in the fall of 2004 to undertake a comprehensive evidence-based review of the influence of food and beverage marketing on the diets and health of children and youth in the United States, including the characteristics of effective marketing of foods and beverages to promote healthful choices. The committee members have expertise in the areas of child and adolescent development, child and adolescent nutrition, psychology, behavioral economics, advertising, consumer marketing and behavior, media, social marketing, program evaluation, education, public health, public policy, industry (e.g., food, beverage, children's entertainment), statistics, constitutional law, and business ethics (Appendix I). The committee was charged with the following six tasks:

1. Assess what is known about the scope, amount, venues, and types of food and beverage product marketing (including market segmentation strategies) to children and youth;

2. Conduct a comprehensive review of the available evidence about the extent to which this marketing affects their diets, including their nutrient intake and health;

3. Synthesize lessons learned from relevant research and experience from other marketing-oriented health promotion efforts (e.g., youth to-

bacco prevention, underage drinking prevention, obesity prevention, and the promotion of physical activity) that can contribute to the development of marketing strategies to promote healthful food choices among children and youth;

4. Identify gaps in the knowledge base related to the impact of marketing on the diets and health of children and youth;

5. Review the issues and strategic options for public policy and private stakeholders to promote public and commercial marketing strategies that foster healthful food and beverage choices by children and youth; and

6. Prepare a consensus report that describes the state of food and beverage marketing to infants, toddlers, children, and adolescents; offers a coherent understanding about the impact of this exposure on their diets and health; and if feasible, provides benchmarks to evaluate progress toward healthful food and beverage promotion to young consumers.

The committee acknowledges that a variety of interacting factors affect the health and weight of children and youth, including societal norms, culture, socioeconomic factors, race/ethnicity, education, and physical activity (Ebbeling et al., 2002; Goran et al., 1999; IOM, 2005; Kumanyika et al., 2001, 2002; NRC and IOM, 2004, Swinburn and Egger, 2002). Although important, these are not the subject of this report, which specifically examines the role of food and beverage marketing in the diets and diet-related health of children and youth.

An important starting point for the committee was the set of recommendations regarding the marketing of foods and beverages to children and youth presented in the IOM report, *Preventing Childhood Obesity: Health in the Balance* (2005). This report concluded that concentrated efforts are urgently needed among various sectors and stakeholder groups to change social norms about childhood obesity and to create supportive environments and consistent messages that promote healthy lifestyles—including healthful eating habits and regular physical activity (IOM, 2005). The report recommended in particular that industry develop and strictly adhere to marketing and advertising guidelines that minimize the risk of obesity in children and youth (IOM, 2005).

The work of the current committee was informed by a variety of sources. Four formal meetings were held during the study. The committee conducted a systematic literature review of evidence that addresses the linkages from food and beverage marketing to young people's diets and diet-related health (Appendixes C, E, and F; Chapters 4 and 5). It also commissioned three papers: a synthesis of the literature on marketing to children over the past three decades; insights into future marketing techniques; and insights about the effectiveness of social marketing campaigns and its application to this issue.

One committee meeting included a public workshop held in January 2005. The workshop, *Marketing Strategies that Foster Healthy Food and Beverage Choices in Children and Youth*, had two goals: to identify effective processes, actions, and campaigns for promoting healthful food and beverage choices and behaviors in children and youth, and to provide a public forum for interested individuals and groups to share their perspectives to the committee. Ten invited speakers presented their views on the food, beverage, and quick serve restaurant[5] industries; youth-focused media and marketing approaches; and research. The public forum included 16 presenters who represented nonprofit organizations, trade organizations, professional associations, and interested individuals (Appendix H).

FOCUS AND CONCEPTS

Target Population

The focus of the committee's study was on children and youth from birth to 18 years of age. The committee recognized that among researchers, policy makers, and marketers, different age groups and terms are used to define this diverse population. In general, the committee used the terms "children," "youth," "young people," "teenagers," and "adolescents." When greater precision was needed, the following age categories and terms were used throughout the report: infants and toddlers (children under 2 years of age), younger children (ages 2–5 years), older children (ages 6–11 years), and teens (ages 12–18 years). In selected sections of the report, particularly those drawing from the marketing literature, "tween" is used to describe young people ages 9–13 years.

Marketing

The focus of the committee's inquiry was on the marketing of foods and beverages to children and youth. As discussed in greater depth in Chapter 4, marketing is a process by which a variety of strategies are used to stimulate consumer demand, promote frequency of purchases, build brand awareness and brand loyalty, and encourage potential or existing customers to try new foods and beverages. Marketing is defined as an

---

[5]Quick serve restaurants are commonly known as "fast food restaurants" and represent a category of restaurants that supply food quickly after ordering with minimal service.

"organizational function and a set of processes for creating, communicating, and delivering value to customers and for managing customer relationships in ways that benefit an organization and its stakeholders" (AMA, 2005). Marketing involves conducting research, defining the target market, analyzing the competition, and implementing the basic processes that constitute the marketing mix or drivers of business (McCarthy, 1975). The key components are the following:

- *Product* (i.e., features, quality, quantity, packaging)
- *Place* (i.e., location, outlets, distribution points used to reach the target market)
- *Price* (i.e., strategy, determinants, levels)
- *Promotion* (i.e., advertising, sales promotion, public relations, trade promotion)

Advertising is a form of paid nonpersonal public presentation and the promotion of ideas, goods, or services by a sponsor (Kotler and Armstrong, 2004). It is a specific type of marketing that brings a product to the attention of consumers and may be delivered through a variety of media channels such as television, radio, print, billboards, personal contact, and the Internet (Boone and Kurtz, 1998). Advertising is the most visible form of marketing that contributes to the success of other strategies by (1) providing the conditions for developing a company's brand image by building brand awareness and brand loyalty among potential consumers, and (2) creating perceived value by persuading consumers that they are getting more than the product itself (e.g., a meal, food, or beverage product).

Ecological Perspective

Consistent with the committee's charge, the primary focus of this report is the evaluation of the available evidence for assessing the nature of the relationship between marketing and the diets and health of children and youth. The committee used a simplified ecological perspective to conceptualize the relationship of food marketing to other important influences on the diets and related health outcomes of children and youth (Figure 1-1; see also Chapter 3). This perspective places food and beverage marketing influences within a context that recognizes the multiple interactions among factors that also affect children's and adolescents' food preferences and choices, eating behaviors, total calorie intake, diet quality, and health outcomes. The use of an ecological perspective requires an understanding of processes and intertwining interactions among individuals, communities, and their social, economic, cultural, and physical environments over time (IOM, 2001). This approach considers the relative strengths of the multiple

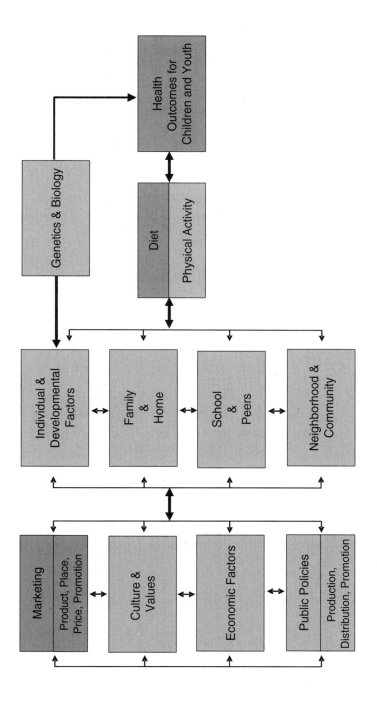

FIGURE 1-1 Influences on the diets and related health outcomes of children and youth.

factors influencing diet, including the role of marketing in overall diet quality and quantity of foods consumed.

The committee's perspective views children, adolescents, and their families as functioning within broader social, economic, and political systems— including the food and agricultural system and the marketplace where products and services are exchanged. These systems also influence behaviors and may facilitate or impede availability and access to nutritious foods and beverages and to the resources necessary to maintain good health. Included among the systemic forces are the four components of the marketing mix— product, place, price, and promotion (discussed in more detail in Chapter 4); culture and values that influence societal norms and behaviors (Chapter 3); economic factors that influence food and beverage choices and consumption patterns including family income, food security status, and affordability (Chapter 3); and a broad range of policies that affect food and beverage availability, access, affordability, preferences, choices, and purchases (Chapters 4 and 6).

These systematic factors interact with each other and with individual and developmental factors, family and home, school and peers, and neighborhood and community to influence children's and youths' diet and physical activity patterns (Chapter 3). Genetic and biological factors also influence these patterns and moderate the ways in which these patterns affect health outcomes for a given individual (Chapter 3). An important note is that this committee recognizes the fundamental nature of the interaction between diet and physical activity for children and youth to achieve energy balance at a healthy weight; however, an examination of marketing related to promoting physical activity and reducing sedentary behaviors was beyond the study charge. A review of this issue may be found in the IOM report, *Preventing Childhood Obesity: Health in the Balance*.

RELATED BACKGROUND AND PERSPECTIVES

Advertising and marketing play a central role in shaping the profile and vitality of the U.S. economy and culture (Klein and Donaton, 1999). Market forces create, modify, and respond to consumer demand; they influence the choices and preferences of individuals and populations, as well as the attitudes, opinions, and behaviors of consumers, industries, and governments. The pace at which change occurs is influenced by cultural and social norms and values that support or reject new private-sector offerings and innovations.

Industry develops new products, ideas, and services in response to changing consumer demand and market forces (Kotler and Armstrong, 2004), and it also creates consumer demand for products, including foods and beverages consumed by individuals and populations over the long term

(Hawkes, 2002). For this reason the issues often emphasized by industry—sales trends, marketing opportunities, product appeal, advertising exposure, brand awareness, brand recognition, brand loyalty, brand equity, and expanding market share for specific product categories and product brands (Barbour, 2003; Moore et al., 2002; Roberts, 2004)—can also be important issues for healthier and more active lifestyles, including the promotion of healthful foods and beverages, more nutritious diets, more vigorous activity patterns, and healthier weights.

Although food manufacturers and producers have not historically or predominantly viewed their roles and responsibilities in terms of changing consumers' preferences toward healthier choices, the recent trend toward heavier children and youth—and the broader increased prevalence of obesity-related chronic disease among adults—places a compelling priority on industry's work with other groups and sectors to play a central role in achieving this goal (IOM, 2005). This is a complex challenge in a marketplace driven by profit margins and market shares. There are encouraging examples of food and beverage companies that are making changes to their product portfolios. However, shifting the proportion of companies' overall product portfolios from high-calorie and low-nutrient options to more healthful foods and beverages will require substantial change and evaluation of these efforts to understand if they can retain market share for their products (Chapters 4 and 6).

Also complex is the potential use of policy levers to guide marketing practices when it comes to children and youth. Our legal traditions balance the protection of the right to advertise and promote products and ideas through various communication channels with the duty to protect the welfare of children and youth. For example, with increasing understanding of the lifelong and life-threatening consequences of tobacco use, restrictions have been imposed on tobacco advertising and promotion directed to youth. Yet tobacco companies have continued to use an extensive array of marketing communication practices that reach youth. In this case, the compelling state interest in promoting public health by protecting children has generally prevailed over protecting the right to advertise as a form of free speech.

The Federal Trade Commission Case and Beyond

With respect to foods and beverages, Congress has been reluctant to impose mandatory constraints on advertising to children. The illustrative case is a Federal Trade Commission (FTC) exploration through a rule-making process more than 25 years ago on restricting or banning advertising to young children (Beales, 2004; Elliott et al., 1981; Ratner et al., 1978).

In the late 1970s, consumer groups and members of a concerned American public engaged Congress, industry representatives, and other stakeholders in a multiyear FTC deliberation to consider the possible need for government intervention to regulate advertising because of the perceived adverse effects of television advertising directed to young children. At that time, strong scientific evidence connected the consumption of sugar to the development of dental caries, which became a public health concern. The argument favoring regulation focused on the increased number of sweetened food and beverage advertisements that were reaching children through television (the primary media channel at that time), combined with the social concern that young children were unable to discern the difference between television advertisements and educational programming (Beales, 2004; Ratner et al., 1978).

The FTC proposed a rulemaking process in 1978—known as "Kidvid" —that would either restrict or ban advertising to young children as a protective measure, and FTC staff sought public comment on the issues, including three proposed alternative actions (Ratner et al., 1978). During this process, the FTC provisionally concluded, based upon its review of scientific evidence, that television advertising directed at young children was unfair and deceptive (Elliott et al., 1981). Congress subsequently objected to intrusions on private-sector advertising and pressured the FTC to withdraw its proposed rule and to conclude that evidence of adverse effects of advertising on children was inconclusive (Elliott et al., 1981). Acknowledging that there was some cause for concern, the FTC stated that it would be difficult to develop a workable rule that would alleviate harm without also infringing on First Amendment rights. Congress barred any rule based on unfairness, and the FTC terminated the rulemaking process in 1981 (Beales, 2004; Elliott et al., 1981).

In the agency's final report to Congress (Elliott et al., 1981), the FTC concluded that young children lack the capacity to distinguish between persuading and informing. The American Psychological Association Task Force on Advertising and Children reiterated the same conclusion in a report nearly a quarter of a century later (Kunkel et al., 2004). Although some have called for extension of the FTC conclusions on television advertising to vulnerabilities from other sources of marketing to children, the influence of other forms of consumer promotion and marketing strategies to children has not been systematically studied, in part because of the newness of the techniques and also because of the lack of peer-reviewed evidence and difficulties in accessing propriety data.

Common issues raised include not only concern with the content and integrated nature (i.e., multiple channels and venues) of advertising and other forms of marketing to children and adolescents, but also the types and overall quality of foods and beverages that are advertised and marketed to young consumers and their parents. Branding, for example, has become a routine part of children's lives. Some believe that parental ability to guide their children's consumption of food and beverages has been compromised by an environment that exposes children to an array of advertising and marketing messages for junk food[6] (CSPI, 2003; IACFO, 2003; Schor, 2004).

Market research shows that children as young as 2 years have beliefs about specific brands that are promoted by television advertising and parental usage (Hite and Hite, 1995). Young children ages 3 to 6 years recognize brand logos for all types of products, and this recognition increases with television viewing, age, and the use of visual cues in advertising (Fischer et al., 1991; Henke, 1995; Macklin, 1994; Chapter 5). Brand choices are intergenerationally influenced (Moore et al., 2002). Thus, it has been asserted that commercialism and consumerism pervade the daily life of young children to an extent that is far greater than that experienced by previous generations. Children's consumer desires are now considered natural even though children and youth in previous generations and in different cultures vary widely in how much they care about consumer trends and engage in consumer activities (Schor, 2004).

Since the FTC case was initiated in the 1970s, a lively debate has persisted about the nature and extent of the influence of marketing on children's food and beverage choices, eating behaviors, and diet-related health conditions. This debate has intensified recently in the face of growing concern over childhood obesity, and reflects diverse values and strongly discordant viewpoints. It has been difficult to reconcile among these distinct viewpoints, partly because of the paucity of robust evidence on causal relationships among advertising, other forms of promotion, and consumption patterns.

Some view marketing as a form of information that contributes to consumer choice in the marketplace. For adults the differentiation of brands creates choices that provide the opportunity for individuals to make decisions based on their own needs, preferences, desires, and lifestyles. To the extent that children are to be educated and socialized into the autonomous practices of adults, certain groups believe that they must learn to make such decisions for themselves. Proponents of an unrestricted advertising perspective, such as the Alliance for American Advertising, created by the food and beverage, advertising, and media industries (ANA, 2005; Office of the Clerk and U.S. House of Representatives, 2004), have asserted that the First Amendment protects their rights to advertise to children (ANA, 2005; Egerstrom, 2005; Ellison, 2005).

---

[6]There is no widely accepted definition for *junk food* although it is often used by popular culture to describe high-calorie (e.g., high fat, high sugar), and low-nutrient foods and beverages. In this report, *fast food* is defined as any food designed for ready availability, use, or consumption and sold at eating establishments for quick availability or takeout.

Others are concerned about the ways marketing might undermine parental authority and social morality, and the promotion of less healthful lifestyles (Bjurstrom, 1994; Haefner, 1991; Schor, 2004). Contemporary thinking about the long-term socialization effects of media suggests that children's unintended exposure to advertisements intended for other target audiences (e.g., older teens and adults) may influence their expectations, values, and world views (Haefner, 1991). Prompted by concerns about the possible adverse health impact of food and beverage marketing to children and youth, a variety of states, localities, and school districts have taken steps to restrict marketing and distribution of certain foods and beverages in schools, and various advocacy groups and legislative bodies have turned stronger attention to the issues in the United States (Chapter 6).

International Perspectives

The rising concern about obesity in children and youth has prompted some groups to call for collective international action among many stakeholder groups and changing behaviors across multiple sectors. The World Health Organization's *Global Strategy on Diet, Physical Activity and Health* was endorsed by the 57th World Health Assembly in 2004 (WHO, 2004). The Global Strategy provides member states with a range of policy options to address less healthful dietary practices and physical inactivity, including provisions for marketing, advertising, sponsorship, and promotion to support international public health goals. These provisions recommended that "food and beverage advertisements should not exploit children's inexperience or credulity," should discourage messages that promote less healthful dietary practices, and should encourage positive healthful messages (WHO, 2004).

The European Heart Network, concerned about the 20 percent of school-aged European children who are either obese or at risk for obesity, documented marketing trends for children in 20 European countries. The Network is developing an action plan to address childhood obesity throughout the region of the European Union. The plan includes protection of children from less healthful food marketing as one of many interventions to address childhood obesity (Matthews et al., 2005).

Several strong government and professional positions have been taken on the issue of advertising and marketing to children. Bans on television advertising were adopted in the Canadian province of Quebec in 1980, Sweden in 1991, and Norway in 1992. The prevailing principle in these countries is that children should have the right to grow up in a commercial-free environment, especially younger children who are trusting and do not understand the difference between information and the persuasive intent of advertisements or commercials (Bjurstrom, 1994; Government of Quebec, 2005; Haefner, 1991; Jarlbro, 2001; Norwegian Ministry of Children and Family Affairs, 2005; The Consumer Ombudsman, 1999; Chapter 6). However, comprehensive evaluations of the effects of the television advertising bans are currently not available to assess their impact (Chapter 6). The Australian obesity prevention action plan supports stricter national regulations on food advertising directed at children, and is considering a ban during children's television viewing time (NSW Centre for Public Health Nutrition, 2005). The British Medical Association recommended a ban on advertising of less healthful foods, including certain sponsorship programs targeted at school children, and a ban on less healthful foods and beverages purchased from school vending machines (British Medical Association and Board of Science, 2005).

REVIEW OF THE EVIDENCE

The committee drew from several sources of evidence that were directly relevant to the committee's charge—*What is the effect of food and beverage marketing on the diets and health of children and youth?* In order to be comprehensive, the committee reviewed a broad range of material drawn from both academic, peer-reviewed literature and industry and marketing sources. In addition, the committee commissioned papers examining past, present, and future food and beverage marketing trends affecting children and youth and describing effective elements of social marketing campaigns. The committee also reviewed presentations and comments provided during the January 2005 public workshop, as well as documents received and placed in the National Academies' public access file.

Particular attention was given to the process of gathering and considering the relevant scientific, peer-reviewed literature. Prior to this IOM study, the most recent systematic review of such literature was the report of Hastings et al. (2003). That review, sponsored by the Food Standards Agency in the United Kingdom, found that food advertising to children affected their preferences, purchase behaviors, and consumption, not just for different brands but also for different food categories.

The committee's search for relevant literature included an online bibliographic search of several databases, outreach to experts in relevant fields, examination of published literature reviews, and acquisition of references cited in articles found to be relevant (Appendix C). From this search, the committee selected 123 empirical studies that were subjected to a systematic evidence review using a committee-established protocol. Each study was coded on several dimensions, including the relationship of marketing to diet, cause and effect variables, methods of research, and the comparative quality of the evidence. Both the process and the results are described in detail in Chapter 5 and Appendix F.

In order to fully understand the status and influences of food and beverage marketing in U.S. children and youth, the committee also drew on publicly available industry and commercial marketing research. This material was acquired through marketing, advertising, or industry trade journals; food and beverage companies' annual reports; foundation and nonprofit organization reports and briefs; government, company, and trade organization materials; popular magazines and books relevant to advertising and marketing; news releases; government, company, and trade organization websites; and selected marketing research briefs, executive summaries, or full reports that were requested by and provided to the committee. Much of this material focused on specific brands and products in target markets, including brand or product awareness, product purchases, brand loyalty, perceived differentiation from competitors, marketing costs, and scalability. A discussion of this material is presented in Chapter 4.

The committee faced several notable challenges to acquiring and using this commercial marketing research. Businesses are increasingly using integrated marketing strategies to ensure that young consumers are exposed to messages that will stimulate demand, build brand loyalty, and encourage potential or existing customers to purchase new products. A variety of measured media channels (e.g., television, radio, magazines, Internet) and unmeasured media channels (e.g., product placement, video games, advergames, in-store promotions, special events) and other venues (e.g., schools) are used to deliver promotional messages to young consumers. Many of these strategies are new, and are not well researched or evaluated. Additionally, a large proportion of this research is conducted for paying clients and is therefore considered to be proprietary information that is not publicly accessible or is available only for purchase at considerable cost to the committee and with prohibitive constraints on public availability of the data.

Another challenge faced by the committee was understanding and reconciling the differences in the evidence derived from the various sources of information presented in Chapters 4 and 5. For instance, in general, the industry and marketing information presented in Chapter 4 is of short-term duration, the analyses tend to be descriptive, and they only rarely use multivariate statistical designs. The peer-reviewed literature reviewed in Chapter 5, on the other hand, uses distinct research methodologies to answer different research questions than those questions explored by marketing research firms. The committee considered both of these sources in developing its findings and recommendations.

GUIDE TO THE REPORT

This report describes the committee's findings and conclusions, identifies promising strategies, and offers recommendations for public and private stakeholders to foster healthful food and beverage choices in children and youth. Chapter 2 provides a summary of the health, diet, and eating patterns of children and youth. Chapter 3 reviews the factors shaping the food and beverage consumption of children and youth, including age-related developmental factors involved in consumer socialization—the process by which children acquire skills, knowledge, and attitudes relevant to functioning as consumers in the marketplace. Chapter 4 describes the status and trends of food and beverage marketing to children and youth and draws from a range of evidentiary sources. Chapter 5 systematically considers the evidence from peer-reviewed literature on the influence of food and beverage marketing on the diets and diet-related health of children and youth. Chapter 6 considers relevant public policy issues. Chapter 7 summarizes the committee's findings, conclusions, recommendations, and priorities for moving forward. For reference throughout the report, a list of acronyms and a glossary of terms are provided in Appendixes A and B.

REFERENCES

AMA (American Marketing Association). 2005. *Marketing Definitions.* [Online]. Available: http://www.marketingpower.com/content4620.php [accessed August 4, 2005].

ANA (Association of National Advertisers). 2005. *ANA Compendium of Legislative, Regulatory, and Legal Issues 2004.* New York: Association of National Advertisers, Inc.

Barbour J. 2003. *The U.S. Market for Kids' Food and Beverages—5th Edition.* [Online]. Available: http://www.marketresearch.com/product/display.asp?productid=849192&SID =46320173-327969985-290367212/ [accessed August 4, 2005].

Beales JH. 2004. *Advertising to Kids and the FTC: A Regulatory Retrospective that Advises the Present.* [Online]. Available: http://www.ftc.gov/speeches/beales/040802adstokids. pdf [accessed October 3, 2005].

Benton D. 2004. Role of parents in the determination of the food preferences of children and the development of obesity. *Int J Obes Relat Metab Disord* 28(7):858–869.

Birch LL. 1999. Development of food preferences. *Annu Rev Nutr* 19:41–62.

Bjurstrom E. 1994. *Children and Television Advertising.* Report No. 1994/95:8. Stockholm, Sweden: Swedish Consumer Agency.

Boone LE, Kurtz DL. 1998. *Contemporary Marketing Wired.* 9th ed. Orlando, FL: Harcourt Brace College Publishers.

British Medical Association and Board of Science. 2005. *Preventing Childhood Obesity.* London, UK: British Medical Association.

Brucks M, Armstrong GM, Goldberg ME. 1988. Children's use of cognitive defenses against television advertising: A cognitive response approach. *J Consum Res* 14:471–482.

Chaplin H. 1999. Food fight! *Am Demographics* 21(6):64–65.

Cleeremans A, Destrebecqz A, Boyer M. 1998. Implicit learning: News from the front. *Trend Cogn Sci* 2(10):406–416.

CSPI (Center for Science in the Public Interest). 2003. *Pestering Parents: How Food Companies Market Obesity to Children.* Washington, DC: CSPI.

Ebbeling CB, Pawlak DB, Ludwig DS. 2002. Childhood obesity: Public-health crisis, common sense cure. *Lancet* 360(9331):473–482.

Egerstrom L. 2005, January 27. General Mills exec to defend ads for kids; Hearing to focus on how food is marketed to children. *Saint Paul Pioneer Press*. P. 1C.

Elliott S, Wilkenfeld JP, Guarino ET, Kolish ED, Jennings CJ, Siegal D. 1981. *FTC Final Staff Report and Recommendation That the Commission Terminate Proceedings for the Promulgation of a Trade Regulation Rule on Children's Advertising*. TRR No. 215-60. Washington, DC: Federal Trade Commission.

Ellison S. 2005, January 26. Divided, companies fight for right to plug kids' food. *The Wall Street Journal Online*. P. B1.

Fagot-Compagna A, Pettitt DJ, Engelgau MM, Burrows NR, Geiss LS, Valdez R, Beckles GL, Saaddine J, Gregg EW, Williamson DF, Narayan KM. 2000. Type 2 diabetes among North American children and adolescents: An epidemiologic review and a public health perspective. *J Pediatr* 136(5):664–672.

Fischer PM, Schwartz MP, Richards JW Jr, Goldstein AO, Rojas TH. 1991. Brand logo recognition by children aged 3 to 6 years. Mickey Mouse and Old Joe the Camel. *J Am Med Assoc* 266(22):3145–3148.

Freedman DS, Khan LK, Dietz WH, Srinivasan SR, Berenson GS. 2001. Relationship of childhood obesity to coronary heart disease risk factors in adulthood: The Bogalusa Heart Study. *Pediatrics* 108(3):712–718.

Freedman DS, Khan LK, Serdula MK, Galuska DA, Dietz WH. 2002. Trends and correlates of class 3 obesity in the United States from 1990 through 2000. *J Am Med Assoc* 288(14):1758–1761.

Freedman DS, Khan LK, Serdula MK, Dietz WH, Srinivasan SR, Berenson GS. 2005. The relation of childhood BMI to adult adiposity: The Bogalusa Heart Study. *Pediatrics* 115(1):22–27.

Gamble M, Cotugna N. 1999. A quarter century of TV food advertising targeted at children. *Am J Health Behav* 23(4):261–267.

Goran MI, Reynolds KD, Lindquist CH. 1999. Role of physical activity in the prevention of obesity in children. *Int J Obesity* 23(S3):S18–S33.

Government of Quebec. 2005. *Consumer Protection Act P-40.1*. [Online]. Available: http://www2.publicationsduquebec.gouv.qc.ca/home.php [accessed July 27, 2005].

Gunter B, Oates C, Blades M. 2005. *Advertising to Children on TV. Content, Impact, and Regulation*. Mahwah, NJ: Lawrence Erlbaum Associates.

Haefner MJ. 1991. Ethical problems of advertising to children. *J Mass Media Ethics* 6:83–92.

Hastings G, Stead M, McDermot L, Forsyth A, MacKintosh AM, Rayner M, Godfrey C, Caraher M, Angus K. 2003. *Review of Research on the Effects of Food Promotion to Children*. Glasgow, UK: Centre for Social Marketing.

Hawkes C. 2002. Marketing activities of global soft drink and fast food companies in emerging markets: A review. In: *Globalization, Diets, and Non-Communicable Diseases*. Geneva: World Health Organization.

Henke LL. 1995. Young children's perceptions of cigarette brand advertising symbols: Awareness, affect, and target market identification. *J Advertising* 24(4):13–28.

Hite CF, Hite RE. 1995. Reliance on brand by young children. *J Market Res Soc* 37(2): 185–193.

IACFO (International Association of Consumer Food Organizations). 2003. *Broadcasting Bad Health. Why Food Marketing to Children Needs to Be Controlled*. London, UK: IACFO.

IOM (Institute of Medicine). 2001. *Health and Behavior: The Interplay of Biological, Behavioral, and Societal Influences*. Washington, DC: National Academy Press.

IOM. 2005. *Preventing Childhood Obesity: Health in the Balance*. Washington, DC: The National Academies Press.

Jarlbro G. 2001. *Children and Television Advertising. The Players, the Arguments, and the Research During the Period 1994–2000*. Stockholm, Sweden: Swedish Consumer Agency.

John D. 1999. Consumer socialization of children: A retrospective look at twenty-five years of research. *J Consum Res* 26(3):183–213.

Klein D, Donaton S. 1999. Letter from the editors. *Advertising Age* 70(13):3.

Kotler P, Armstrong G. 2004. *Principles of Marketing*. 10th ed. Upper Saddle River, NJ: Prentice Hall.

Kuczmarski RJ, Ogden CL, Grummer-Strawn LM, Flegal KM, Guo SS, Wei R, Mei Z, Curtin LR, Roche AF, Johnson CL. 2000. CDC growth charts: United States. *Adv Data* (314): 1–27.

Kumanyika SK, Krebs-Smith SM. 2001. Preventive nutrition issues in ethnic and socioeconomic groups in the United States. In: Bendich A, Deckelbaum RJ, eds. *Primary and Secondary Preventive Nutrition*. Totowa, NJ: Humana Press. Pp. 325–356.

Kumanyika S, Jeffery RW, Morabia A, Ritenbaugh C, Antipatis VJ, Public Health Approaches to the Prevention of Obesity (PHAPO) Working Group of the International Obesity Task Force (IOTF). 2002. Obesity prevention: The case for action. *Int J Obes Relat Metab Disord* 26(3):425–436.

Kunkel D. 2001. Children and television advertising. In: Singer DG, Singer JL, eds. *Handbook of Children and the Media*. Thousand Oaks, CA: Sage Publications. Pp. 375–393.

Kunkel D, Wilcox BL, Cantor J, Palmer E, Linn S, Dowrick P. 2004. *Report of The APA Task Force on Advertising and Children. Section: Psychological Issues in the Increasing Commercialization of Childhood*. [Online]. Available: http://www.apa.org/releases/childrenads.pdf [accessed August 4, 2005].

Li X, Li S, Ulusoy E, Chen W, Srinivasan SR, Berenson GS. 2004. Childhood adiposity as a predictor of cardiac mass in adulthood: The Bogalusa Heart Study. *Circulation* 110(22):3488–3492.

Macklin MC. 1994. The effects of an advertising retrieval cue on young children's memory and brand evaluations. *Psychol Marketing* 11(3):291–311.

Matthews A, Cowburn G, Rayner M, Longfield J, Powell C. 2005. *The Marketing of Unhealthy Food to Children in Europe. A Report of Phase 1 of "The Children, Obesity and Associated Avoidable Chronic Diseases" Project*. Brussels: European Heart Network.

McCarthy EJ. 1975. *Basic Marketing: A Managerial Approach*. 5th ed. Homewood, IL: R.D. Irwin.

McNeal JU. 1999. *The Kids Market Myths and Realities*. Ithaca, NY: Paramount Market Publishing.

Mennella JA, Beauchamp GK. 1998. Early flavor experiences: Research update. *Nutr Rev* 56(7):205–211.

Moore ES. 2005, January 27. *An Overview of Academic Marketing Research on Children's Issues*. Presentation at the Institute of Medicine Workshop on Marketing Strategies that Foster Healthy Food and Beverage Choices in Children and Youth, Washington, DC. Committee on Food Marketing and the Diets of Children and Youth.

Moore ES, Lutz RJ. 2000. Children, advertising, and product experiences: A multimethod inquiry. *J Consum Res* 27(1):31–48.

Moore ES, Wilkie WL, Lutz RJ. 2002. Passing the torch: Intergenerational influences as a source of brand equity. *J Marketing* 66(2):17–37.

MPA (Magazine Publishers of America). 2004. *Teen Market Profile*. [Online]. Available: http://www.magazine.org/content/files/teenprofile04.pdf [accessed August 4, 2005].

Nickelodeon. 2005. *All Nick TV Shows*. [Online]. Available: http://www.nick.com/all_nick/ [accessed August 4, 2005].

Norwegian Ministry of Children and Family Affairs. 2005. *The Norwegian Action Plan to Reduce Commercial Pressure on Children and the Young People.* [Online]. Available at: http://odin.dep.no/bfd/english/doc/handbooks/004061-990036/dok-bn.html [accessed July 27, 2005].

NRC (National Research Council) and IOM. 2004. *Children's Health, the Nation's Wealth: Assessing and Improving Child Health.* Washington, DC: The National Academies Press.

NSW Centre for Public Health Nutrition. 2005. *Best Options for Promoting Healthy Weight and Preventing Weight Gain in NSW.* Sydney, Australia: NSW Department of Health.

Office of the Clerk and U.S. House of Representatives. 2004. *Alliance for American Advertising House ID Numbers.* [Online]. Available: http://clerk.house.gov/pd/houseID.html?reg_id=37455/ [accessed July 27, 2005].

Peters JC, Wyatt HR, Donahoo WT, Hill JO. 2002. From instinct to intellect: The challenge of maintaining healthy weight in the modern world. *Obes Rev* 3(2):69–74.

Ratner EM, Hellegers JF, Stern GP, Ogg RC, Adair S, Zacharias L. 1978. *FTC Staff Report on Television Advertising to Children.* Washington, DC: Federal Trade Commission.

Reilly JJ, Armstrong J, Dorosty AR, Emmett PM, Ness A, Rogers I, Steer C, Sherriff A. 2005. Early life risk factors for obesity in childhood: Cohort study. *Br Med J Online* 330(7504):1357–1364.

Roberts DF, Foehr UG, Rideout V. 2005. *Generation M: Media in the Lives of 8–18 Year Olds.* Menlo Park, CA: Henry J. Kaiser Family Foundation.

Roberts K. 2004. *The Future Beyond Brands: Lovemarks.* New York: PowerHouse Books.

Schlosser E. 2001. *Fast Food Nation. The Dark Side of the All-American Meal.* Boston, MA: Houghton Mifflin Company.

Schor JB. 2004. *Born to Buy: The Commercialized Child and the New Consumer Culture.* New York: Scribner.

Schudson M. 1986. *Advertising, The Uneasy Persuasion. It's Dubious Impact on American Society.* New York: BasicBooks.

Skinner JD, Carruth BR, Bounds W, Ziegler P, Reidy K. 2002. Do food-related experiences in the first 2 years of life predict dietary variety in school-aged children? *J Nutr Educ Behav* 34(6):310–315.

Srinivasan SR, Myers L, Berenson GS. 2002. Predictability of childhood adiposity and insulin for developing insulin resistance syndrome (syndrome X) in young adulthood: The Bogalusa Heart Study. *Diabetes* 51(1):204–209.

Swinburn B, Egger G. 2005. Preventive strategies against weight gain and obesity. *Obes Rev* 3:289–301.

Taylor JP, Evers S, McKenna M. 2005. Determinants of healthy eating in children and youth. *Canadian J Public Health* 96(Suppl 3):S20–S26.

Teenage Research Unlimited. 2004. *Teens Spent $175 Billion in 2003.* [Online]. Available: http://www.teenresearch.com/PRview.cfm?edit_id=168/ [accessed August 4, 2005].

The Consumer Ombudsman. 1999. *Guidelines on the Consumer Ombudsman's Practice. Marketing in Relation to Children and Young People.* Lysaker, Norway: The Consumer Ombudsman.

Whitaker RC, Wright JA, Pepe MS, Seidel KD, Dietz WH. 1997. Predicting obesity in young adulthood from childhood and parental obesity. *N Engl J Med* 337(13):869–873.

WHO (World Health Organization). 2004. *Global Strategy on Diet, Physical Activity and Health.* Report No. WHA57.17. [Online]. Available: http://www.who.int/gb/ebwha/pdf_files/WHA57/A57_R17-en.pdf [accessed August 5, 2005].

Young BM. 1990. *Television Advertising and Children.* Oxford, U.K.: Clarendon Press.

2

Health, Diet, and Eating Patterns of Children and Youth

INTRODUCTION

Over the past four decades, lower rates of nutrient deficiencies, dental caries, infectious diseases, and injuries have all contributed to lower childhood morbidity and mortality and better health for children. In that same period, a troubling new trend has steadily and dramatically emerged, threatening to reverse many of these gains. From 1963 to 2002, rates of obesity tripled for older children ages 6–11 years and adolescents ages 12–19 years. For consistency between Institute of Medicine (IOM) reports, the term *obesity* is used to refer to children and youth who have a body mass index (BMI) equal to or greater than the 95th percentile of the age- and gender-specific BMI charts developed by the Centers for Disease Control and Prevention (CDC). By this definition, an estimated 9.18 million U.S. children and adolescents ages 6–19 years are considered obese. If obesity levels continue at the current rate, the lifetime risk of being diagnosed with type 2 diabetes at some point in their lives is 30 percent for boys and 40 percent for girls. Moreover, an estimated 1 million 12- to 19-year-old American adolescents have the metabolic syndrome, described later in this chapter.

Health-related behaviors such as eating habits and physical activity patterns develop early in life and often extend into adulthood. They consequently affect risk for a variety of chronic diseases including type 2 diabetes and cardiovascular disease. Parents, communities, government, the public health sector, and health care systems accordingly face the significant challenge of creating a supportive environment in which children can grow up in a way that maximizes their chances for a healthy life. As a result of the distinct trend toward the onset of chronic disease risks much earlier in life, dietary guidance for children and youth has evolved from an historic emphasis on ensuring nutrient and energy (calorie) adequacy to meet basic metabolic needs to the more recent focus on ensuring dietary quality while avoiding calorie excesses. The current goal is to promote a lifestyle for children and youth that incorporates nutrient-dense foods and beverages into their diet, and balances their calorie consumption with levels of physical activity sufficient to create energy balance at a healthy weight.[1]

This chapter provides an overview of the dietary intake, eating patterns, and sources of nutrients for infants and toddlers, younger children, school-aged children, and adolescents. It examines how nutrient and food intakes compare to reference standards and guidelines, and it also addresses regional and income-related differences in food consumption and nutrient intake.

OVERVIEW OF CHILDREN'S HEALTH AND DIET

Public health and technological improvements over the past century have enhanced the survival and health of infants, school-aged children, and adolescents in the United States (NRC and IOM, 2004). Widespread access to potable water, vaccines, and antibiotics has reduced child morbidity and mortality rates attributed to infectious diseases (CDC, 1999; IOM, 2005b). Safety initiatives targeted to motor vehicles and children's home and recreational environments have led to a 39 percent decline in unintentional injury deaths among children ages 14 and under from 1987 to 2000 (National SAFE KIDS Campaign, 2003). The introduction of various fluoride vehicles through municipal water systems and other sources has prompted a substantial decline in dental caries in children over the past two decades (DHHS, 2000b; Dye et al., 2004).

The health and nutritional well-being of millions of Americans have benefited from a number of interventions, including the fortification of the food supply with essential micronutrients such as B vitamins, iron, iodine, and folic acid (Hetzel and Clugston, 1999; Honein et al., 2001; IOM, 2003; Park et al., 2000; Pfeiffer et al., 2005). The diets of low-income families, their infants, and school-aged children have improved through the creation and expanded coverage of domestic food assistance programs to increase

---

[1]Growing children, even those at a healthy body weight, must be in a slightly positive energy balance to satisfy the additional calorie needs of tissue deposition for normal growth. However, for the purpose of simplicity in this report, the committee uses the term energy balance in children and youth to indicate an equality between energy intake and energy expenditure that supports normal growth without promoting excess weight gain and body fat.

food security, such as the Special Supplemental Nutrition Program for Women, Infants, and Children (WIC), the National School Meals Program, and the Food Stamp Program (IOM, 2005b,c; USDA, 2005c); and improved state health insurance coverage for children living in poor families (Cohen and Bloom, 2005; Wise, 2004). The outcomes have been linked to increased birth weights (IOM, 2005c), and a steady decline in the prevalence of micronutrient-deficiency diseases in childhood such as rickets, pellagra, goiter, iron-deficiency anemia, and neural tube defects (CDC, 1999, 2002; Honein et al., 2001).

Obesity

Although the health of children and youth has improved in many respects, they face new diet-related health problems today that were unexpected just a generation ago. The increasing prevalence over the past three decades of children who are obese, defined in this report as children and youth who have a BMI equal to or greater than the 95th percentile of the age- and gender-specific BMI charts developed by the CDC, and those who are at risk for becoming obese, defined in this report as children and youth who have a BMI between the 85th and 95th percentile of the age- and gender-specific CDC BMI charts, makes it the most common serious contemporary public health concern faced by young people in the United States (IOM, 2005b; Land, 2005). The average weight for a 10-year-old boy increased from 74.2 pounds in 1963 to nearly 85 pounds in 2002. The average weight for a 10-year-old girl went from 77.4 pounds to an estimated 88 pounds. The average 15-year-old boy weighed 135.5 pounds in 1966, and 150.3 pounds in 2002. The average weight of a 15-year-old girl rose from 124.2 pounds to 134.4 pounds during the same time frame (Ogden et al., 2004). The trends are similar for American adults. Improved nutrition has helped them grow taller over the past four decades, but it has also made them heavier. Adults are an average of 1 inch taller than they were in the 1960s but about 25 pounds heavier (Ogden et al., 2004).

Obesity has both short- and long-term consequences for children's emotional health and physical and social functioning and well-being (IOM, 2005b; Williams et al., 2005). Obesity also produces significant burdens on the health care system. Obesity-associated annual hospital costs for children and adolescents more than tripled over two decades, rising from $35 million (1979–1981) to $127 million (1997–1999, based on 2001 dollars) (Wang and Dietz, 2002). After adjusting for inflation and converting to 2004 dollars, the national direct and indirect health care expenditures associated with adult overweight and obesity range from $98 billion to $129 billion (IOM, 2005b). If the childhood obesity epidemic continues at its current rate, conditions related to type 2 diabetes, such as blindness, coronary artery disease, stroke, and kidney failure, may become ordinary conditions in middle age (IOM, 2005b).

Between 1999 and 2002, the prevalence of obesity was 10.3 percent for younger children ages 2–5 years, 15.8 percent among children ages 6–11 years, and 16.1 percent among adolescents ages 12–19 years (Hedley et al., 2004). Overall, 31 percent of U.S. children and adolescents are either obese (16 percent) or at risk of becoming obese (15 percent)—figures that are three and six times greater than the Healthy People 2010 goal of 5 percent (DHHS, 2000a; Hedley et al., 2004). Since the 1970s, the rate of obesity has more than doubled for preschool children ages 2 to 5 years (IOM, 2005b; Ogden et al., 2003). As shown in Figure 2-1, between 1963 and 2002, obesity rates tripled for older children ages 6–11 years and youth ages 12–19 years (CDC, 2005). More than 9 million U.S. children and adolescents ages 6–19 years are considered to be obese (CDC, 2004).

Leaner children and youth have remained more or less the same weight,

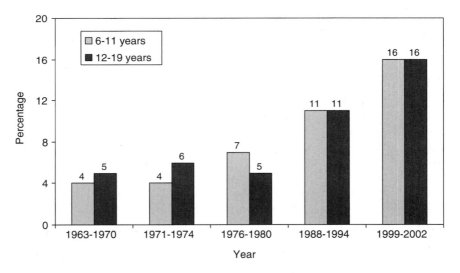

FIGURE 2-1 Prevalence of obesity among U.S. children and adolescents by age group and selected period, 1963–2002.
NOTE: In this report, children with a body mass index (BMI) value at or above the 95th percentile of the CDC age- and gender-specific BMI curves for 2000 are referred to as obese, and children with a BMI value between the 85th percentile and 95th percentile are referred to as at risk for becoming obese. These cut-off points correspond to the terms, overweight and at risk for overweight, used for children and youth by the CDC.
SOURCE: CDC (2005).

but those in the upper percentiles of the BMI charts are heavier. The CDC compiled BMI charts on the basis of combined survey data from several nationally representative cross-sectional samples of the U.S. population that were collected between 1963 and 1980.[2] It is notable that the BMI levels for children in the lower part of the BMI chart distribution (the 5th to the 50th percentiles) remained stable when comparing the national surveys (Flegal and Troiano, 2000). Thus, a child in the 1990s who is at or below the 50th percentile is more likely to have a similar BMI when compared to a child in the 1970s; however, a child in the 1990s who is at or above the 85th percentile is more likely to have a significantly higher BMI when compared to a cohort from the 1970s.

Related Chronic Disease Risk

Even among children and youth who are not obese, diets too high in saturated fats, *trans* fat, and sodium predispose them to the risk of heart disease, stroke, and certain cancers. Moreover, approximately 1 million 12- to 19-year-olds in the United States have the metabolic syndrome (AHA, 2005; Cook et al., 2003), defined as having three or more of the following abnormalities: blood triglyceride level of 110 milligrams per deciliter (mg/dL) or higher; high-density lipoprotein levels of 40 mg/dL or lower; elevated fasting glucose of 110 mg/dL or higher; blood pressure above the 90th percentile for age, sex, and height; and waist circumference at or above the 90th percentile for age and sex.

About 30 percent of obese adolescents will develop the metabolic syndrome, and nearly two-thirds who develop the syndrome are obese (AHA, 2005). In adults, the metabolic syndrome is associated with type 2 diabetes (Cook et al., 2003; Haffner et al., 1992), cardiovascular disease (Cook et al., 2003; Isomaa et al., 2001), and a higher mortality rate (Cook et al., 2003; Lakka et al., 2002). Even among those obese youth who do not yet have clinical diabetes, components of the metabolic syndrome appear to contribute to the development of atherosclerosis (Berenson et al., 1998; Mahoney et al., 1996; McGill et al., 2002). The association of childhood and youth obesity with the metabolic syndrome, rather than exclusively with diabetes, may present the greatest physical health threat of childhood obesity.

---

[2]Because of the increases in bodyweight that occurred in the 1980s and 1990s, the CDC decided not to include the National Health and Nutrition Examination Study (NHANES) III (1988–1994) body weight data in the revised year 2000 charts of BMI standards for children ages 6 years or older. The NHANES III data would have shifted the curves (weight-for-age and BMI-for-age) upward, erroneously conveying a range of appropriateness to the higher weights.

Micronutrient Inadequacies

Although progress has been made in certain areas, subgroups of children and adolescents still experience micronutrient inadequacies that may adversely affect their health, particularly insufficient intakes of vitamins A, E, B_6, and folate as well as calcium, iron, potassium, zinc, and magnesium (DHHS and USDA, 2004; Ganji et al., 2003; IOM, 2005c).

Inadequate dietary calcium intake combined with physical inactivity during childhood, adolescence, and early adulthood compromises peak bone mass and contributes to bone resorption and bone diseases, including osteomalacia and osteoporosis in later adulthood (NIH, 2001). Young adults who do not reach a normal peak bone mass by 20 years of age have the greatest risk of developing osteoporosis in later years (Beck and Shoemaker, 2000). Osteoporosis is a serious health problem for today's youth that has been associated with a decline in calcium intake (NIH, 2001), attributed in part to increased consumption of sweetened beverages (such as carbonated soft drinks, fruit drinks, and sweetened teas) and reduced consumption of milk—the primary source of calcium in U.S. children's and adolescents' diets (AAP, 2004; Fisher et al., 2004; Mrdjenovic and Levitsky, 2003). Studies suggest that a higher consumption of carbonated beverages in adolescent girls may be associated with incidence of bone fracture (Wyshak, 2000). Moreover, rickets among infants is attributed to inadequate vitamin D intake and reduced exposure to sunlight, and remains a problem in the United States. For example, reemergence of nutritional rickets has been reported in some African American infants[3] (Weisberg et al., 2004).

Dental Caries

Diets high in added sugars also predispose to dental caries. Although the prevalence of dental caries has decreased in the United States, in particular due to topical and water supply fluoridation, lack of access to care has contributed to declines in dental visits and increased rates of untreated dental caries for children and adolescents (DHHS, 2000b; Gift et al., 1996). More than one-half of low-income children without health insurance had no preventive dental care visits (Kenney et al., 2005). The Surgeon General's

---

[3]The American Academy of Pediatrics (AAP) recommends that all infants, including those who are exclusively breastfed, receive a minimum intake of 200 international units (IU) of vitamin D daily beginning during the first 2 months of life. Additionally, the AAP recommends that an intake of 200 IU of vitamin D be continued throughout childhood and adolescence because adequate sunlight exposure is not easily determined for an individual (Gartner et al., 2003). Daily sunlight exposure to skin allows the human body to convert vitamin D to a biologically active form that is absorbed by the lower intestine and metabolized with dietary calcium to prevent rickets (IOM, 1997).

Report on Oral Health in America (DHHS, 2000b) has documented that despite progress in reducing dental caries, children and adolescents in families living below the poverty level experience more dental decay than those in higher socioeconomic levels. In addition, the proportion of teeth affected by dental caries varies by age and race/ethnicity. Poor Mexican-American children ages 2–9 have the highest proportion of untreated decayed teeth (70.5 percent), followed by poor African-American children (67.4 percent), as compared to poor white children (57.2 percent). Poor adolescents ages 12–17 years in each racial/ethnic group have a higher percentage of untreated decayed primary teeth than their peers who do not live in poverty (DHHS, 2000b). Changes in dietary patterns of younger children ages 2–5 years (e.g., increased frequency of sweetened snacks) may also contribute to the reversal of oral health benefits of fluoridation observed since the 1980s (Dye et al., 2004).

DIETARY RECOMMENDATIONS AND GUIDELINES

A healthful diet for children and adolescents provides recommended amounts of nutrients and other food components within estimated energy requirements (EER)[4] to promote normal growth and development, a healthy weight trajectory, and energy balance.[5] A healthful diet also reduces the long-term risk for obesity and related chronic diseases associated with aging, including type 2 diabetes and the metabolic syndrome (IOM, 2005b).

Thirty years ago, diet quality for children and youth focused on the consumption of a sufficient and balanced intake of foods providing calories, protein, and micronutrients to prevent deficiency diseases. Today, by contrast, dietary quality emphasizes the principles of adequacy, variety, proportionality, and moderation, as well as reinforcing recommendations for a high intake of fruits, vegetables, and whole grains; nutrient-dense foods providing sufficient calories that are balanced with daily physical activity levels; and limited consumption of total fat, saturated fat, *trans* fatty acids, cholesterol, sodium, and added sugars (DHHS and USDA, 2005).

The average healthy child ages 2 to 5 years gains 4.5 to 6.5 pounds and grows 2.5 to 3.5 inches each year (Story et al., 2003). Child growth continues at a slow and steady rate until the onset of puberty in late middle childhood or early adolescence. A healthy child's appetite and food intake

---

[4]Estimated energy requirements (EER) are available for children and youth ages 2–18 years and calculated based gender, age, and three different activity levels (IOM, 2002–2005; Appendix D-1).

[5]In this report, energy balance in children and youth refers to a state in which energy intake equals energy expenditure; energy balance supports normal growth and development without promoting excess weight gain and body fat.

varies with the rate of growth, which occurs unevenly in spurts and periods of slower growth. The growth that occurs during adolescence is significant and comparable to the growth that occurs during the first year of life. During adolescence, nutrition needs are higher than during any other period of the lifecycle. Puberty is when adolescents gain approximately 50 percent of their adult body weight, accumulate an estimated 40–45 percent of skeletal muscle mass, and achieve the final 15–20 percent of their linear growth (Shils et al., 1999; Story et al., 2003).

National dietary recommendations and guidelines established for the American population have been used to assess the diets of children and youth. These recommendations and guidelines collectively include the Dietary Reference Intakes (DRIs), the Dietary Guidelines for Americans, and the Food Guide Pyramid (FGP) and *MyPyramid*.

Dietary Reference Intakes

The DRIs is a term used for a set of distinct, nutrient-based reference values that are based on scientifically grounded relationships between nutrient intake and indicators of good health and chronic disease prevention (IOM, 1997, 1998, 2001, 2002–2005, 2005a). The DRIs, which replaced the former Recommended Dietary Allowances in the United States (NRC, 1989), include values for the following:

• Estimated Average Requirement (EAR), which is the nutrient intake level estimated to meet the requirements of half the healthy individuals in a given life stage and gender group for a specific indicator or outcome; it is the median of a distribution and can be used to estimate the prevalence of inadequacy in a group;
• Recommended Dietary Allowance (RDA), which is a nutrient intake level estimated to meet the needs of nearly all individuals (97.5 percent) within a given life stage and gender group, and is calculated as two standard deviations above the EAR;
• Adequate Intake (AI),[6] which is a nutrient intake level based on observed or experimentally derived estimates of nutrient intake of healthy

---

[6]Mean usual intake at or greater than the AI is equated with a low prevalence of inadequate nutrient intakes, especially when the AI is based on the mean intake of a healthy group. Unlike an EAR, an AI value cannot be used to estimate the prevalence of nutrient inadequacy in a population. If at least 50 percent of the gender or age group has intakes greater than the AI, then the prevalence of inadequacy should be low. If less than 50 percent have intakes greater than the AI, then no conclusion can be drawn about the prevalence of nutrient inadequacy in a population group.

people and used as a guide for individual intake when there is insufficient scientific evidence to calculate an RDA for a specific nutrient; and

- Tolerable Upper Intake Level (UL), which is based on a risk assessment model and used in the highest average daily intake likely to pose no risk of adverse health effects.

The DRI report series was released by the IOM between 1997 and 2004. The 2002–2005 IOM report provided EER levels, which are suggested calorie[7] intakes based on age, sex, and physical activity level, and DRIs for carbohydrate and fat (including saturated, unsaturated, and *trans* fats), cholesterol, total protein, and individual amino acids (IOM, 2002–2005). This report introduced the concept of an Acceptable Macronutrient Distribution Range (AMDR), representing a range of intakes for carbohydrates, fats, and protein expressed as a percentage of calorie intake. Consumption outside the AMDR is associated with an increased risk of chronic disease and insufficient nutrient intake (IOM, 2002–2005).

Energy intakes based on the EER for proposed food consumption patterns have been developed for boys and girls ages 2 to 18 years for three physical activity levels—sedentary, low active, and active (USDA, 2003a; Appendix D, Table D-1). The DRI report on electrolytes and water provides total water AI levels for children and adolescents of different ages, which can be used as guidelines for total fluid intake obtained from beverages and foods (IOM, 2005a). Macronutrient and micronutrient recommendations for children and adolescents from the DRI reports are summarized in Appendix D, Tables D-2 and D-3. Many EAR, RDA, and AI levels for children and adolescents are estimates or extrapolations from data on adults (IOM, 1997, 1998, 2001, 2002–2005).

Finding: More certain determinations of nutritional requirements for children and adolescents await the development of better techniques and data sets.

Dietary Guidelines for Americans

The Dietary Guidelines for Americans are developed jointly by the U.S. Department of Health and Human Services (DHHS) and the U.S. Department of Agriculture (USDA) and draw from recommendations of a nonfederal Dietary Advisory Committee. The Dietary Guidelines for Americans present summary dietary recommendations for the public based on current scientific evidence and medical knowledge. They represent the government

---

[7]In this report, the term calories is used synonymously with kilocalories.

BOX 2-1
2005 Dietary Guidelines for Americans

- Consume a variety of nutrient-dense foods and beverages within and among the basic food groups while choosing foods that limit the intake of saturated and *trans* fats, cholesterol, added sugars, salt, and alcohol.
- Meet recommended intakes within calorie needs by adopting a balanced eating pattern, such as the U.S. Department of Agriculture Food Guide Pyramid or the Dietary Approaches to Stop Hypertension (DASH) Eating Plan.
- For weight management, maintain body weight in a healthy range and balance calories from foods and beverages with calories expended. To prevent gradual weight gain over time, make small decreases in food and beverage calories and increase physical activity.

SOURCE: DHHS and USDA (2005).

---

policy document on dietary practices and are mandated to be promoted in all federal nutrition education programs. Initially published in 1980, they are revised every 5 years. The sixth edition was released in 2005. The key recommendations of the Dietary Guidelines, summarized in Box 2-1, are based on a preponderance of the scientific evidence of nutritional factors that are important in lowering the risk of chronic disease and promoting health, including specific recommendations for weight management, physical activity, food safety, and consumption patterns among food groups, saturated fats, *trans* fats, cholesterol, sugars, other carbohydrates, sodium and potassium, and alcoholic beverages (DHHS and USDA, 2005).

Food Guide Pyramid and *MyPyramid*

The FGP is an educational tool for the public that was designed by the USDA in 1992 as the graphic representation of the Dietary Guidelines for Americans. It takes the Dietary Guidelines, along with the Recommended Dietary Allowances, and translates them into servings from various food groups with the goal of promoting a healthful diet for the U.S. population. The qualitative dietary guidance depicted by the FGP is based on the principles of balance, variety, proportionality, and moderation (USDA, 1992, 1996). The FGP for Young Children is similar in content to the FGP but was adapted for younger children ages 2 to 6 years, and recommended fewer serving sizes from certain food groups (USDA, 2003b).

In 2005, an interactive food guidance system, *MyPyramid*, was released that replaced the existing FGP (USDA, 2005b). *MyPyramid* is a component of an overall food guidance system that emphasizes a more individualized approach to improving diet and lifestyle. In particular, it offers personalized recommendations for the types and amounts of food for individuals to consume each day, recommends gradual improvement in daily diet and lifestyle habits including physical activity, and underscores the principles of variety, moderation, and proportionality. A child-friendly version of *MyPyramid* was recently released to reach children ages 6–11 years with targeted messages about the importance of making healthful eating and physical activity choices and an interactive computer game to apply these messages (USDA, 2005b).

Linked to *MyPyramid* is the *MyPyramid Tracker*, which has two components—assessment of food intake and physical activity. The food intake assessment component incorporates what was previously the Interactive Healthy Eating Index (HEI) as an online educational tool for individuals who would like to assess their dietary intake according to *MyPyramid* and the Dietary Guidelines for Americans (USDA, 2005a). The USDA and other researchers use the HEI for research and assessment purposes to assess and monitor diet quality of the U.S. population according to the Dietary Guidelines for Americans and to investigate relationships between diet and health (USDA, 2005d). The HEI evaluates food consumption patterns against the FGP recommendations using five food-based components (grains, vegetables, fruits, dairy, and meat) and it uses four nutrient-based components to assess adherence to recommendations in the 2000 Dietary Guidelines for Americans for maximum daily intake of total fat and saturated fat, as well as the IOM recommendations for daily cholesterol and sodium (Basiotis et al., 2002; Lin, 2005).[8]

WHAT CHILDREN AND YOUTH EAT

The Dietary Guidelines Advisory Committee Report (DHHS and USDA, 2004) noted that, based on available food consumption data, children's and adolescents' dietary intakes of saturated fatty acids, *trans* fatty acids, and sodium are higher than recommended (DHHS and USDA, 2004). Additionally, the rising prevalence of obesity in children and adolescents of all ages and across all ethnic groups over the past four decades indicates that their calorie intakes are not balanced with their energy expenditure levels over

---

[8]The HEI is being updated by the USDA Center for Nutrition Policy and Promotion to reflect the 2005 Dietary Guidelines for Americans. It should be completed by early 2006 (USDA, 2005c). The food intake assessment component of *MyPyramid Tracker* will be updated in 2006 to reflect the new HEI.

time (CDC, 2005; IOM, 2005b). The Dietary Guidelines Advisory Committee Report also identified sufficiently low intakes of dietary calcium, potassium, fiber, magnesium, and vitamin E by children and adolescents to raise concern about nutrient adequacy, and highlighted the need for sufficient intake of iron and folic acid by adolescent girls of childbearing age (DHHS and USDA, 2004). Substantial evidence reviewed in this chapter underlies the concern about the intake of certain nutrients and food components in the diets of children and adolescents, the food consumption patterns associated with these intakes, and changes observed over time.

Sources of Nutrient and Food Intake Information

Major sources of information about the food and nutrient intakes of nationally representative groups of children and youth are the USDA's older Nationwide Food Consumption Survey (NFCS) (through 1977) and its more recent Continuing Survey of Food Intakes by Individuals (CSFII) and the DHHS's series of National Health and Nutrition Examination Surveys (NHANES).[9] In general, these cross-sectional surveys are complex stratified samples of the population and sampling weights varied depending on the design and oversampling of selected subgroups. The design, sampling, and methods for collecting dietary data differ among the surveys and have evolved over time, confounding conclusions as to trends. Information about the dates, population, sample size, and methodology for assessing dietary intake for the main surveys referenced in this chapter is summarized in Appendix D (Table D-4).

Challenges of Dietary Assessment Methods

Dietary assessment methods are subject to a variety of reporting errors, including problems associated with individuals accurately recalling the types and quantities of foods and beverages consumed; estimating portion sizes; general misreporting according to what is considered socially desirable, especially among individuals who are overweight or obese; and selective underreporting of specific foods (e.g., foods high in fat, sugars, and refined carbohydrates) (Huang et al., 2004; IOM, 2002–2005, 2005b).

To compensate for these methodological limitations, multiple passes were added to the 24-hour dietary recall starting with CSFII 1994–1996, including detailed questions addressing food preparation and frequently unreported foods. These have improved the completeness of data collec-

---

[9]The dietary component of NHANES is called *What We Eat in America*, a joint effort of the USDA and DHHS.

tion. The combination of improved methodology for collecting dietary information and the pervasive problems of underreporting total food and calorie intake confound the assessment of an individual's actual dietary intake as well as trends in dietary intake over time. However, the dietary data from each survey provide the best estimate of a group's intake at that point in time. The assessment of children's dietary intake poses additional problems due to the nature, extent, and determinants of underreporting or overreporting for children and adolescents because the combination of methodological limitations are not well understood (Livingstone and Robson, 2000). Additionally, food intake for younger children is provided by proxy. Although the primary caregiver may be a reliable reporter of a child's food intake in the home setting, that may not be the case for foods and beverages consumed away from home.

In NFCS 1977–1978 and CSFII 1989–1991, an adult household member reported information for children younger than age 12 years (Enns et al., 2002). In CSFII 1994–1996 and 1998, children ages 6–11 years were interviewed directly when asked to describe their individual food intake and were assisted as necessary by an adult household member (Enns et al., 2002). When needed, additional information was obtained from the school cafeteria personnel or care providers to improve completeness of data collected. In NHANES III, proxy respondents provided information for 97 percent of the children younger than age 6 years; children ages 6–11 years were permitted to report their own intake but only 55 percent did so, with the remaining respondents either completed by proxy (23 percent) or by both a child and a proxy (23 percent) (Troiano et al., 2000). Children ages 12 years and older typically reported their own dietary intake information (Enns et al., 2002; Troiano et al., 2000).

Huang and colleagues (2004) estimated that 55 percent of children and adolescents in CSFII 1994–1996 and 1998 had reported calorie intakes that were not scientifically reliable or plausible. In children with plausible data, calorie intake tended to be overreported for younger children and underreported more often in obese older children, thereby concluding that it is necessary to exclude implausible dietary reports to draw dietary associations between children's dietary intake and BMI percentiles. Experimental studies in children and adolescents have shown that mean daily calorie intakes can be underreported by as much as 17 to 33 percent of energy expenditure and that underreporting tends to increase with age (Bandini et al., 2003; Champagne et al., 1998). Similar methodological challenges exist for conducting research on children's physical activity levels (IOM, 2005b).

Finding: More accurate methods are needed to assess the dietary intakes of children and youth, including calorie intakes and expenditures.

Nutrient Intakes of Children and Youth

Mean Nutrient Intakes and Changes Between the 1970s and 1990s

Data from different sources on calorie intakes present variable results by age and gender. Substantial overall increases were reported in the mean calorie intakes of children and youth from the mid-1970s to the mid-1990s. Average calorie intakes by younger children ages 2–5 years increased by 172 calories (Kranz et al., 2004), among adolescent boys by 243 calories (Enns et al., 2003), and among adolescent girls by approximately 113 calories (Enns et al., 2003). Detailed data on the nutrient intakes of different racial/ethnic groups is limited; thus, there is a need to be cautious when extrapolating the results to the various groups of U.S. ethnic minority children and youth.

Finding: Total calorie intake appears to have increased substantially over the past 25 years for preschool children and adolescent boys and girls, with more modest changes for children ages 6–11 years.[10]

Trends in percentage of calorie intake of specific foods and beverages in U.S. children and adolescents, ages 2–18 years, are available from 1977–1978 to 1994–1996 (Nielsen et al., 2002b). Some foods, such as low- and medium-fat milk, and medium- and high-fat beef and pork, declined as a percentage of overall calorie intake from 1977–1978 to 1994–1996. Other foods and beverages revealed a modest increase in percentage of total calorie intake during this period, such as carbonated soft drinks (3 percent to 5.5 percent), fruit drinks (1.8 percent to 3.1 percent), candy (1.1 percent to 2.1 percent), french fries (1.7 percent to 2.6 percent), and pizza (1.4 percent to 3.4 percent) (Nielsen et al., 2002b). In this data analysis, mean calorie intake increased 118 calories (6.4 percent), from 1,840 calories in 1977–1978 to 1,958 calories in 1994–1996.

Another analysis of CSFII 1989–1991 data examined major food sources of nutrients and dietary constituents in 4,008 U.S. children ages 2–18 years (Subar et al., 1998). Milk, yeast breads/donuts, beef, and cheese were ranked among the top 10 sources of total calories, fat, and protein in children's and youths' diet. Many of the top 10 sources of carbohydrates and fat contributed more than 2 percent each to children's calorie intake

---

[10]Although there are methodological challenges in accurately assessing both calorie intake and physical activity levels, an in-depth discussion about physical activity is beyond the committee's charge. An extensive discussion of trends in the physical activity of children and youth, and its relationship to energy balance, may be found in the report, *Preventing Childhood Obesity: Health in the Balance* (IOM, 2005b).

(Subar et al., 1998; Appendix D, Table D-6). Carbohydrate sources include yeast breads, soft drinks, sodas, milk, ready-to-eat (RTE) cereals, cakes/cookies/quick breads/donuts, sugars/syrups/jams, fruit drinks, pasta, and white potatoes. Fat sources include milk, cheese, cakes/cookies/quick breads/donuts, potato chips/corn chips, and ice cream/sherbet/frozen yogurt. Based on this analysis, low-nutrient foods are a significant contributor to the total calorie, fat, and carbohydrate intake of children and youth (Subar et al., 1998). These results were confirmed in a more recent analysis of NHANES III and NHANES 1999–2000 that examined foods and food groups contributing the most to population intake of calories (Block, 2004). Although the analysis did not report percentage of calorie intake by age, it found that the top 10 food items that contributed the most to calorie intake in the entire U.S. population were high-calorie, low-nutrient foods and beverages (e.g., sweets and carbonated soft drinks), which contributed nearly one third of all the calories consumed (Block, 2004; Appendix D, Table D-7).

Finding: Children and youth consume a large proportion of their total calories from foods and beverages that are of high-calorie and low-nutrient content.

Obesity may develop from a relatively small excess of daily calories consumed (e.g., 50 to 100 calories/day) versus calories expended over several months and years (IOM, 2005b). Both excessive calorie intake and physical inactivity are likely contributors to the calorie imbalance that leads to obesity. Further study is needed on the relative contribution to childhood obesity of excess calorie intake versus insufficient calorie expenditure (IOM, 2005b).

NFCS and CSFII data indicate changes in the macronutrient sources of calories for children (6–11 years) and adolescents (12–19 years) over time, suggesting a possible decrease in the gram (g) amounts of fat and protein and an increase in the gram amounts of carbohydrate (Enns et al., 2002, 2003) with associated changes in the percentage of calorie intake from protein, fat, and carbohydrates (Appendix D, Table D-5) (Enns et al., 2002, 2003).

Carbohydrate intake increased both in total amount and as a percent of calories for boys, ages 6–11 years, from 226 g in 1977–1978 to 280 g in 1994–1996 and 1998 (representing an increase from 46.8 percent to 54.8 percent of carbohydrates as a percent of total calories) and for girls, ages 6–11 years, an increase from 212 g in 1977–1978 to 250 g in 1994–1996 and 1998 (representing an increase from 47.4 percent to 54.9 percent of carbohydrates as a percent of total calories) (Enns et al., 2002). An analysis of the same data showed similar increased trends in carbohydrate intake for adolescent boys, ages 12–19 years, from 279 g in 1977–

1978 to 366 g in 1994–1996 and 1998 (representing an increase from 44.6 percent to 53.2 percent of carbohydrates as a percent of total calories) and for girls, ages 12–19 years, an increase from 45.4 g in 1977–1978 to 55 g in 1994–1996 and 1998 (representing an increase from 45.4 percent to 55 percent of carbohydrates as a percent of total calories) (Enns et al., 2002).

Finding: Carbohydrate intake has increased substantially among children and youth over approximately the past two decades.

Total fat intake of children and adolescents was 38–40 percent of calories in 1977–1978 (Enns et al., 2002, 2003). Based on data from CSFII 1994–1996 and 1998, total fat intake in children and adolescents (ages 6–18 years) was 32 percent of calories (Enns et al., 2002, 2003). Only an estimated 25 percent of children and adolescents had usual total fat intakes that were 30 percent of energy or less (Gleason and Suitor, 2001). Non-Hispanic black adolescents had slightly higher fat intakes (36 percent of calories) than non-Hispanic white adolescents (33 percent of calories) and Mexican American adolescents (34 percent of calories) (Troiano et al., 2000).

Another study based on CSFII 1994–1996 and 1998 showed a decline in fat and saturated fat intake as a percentage of calories for younger children (ages 2–5 years) (Kranz et al., 2004). Fat intake decreased from 36 percent of calories in 1977–1978 to 32 percent of calories in 1994–1996 and 1998, and saturated fat intake decreased from 14 percent of calories to 12 percent. However, the absolute amount of fat intake (measured by grams/day) in younger children increased slightly (Kranz et al., 2004). Although children and youth may have reduced their fat intake and saturated fat intake over the past 25 years, a large proportion still consume amounts that exceed recommended levels.

Mean intakes of cholesterol ranged from 257 mg in younger children (ages 2–5 years) to 340 mg in youth (ages 12–19 years) in NHANES I, and intakes were highest in adolescent boys (411 mg) (Troiano et al., 2000). The higher cholesterol intake in adolescent boys is consistent with their higher calorie intake. Cholesterol intakes declined consistently between NHANES I, II, and III across all age, race, and sex groups to 193–211 mg, except for adolescent African American boys whose cholesterol intake remained at about 355 mg.

Of the vitamins and minerals reported in NFCS 1977–1978 and CSFII 1994–1996 and 1998, the mean intake of vitamin B_{12} decreased significantly; thiamin and iron increased; and calcium, phosphorus, magnesium, and vitamin A did not change for children or adolescents (Enns et al., 2002, 2003; Appendix D, Table D-5). Intakes of vitamin C, riboflavin, niacin, and vitamin B_6 either increased or did not change significantly, depending on age and sex. The nutrient intakes of girls did not appear to differ appreciably between 6- to 11-year-olds and 12- to 19-year-olds, except for 8 percent lower riboflavin and 10 percent lower calcium intakes in adolescents despite a higher calorie intake. Vitamin and mineral intakes for adolescent boys were higher than for the younger boys, and were most likely related to the overall higher calorie intake of older boys. Iron intakes in younger children (ages 2–5 years) increased between 1977–1978 and 1994–1996 and 1998 from 9.9 mg to 12.3 mg (Kranz et al., 2004).

Sodium intake data from the NHANES series reveal an increase in mean intake among all age groups of children and adolescents between 1971–1974 and 1999–2000 (Briefel and Johnson, 2004; Appendix D, Table D-8). For example, sodium intake in older adolescent boys (ages 16–19 years) increased 34 percent between 1971–1977 and 1999–2000 from 3,219 mg to 4,415 mg. Mean intakes increased 32–36 percent for children (ages 3–11 years) and younger adolescent boys (ages 12–15 years) and 45–68 percent for adolescent girls (ages 12–19 years). Assessment of sodium intakes and trends is difficult because sources include salt added in cooking, salt added at the table, and processed foods, and there are uncertainties associated with the exact sodium content of each source. Nonetheless increased consumption of processed foods and a greater frequency of eating away from home have contributed to the increased sodium intakes observed over the past three decades.

Nutrient Intakes Compared with the Dietary Reference Intakes and Dietary Guidelines

Usual nutrient intakes of U.S. children and adolescents (ages 1–18 years) from the dietary interview component of the NHANES 2001–2002 have been compared to the DRIs (Moshfegh et al., 2005). In general, less than 4 percent of 1- to 8-year-old children had nutrient intakes less than the EAR. Nutrients identified as potential problems in comparison with the EAR for boys and girls ages 9–18 years include vitamin A (13 percent to 55 percent),[11] vitamin E (80 percent to >97 percent), vitamin C (8 percent to 42 percent), and magnesium (14 percent to 91 percent). Adolescent girls were at highest risk for having nutrient intakes below the EAR, especially for folate (19 percent), phosphorus (49 percent),[12] vitamin B_6 (16 percent), zinc (26 percent), and copper (16 percent).

Although the AI cannot be used to estimate the prevalence of inad-

---

[11]Lowest and highest percent less than the EAR for the age range.
[12]Also of concern for girls 14–18 years with 42 percent less than the EAR.

equate nutrient intakes in a group, the prevalence of inadequacy should be low if at least 50 percent of a group has intakes greater than the AI. More than 50 percent of 1- to 8-year-olds had calcium intakes above the AI, but less than 5 percent of 9- to 18-year-old girls had usual calcium intakes above the recommended AI. The difference between the younger children and older girls is related primarily to the difference in the calcium AI values for the two age groups (800 mg for 4- to 8-year-olds versus 1,300 mg for 9- to 18-year-olds), but is also related to the lower calcium intakes observed in adolescent girls. Only 6 percent of girls, ages 9–13 years, and 9 percent of girls, ages 14–18 years, had calcium intakes greater than the AI (Moshfegh et al., 2005).

Other analyses of foods indicate that dairy foods and ingredients contribute more than 60 percent of the dietary calcium, nearly 25 percent of total fat, 39 percent of saturated fat, and 31 percent of cholesterol to the total dietary intakes of children and adolescents from birth to 19 years of age (Weinberg et al., 2004). Several studies have demonstrated that higher intakes of total dairy and milk are not only associated with increases in the intake of calcium but also often with significant increases in other essential nutrients, including magnesium, potassium, zinc, iron, vitamin A, riboflavin, and folate (Subar et al., 1998; Weinberg et al., 2004).

An analysis of calorie intakes in relation to the EER was not available. An older analysis compared calorie intakes with the 1989 Recommended Energy Allowances (REA) (NRC, 1989). Calorie intakes were above the REA for more than half the children, but technically below the REA for the remainder of the children studied (Suitor and Gleason, 2002). Factors discussed earlier that may explain why such a large proportion of children were below the REA include underreporting of food intake, a level of physical activity that is below the REA, or a combination of both factors (Suitor and Gleason, 2002). Additionally, the REA for children and adolescents was based on a theoretical estimation of total energy expenditure for a defined activity pattern rather than on measured energy expenditure. As a result the 1989 REA levels were based on a low to moderate activity level that is higher than the EER calculated for a sedentary activity level for the same age groups reported in the DRI report on macronutrients (IOM, 2002–2005) (Figure 2-2). The differences between the REA and EER suggest that children's calorie needs were overestimated from the 1970s to 2002. Some have suggested that decreased physical activity was likely more important than increased calorie intake as a contributor to the increase in obesity prevalence (Troiano et al., 2000). If children and adolescents were more sedentary over the past 20–30 years, then their REA levels should have been adjusted accordingly to account for the lower energy expenditure levels.

The current EER allows calorie requirements to be calculated based on

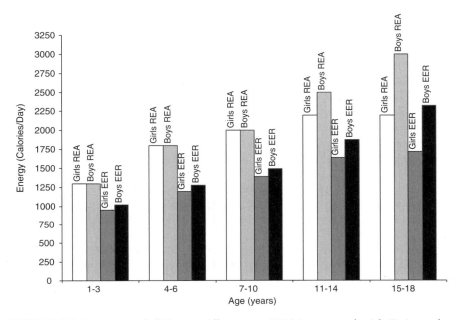

FIGURE 2-2 Recommended Energy Allowances (REA) compared with Estimated Energy Requirements (EER) for U.S. children and adolescents, ages 1–18 years, 1989 and 2002.
NOTE: The REA for girls and boys, ages 1–18 years, were calculated based on a low to moderate activity level that is higher than the EER calculated for a sedentary activity level for the same age groups reported in the DRI report on macronutrients.
SOURCES: IOM (2002–2005), NRC (1989).

several different physical activity levels and the corresponding DRI report provides guidance for using the EER to maintain body weight, to prevent weight gain, and assess intake in individuals and groups (IOM, 2002–2005).

A total fat intake of 30–40 percent of calories is recommended for children ages 1–3 years and 20–35 percent of calories for ages 4–18 years (IOM, 2002; Appendix D, Table D-2), and saturated fat intakes should be as low as possible—less that 10 percent of calories according to the Dietary Guidelines for Americans (DHHS and USDA, 2005). Data from CSFII 1994–1996 found the mean usual intake of saturated fat among school-aged children to be 12 percent of calories (Gleason and Suitor, 2001). Only an estimated one-quarter of girls (23 percent) and boys (25 percent) ages 6–11 years and about one-third of girls (34 percent) and boys (28 percent) ages 12–19 years had saturated fat intakes less than 10 percent of calories (USDA, 1999).

Based on percent of calories, the majority of children and adolescents ages 6–18 years met the intake recommendations for total fat (74 percent) and saturated fat (53 percent) during breakfast; however many fewer children met the recommendations (24 percent and 21 percent, respectively) during their lunch meals (Gleason and Suitor, 2001). Less Hispanic (17 percent; 10 percent) and African American (7 percent; 6 percent) children and adolescents achieved intakes within the recommendations for total fat and saturated fat, respectively, compared to 29 percent and 18 percent of non-Hispanic whites (Gleason and Suitor, 2001). The overall mean saturated fat intake reported in NHANES III (1988–1994) also was 12 percent of calories, varied little by sex and age, and displayed no consistent pattern by race or ethnicity (Troiano et al., 2000). Data from 1988–1994 showed an improvement in that about one-quarter of individuals under age 20 years had saturated fat intakes less than the recommended 10 percent of total calories (Carriquiry et al., 1997).

Similar to saturated fats, the intake of *trans* fatty acid should be kept as low as possible within the context of a nutritionally adequate diet (DHHS and USDA, 2005; IOM, 2002). *Trans* fatty acid intakes estimated from food intake data reported in CSFII 1989–1991 was 2.6 to 2.8 percent of calorie intake for children and adolescents ages 3–19 years (Allison et al., 1999). Approximately 80 percent of *trans* fatty acid intake in the U.S. diet is attributed to partially hydrogenated vegetable oil, which is used in products such as cakes, cookies, crackers, pies, and breads; margarine; fried potatoes; and potato chips, corn chips, and popcorn. *Trans* fatty acids also occur naturally in animal products, which account for 20 percent of intake.

Cholesterol intake also should be as low as possible within the context of a nutritionally adequate diet (IOM, 2002) with less than 300 mg/day recommended by the Dietary Guidelines for Americans (DHHS and USDA, 2005). Mean and median cholesterol intakes from NHANES III (1988–1994) were below 300 mg/day, except for adolescent boys (Troiano et al., 2000); between 50 to 75 percent of individuals under age 20 years had mean intakes below 300 mg/day (Carriquiry et al., 1997). Data from CSFII 1994–1996 and 1998 indicate that at least 80 percent of children and adolescents ages 6–19 years had cholesterol intakes below 300 mg, except adolescent boys, 56 percent of whom achieved desirable intakes below 300 mg/day (USDA, 1999).

Finding: Total fat and saturated fat intakes among children and youth remain at levels that exceed dietary recommendations.

A fiber intake of 14 g/1,000 calories is recommended as adequate (IOM, 2002). This translates to a daily total fiber intake of 19 to 38 grams for children and adolescents depending on age and sex (Appendix D, Table D-2). However, mean dietary fiber intakes based on CSFII 1994–1996 and 1998 were 12–13 g for girls and 14–17 g for boys (Enns et al., 2002, 2003), suggesting that most children and adolescents are not consuming recommended amounts of dietary fiber. In this same survey, with the exception of vitamin B_{12} and calcium, nutrient and food group consumption was better in younger children ages 2–5 years who consumed higher levels of dietary fiber, indicating a higher quality diet (Kranz et al., 2005a).

There is no DRI for added sugars[13] because there was insufficient evidence to set a UL (IOM, 2002–2005). However, the suggested limit for added sugars is that they should not exceed 25 percent of total calories to ensure adequate micronutrient intakes (IOM, 2002–2005, 2005). The 2005 Dietary Guidelines for Americans recommend that consumers choose and prepare foods and beverages with little added sugars, in amounts suggested by the USDA food guidance system, *MyPyramid*, and the DASH Eating Plan (DHHS and USDA, 2005). The actual amount of added sugars that is consistent with these eating plans varies and depends on total calorie intake and the amount of discretionary fat[14] consumed. The FGP suggested the following daily amounts of added sugars intake: 6 teaspoons for a 1,600-calorie diet, 12 teaspoons for a 2,200-calorie diet, and 18 teaspoons for a 2,800-calorie diet; these amounts are approximately 6, 9, and 10 percent of calories, respectively (USDA, 1996). A recent analysis that joined data from CSFII 1994–1996 and 1998 and from the U.S. sweetener supply and utilization information indicate that sweetener consumption varies with age (Haley et al., 2005). At an average of over 135 pounds per year, adolescent boys and girls, ages 12–19 years had the highest per capita sweetener consumption (including refined sugar and corn sweeteners) compared to younger children and adults (Haley et al., 2005). USDA dietary intake and survey data show that on average, older children ages 6–11 years consumed 21–23 teaspoons per day of added sugars in diets that provided 1,800–2,000 calories, adolescent girls ages 12–19 years consumed 23 teaspoons in an 1,800-calorie diet, and adolescent boys consumed 34 teaspoons in a 2,700–calorie diet (Enns et al., 2002, 2003). These amounts of added sugars provided approximately 20 percent of total calorie intake. Only 28 per-

---

[13]Added sugars, also known as caloric sweeteners, are sugars and syrups that are added to foods at the table or during processing or preparation, which supply calories but few or no nutrients.

[14]Discretionary fat is the amount of dietary fat remaining in a child's or adolescent's "energy" allowance after consuming sufficient amounts of high-nutrient foods to meet one's energy and nutrient needs while promoting a healthy weight gain trajectory. Examples of discretionary fat include the fat in higher fat meats and dairy products, butter, shortenings, and hard margarine.

cent of younger preschoolers and 21 percent of older preschoolers had added sugar intakes below 10 percent of total calories; 11 percent and 12 percent, respectively, had intakes greater than 25 percent of calories which is the maximal intake level (Kranz et al., 2005b).

Data comparing the sugar consumption of 743 sixth graders, ages 11–13 years, who had purchased and consumed school lunches in middle school cafeterias in Kentucky found that the mean sugar intake for students consuming only the school lunch was 14.1 g, whereas students consuming one or more food items in addition to the school lunch had a mean sugar intake of 30.7 g (Templeton, 2005; Templeton et al., 2005). Chapters 3 and 6 have a more extensive discussion about such supplemental or "competitive" foods.

Finding: Most preschool children consume added sugars well above suggested limits, and older children and adolescents consume about double the suggested limit of added sugars in their diets.

Adequate intakes of potassium for children and adolescents range from 3,000 mg/day (ages 1–3 years) to 4,700 mg/day (ages 14–18 years) (DHHS and USDA, 2005; IOM, 2005a). Virtually all children and adolescents ages 4–19 years had a potassium intake that exceeded their AI (Moshfegh et al., 2005).

The AI for sodium in children and adolescents ranges from 1,000 mg (1–3 years) to 1,500 mg (9–18 years), and the UL ranges from 1,500 mg (1–3 years) to 2,300 mg (14–18 years) (IOM, 2005a). An intake of less than 2,300 mg is recommended by the Dietary Guidelines for Americans (DHHS and USDA, 2005). However, according to data from NHANES III (1988–1994), mean sodium intakes ranged from 2,114 mg (ages 1–3 years) to 4,598 mg (adolescent boys ages 14–18 years) (Briefel and Johnson, 2004). All of the children and adolescents—100 percent—ages 4–18 years exceeded the AI for sodium (IOM, 2005a; Appendix D, Table D-8). Approximately 75 percent (children ages 4–6 years and adolescent girls ages 14–18 years) to more than 91 percent (adolescent boys ages 14–18 years) had sodium intakes greater than 2,300 mg/day (Briefel and Johnson, 2004). In general, non-Hispanic whites, non-Hispanic blacks, and Mexican Americans consume similar amounts of dietary sodium (DHHS, 2000a). The estimates of sodium intake did not include discretionary intake—what children and adolescents added to their meals at the table. Mean sodium intakes reported in NHANES 1999–2000 are even higher than NHANES III (1988–1994) for children ages 1–2 years and 6–11 years; however intakes seem to decline slightly for all other age groups during that time period (Briefel and Johnson, 2004; Appendix D, Table D-8).

Finding: Mean sodium intake of children and youth has increased over the past 35 years, and the majority of children and adolescents are consuming sodium in greater amounts than recommended levels.

Dietary Supplement Use

Although essential nutrients can be obtained from a balanced diet, many individuals take dietary supplements. NHANES III (1988–1994) collected data on supplement use for all individuals including children (ages 2 months–11 years) and adolescents (ages 12–19 years). About 40 percent of children and 25 percent of adolescents took some type of supplement (Ervin et al., 2004). Of those taken, multivitamins plus vitamin C (47 percent) was the leading supplement reported for children, followed by multivitamins/multiminerals (13 percent), multivitamins plus iron (10 percent), vitamin C (7 percent), and multivitamins plus fluoride (6 percent). The supplements reported by adolescent boys included vitamin C (24 percent); multivitamins/multiminerals (21 percent); multivitamins plus vitamin C (17 percent); supplements such as herbs, botanicals, and sport drinks (8 percent); and all other supplements such as single vitamins or minerals (29 percent). Those reported by adolescent girls included multivitamins/multiminerals (23 percent), multivitamins plus vitamin C (20 percent), vitamin C (16 percent), iron (6 percent), vitamin E (5 percent), and a mixture of assorted other supplements (30 percent). The contribution of dietary supplements usually is not included in past assessments of nutrient intakes from dietary survey data.

Dietary Intake and Eating Pattern Trends

Mean Food Intakes and Changes Between the 1970s and 1990s

Children's and adolescents' nutrient intakes reflect their food and beverage choices, which have changed substantially over time. In general, there have been increases in consumption of sweetened carbonated soft drinks, noncitrus juices/nectars, and fruit drinks/ades; grain mixtures such as pasta with sauces, rice dishes, and pizza; salty snacks; fried potatoes; candy; low-fat and skim milk; and cheese. Intakes have decreased for total milk and whole milk; yeast breads and rolls; green beans, corn, peas, and lima beans; and beef and pork (Enns et al., 2002, 2003). For younger children (ages 2–5 years) between 1977 and 1998, the percentage of total calories from added sugars increased during the same time period (Kranz et al., 2004). There has been a small improvement in dietary quality since 1977. Preschoolers had an increased number of servings of grains, dairy products, juice, and fruits and vegetables, although the types of fruits and vegetables were not reported (Kranz et al., 2004). The improvements in fruit and vegetable consumption may be marginal. Data from the Feeding Infants and Toddlers Study (FITS) found that up to one-third of infants and toddlers ages 7–24 months did not consume a discrete serving of vegetables; fewer than 10 percent consumed dark green leafy vegetables; and consumption of potatoes and starchy vegetables consumption increased with age (Fox et al., 2004; Skinner et al., 2004b). Up to one-third of infants and toddlers in this age group did not consume a discrete serving of fruit and 46–62 percent consumed fruit juice (Fox et al., 2004; Skinner et al., 2004b).

Food Intakes Compared with the Food Guide Pyramid

Although the FGP was updated and replaced with *MyPyramid* in 2005, a comparison of intakes with FGP servings still provides a general picture of food consumption patterns. In CSFII 1994–1996 and 1998, less than half of children ages 6–11 years consumed the number of servings recommended by the FGP for any one food group (Enns et al., 2002; USDA, 1996). In CSFII 1994–1996 and 1998, less than half of children ages 6–11 years consumed the number of servings recommended by the FGP for any one food group (Enns et al., 2002; USDA, 1996). On average, children in this age group consumed only one serving of whole grains per day, compared to the recommended three servings per day (DHHS and USDA, 2004); 80 percent did not meet the recommended servings for vegetables or legumes; and about a quarter met the recommendation for fruit intake (Enns et al., 2002). These dietary patterns contribute to the reported low dietary fiber, potassium, and magnesium intakes. Only 29 percent of girls and 40 percent of boys ages 6–11 years consumed the recommended daily servings of dairy products, which explains the low calcium intakes in this group (Enns et al., 2002). Twelve percent of girls and 21 percent of boys consumed the recommended servings from the meat and meat alternatives group, but this may reflect methodological problems with assessing the meat content of meals such as casseroles in which overall protein intake is adequate (Enns et al., 2002). Low intakes of nuts, dark green leafy vegetables, and vegetable oils account for children's low vitamin E intakes. While overall reported energy intakes were below the REA, children ages 6–11 years had intakes of discretionary fat and added sugars that were higher than levels consistent with the healthy eating pattern suggested by the FGP. These food intake patterns reveal that children are not achieving optimal diet quality and nutrient density.

Similar proportions of adolescents (ages 12–19 years) as younger children consumed the recommended servings of whole grains, vegetables, and legumes, and had intakes of discretionary fat and added sugars that exceeded the FGP healthy eating pattern (Enns et al., 2003). Fewer adolescents than children consumed the recommended servings of fruits (18 percent of adolescent girls and 14 percent of adolescent boys) and dairy products (12 percent of adolescent girls and 30 percent of adolescent boys), whereas a slightly higher percentage consumed the recommended servings of meat and meat alternatives (22 percent of adolescent girls and 44 percent of adolescent boys) (Enns et al., 2003).

Dietary quality scores for intakes of grains (8–9), fruits and vegetables (6–7), and dairy products (6) by younger children in CSFII 1994–1996 and 1998 were below the maximum possible for each group (10), and the amount of fruit juice consumed exceeded recommendations by the AAP by approximately one 6-ounce (oz) serving (Kranz et al., 2004).[15] In general, younger preschoolers (ages 2–3 years) had better dietary quality scores than older preschoolers (ages 4–5 years).

Finding: Over the past decade, most children and youth have not met the daily recommended servings for vegetables, fruits, or whole grains.

Low-Nutrient Foods

Dietary calorie density is the calorie content in a given weight of food (calories/gram) and influences the calorie intake of individuals (Ledikwe et al., 2005). Low-nutrient foods contribute a relatively low amount of essential nutrients when expressed per serving or calorie content. Low-nutrient foods are high in calorie density; they include fats, oils, and sugars (e.g., sweets and confectionery), desserts (e.g., ice cream, puddings, cheesecakes, pastries, cookies, cakes, pies), and salty snacks (e.g., potato, corn, tortilla chips), which are included in the dairy or grain groups of the FGP (Kant, 2004; Kant and Graubard, 2003). Carbonated soft drinks are low in nutrient density but are not particularly calorie dense because of their high water content. Fruits and vegetables are relatively nutrient dense, but not calorie dense, because of their high water content (Rolls et al., 2004).

Low-nutrient foods contributed more than 30 percent of daily calories to the diets of children and adolescents ages 8–18 years who participated in NHANES III (1988–1994) (Kant and Graubard, 2003). Of the low-nutrient foods, sweets (e.g., sugar, syrup, candy, carbonated soft drinks) and desserts (e.g., cookies, cakes, ice cream) accounted for nearly 25 percent of total calorie intake (Kant and Graubard, 2003; Figure 2-3). The

---

[15]The AAP has recommended not giving fruit juices to infants less than 6 months of age, and limiting 100 percent fruit juice consumption to one serving (4–6 oz/day) for children ages 1–6 years, and two servings (8–12 oz/day) to children and youth ages 7–18 years (AAP, 2001).

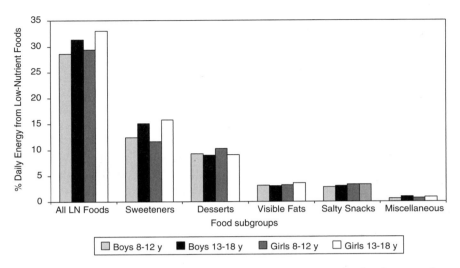

FIGURE 2-3 Percentage of daily calories from low-nutrient food subgroups for U.S. children and adolescents, ages 8–18 years, from National Health and Nutrition Examination Survey (NHANES) III, 1988–1994.
SOURCE: Kant and Graubard (2003).

reported number of low-nutrient foods was positively related to total calorie intake and the percentage of calories from carbohydrate and fat, and was negatively related to the intakes of fiber, vitamins A and B_6, folate, calcium, magnesium, iron, and zinc. The strongest negative predictor of the reported number of low-nutrient foods was the amount of nutrient-dense foods consumed from the five major food groups (Kant and Graubard, 2003). Weekly consumption of a complete school lunch also was a negative predictor, whereas the number of reported eating occasions was a positive predictor.

Stated another way, those children who consumed fewer low-nutrient foods had better quality diets as reflected by fewer eating occasions reported, eating school lunch more regularly, and consuming more foods from the major food groups. Gender- and age-adjusted BMI, sociodemographic and family characteristics, and the reported hours spent in physical activity or watching television were not associated with the number of low-nutrient foods reported. The data suggest that increased access and availability of nutrient-dense foods and decreased access to low-nutrient foods in schools, homes, and other places will moderate low-nutrient food and calorie intake.

Increasing added sugars intake in younger children ages 2–5 years from CSFII 1994–1996 and 1998 was associated with decreasing intakes of several micronutrients (e.g., calcium, iron, folate, and vitamins A and B$_{12}$) and food groups (e.g., grains, vegetables, fruits, and dairy), and increasing proportions of children with intakes below the EAR or decreasing proportion above the AI for selected nutrients (Kranz et al., 2005b). Younger children at the lowest level of added sugars intake (<10 percent of total calories) consumed approximately one serving more of grains, fruits, and dairy compared to those in the highest added sugar intake group (>25 percent of total calories). Approximately 75 percent of younger preschoolers (ages 2–3 years) and 50 percent of older preschoolers (ages 4–5 years) had calcium intakes above the AI with added sugar intakes of 16–25 percent of total calories; 60 percent and 30 percent of younger and older preschoolers, respectively, had calcium intakes above the AI when added sugars exceeded 25 percent of total calories.[16] The main sources of added sugars were fruit drinks (19–20 percent), sweetened carbonated soft drinks (14–16 percent), and high-fat desserts (15–16 percent).

Beverages

The potential calorie and nutrient composition of beverages in the diets of children and youth have important implications for diet-related health risks such as obesity and osteoporosis. Data from the national dietary surveys indicate that beverage consumption habits have changed for children and adolescents over the past 35 years. Between 1965 and 2001, the intake of sweetened beverages (e.g., carbonated soft drinks and fruit drinks) by children and adolescents ages 2–18 years increased and milk decreased—whether expressed as percentage of per capita total calorie intake, percentage of consumers, mean servings per day, or mean portions (Cavadini et al., 2000; Nielsen and Popkin, 2004; Appendix D, Table D-9). Milk consumption decreased from 13.2 percent of total calories in 1977–1978 to 8.3 percent in 2001 for children and youth ages 2–18 years (Nielsen and Popkin, 2004). During this same time period, soft drink consumption in this age group increased from 3 to 6.9 percent, and fruit drink consumption increased from 1.8 to 3.4 percent (Nielsen and Popkin, 2004).

The decline in total milk consumption over time by children (ages 6–11 years) and adolescents (ages 12–19 years) is related to a decline in the consumption of whole milk that is not offset by a commensurate increase in consumption of low-fat milk and skim milk (Enns et al., 2002, 2003). From 1965 to 1996, low-fat milk replaced higher-fat milk intake in 11- to 18-

---

[16]As noted previously, although the AI cannot be used to estimate the prevalence of inadequate nutrient intakes in a group, the prevalence of inadequacy should be low if at least 50 percent of a group has intakes greater than the AI.

year-olds, yet total milk consumption decreased by 36 percent, and was accompanied by a three-fold increase in the consumption of sweetened carbonated soft drinks and a two-fold consumption of fruit-flavored beverages (Cavadini et al., 2000; Huang and McCrory, 2005; Figure 2-4).

A recent study of more than 3,000 children and youth ages 2–18 years using NHANES 1999–2000 data found that sweetened beverages provided approximately 13 percent of adolescents' total caloric intake and represented the single leading source of added sugars in adolescents' diets (Murphy et al., 2005). The study also found that the consumption of carbonated soft drinks and sweetened fruit drinks increased and milk decreased in a step-wise direction as children aged (Murphy et al., 2005).

Diet carbonated soft drinks and water consumption have not been systematically evaluated in national consumption surveys for children and youth, although databases are available to assess nutrient availability per capita of beverages by nationally representative samples of U.S. household purchases. Understanding the beverage choices made by households is important to assess the contribution of caloric beverages to total calorie intake. A USDA analysis used the 1999 ACNielsen Homescan Consumer Panel, which tracked household purchases of beverages over an entire year, to assess the nutrient availability for nonalcoholic beverages consumed at home. The analysis reflected only the purchasing patterns of households and the total household availability of nutrients, and did not disaggregate the findings into intrahousehold differences (Capps et al., 2005). However,

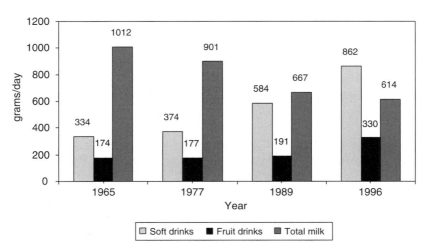

FIGURE 2-4 Trends in milk consumption versus carbonated soft drinks and fruit-flavored beverage consumption in U.S. adolescents, ages 11–18 years, 1965 to 1996. SOURCES: Cavadini et al. (2000); Huang and McCrory (2005).

the analysis found that the average available calcium, vitamin C, and caffeine intakes from nonalcoholic beverages per person per day were lower in households with children younger than 6 years, ages 6–12 years, and 13–17 years (Capps et al., 2005). Additionally, households with children ages 13–17 years had higher daily available calorie intakes per person than did households with no children, though the analysis was unable to identify the reasons for this observation (Capps et al., 2005).

Data from the National Family Opinion Research/Beverage Unit's Share of Intake Panel (SIP) show positive trends in beverage consumption by younger children (ages 1–5 years) during the periods of 1987–1988, 1992–1993, and 1997–1998 (Park et al., 2002). There was a decrease in the percentage of children who consumed carbonated soft drinks (84, 78, and 72 percent), powdered soft drinks[17] (54, 51, and 45 percent), and tea (33, 21, and 17 percent); an increase in those who consumed fruit drinks (53, 55, and 61 percent); and no consistent change in juice (77, 77, and 79 percent) or milk consumption (94, 95, and 91 percent). There was also a decrease in the daily consumed quantity of carbonated soft drinks (from 5.2 to 3.7 oz) and powdered soft drinks (from 4 to 3.5 oz), and an increase in milk (from 11.6 to 13.5 oz), juices (from 5 to 7 oz), and fruit drinks (from 2.1 to 2.9 oz).

The age, gender, and race/ethnicity of children and adolescents affect beverage consumption patterns (Storey et al., 2004). In CSFII 1994–1996 and 1998, milk product consumption in general increased in boys and decreased in girls between ages 2–3 years and 14–18 years. Boys consumed more milk products than girls at all ages, with the difference widening as age increased; white boys drank more milk products than African American boys at all ages and more than Hispanic/Latino boys ages 4–8 years (Storey et al., 2004). White girls consumed similar amounts of milk products as Hispanic/Latina girls until ages 9–18 years when white girls consumed more milk products. African American girls consumed fewer milk products than white or Hispanic/Latino girls at all ages. Sweetened carbonated soft drinks and fruit drinks/ades consumption generally increased with age in both genders, with boys increasingly consuming more than girls as age increased (Storey et al., 2004). African American children and adolescents generally consumed more fruit drinks/ades and less sweetened carbonated soft drinks than whites (Storey et al., 2004). The amount of diet carbonated soft drinks consumed was insignificant at ages 2–3 years and increased slightly with age, but was relatively low compared to other beverage sources (Storey et al., 2004). Similar age and gender patterns in beverage intakes have been observed with data from SIP (Park et al., 2002).

---

[17]Powdered soft drinks are flavored powders that are reconstituted with water.

Sweetened beverages (as a percentage of total calories in 1994–1996) were consumed by children and adolescents ages 2–18 years mostly at home (3.9 percent), followed by restaurants and quick serve restaurants (QSRs) (1.7 percent), obtained from a store but not eaten at home or ever brought into the home (0.7 percent), and vending machines (0.3 percent) (Nielsen and Popkin, 2004). Using a slightly different approach to analyzing the data, French et al. (2003) also reported an increase in the prevalence of sweetened carbonated soft drinks consumption and portion size among youth—with the largest source of consumption at home, followed by restaurants and QSRs, other locations (e.g., friends' homes and entertainment venues), school cafeterias, and vending machines. Sweetened beverages were the largest contributors to added sweeteners in the diets of children and adolescents ages 2–18 years, from 34–52 percent depending on age and sex in 1994–1996 to 35–58 percent in 1999–2000 (Guthrie and Morton, 2000; Murphy et al., 2005). Sweetened beverages represent approximately 10 percent of their total calorie intake.

Finding: Sweetened beverage consumption (e.g., carbonated soft drinks and fruit drinks) by children and adolescents has increased considerably over the past 35 years and is now a leading source of added sugars, especially in adolescents' diets. The consumption of milk, a major source of dietary calcium, has decreased among children and adolescents over the same period, and most have calcium intakes below the recommended adequate intake level.

Breakfast Consumption

Breakfast consumption also has changed over time. In NFCS 1965, 90 percent of boys and 84 percent of girls consumed a food, beverage, or both between 5 am and 10 am compared with 75 percent and 65 percent, respectively, in CSFII 1989–1991 (Siega-Riz et al., 1998). Consumption declined approximately 5 percentage points in younger children, 9 points in older children ages 8–10 years, and 13–20 points in adolescents. The greatest decline was among adolescent girls ages 15–18 years, who dropped from 84 percent in 1965 to 65 percent in 1991. Frequency of breakfast consumption declines with age. In 1965, African Americans and whites had similar breakfast consumption patterns; however, African American adolescents were less likely to consume breakfast by 1989–1991 (Siega-Riz et al., 1998). Data from the National Heart, Lung, and Blood Institute Growth and Health Study, a 9-year longitudinal biracial cohort of 2,379 girls, found that white girls reported more frequent breakfast consumption than African American girls, but the racial differences decreased with age

(Affenito et al., 2005). Beginning in 1977, more children attending school (preschool ages to 14 years) consumed breakfast than those not in school.

Breakfast consumption has been generally associated with higher parental income (Siega-Riz et al., 1998). Eating this meal also has been correlated with higher calcium and fiber intakes, and the number of days eating breakfast is predictive of lower BMI levels (Affenito et al., 2005). Breakfast food choices in 1989–1991 generally reflected fewer sources of dietary fat, especially lower consumption of whole milk, eggs, and bacon (Siega-Riz et al., 1998). Regular consumption of fortified RTE cereals with low-fat milk for breakfast has been correlated with (1) higher nutrient intakes (e.g., fiber, calcium, iron, folic acid, vitamin C, and zinc) (Barton et al., 2005; Subar et al., 1998), (2) decreased intake of fat and cholesterol (Barton et al., 2005), and (3) lower BMI levels in children ages 4–12 years (Albertson et al., 2003) and girls ages 9–19 years (Barton et al., 2005).

Finding: Breakfast consumption by children and adolescents has decreased considerably over the past 40 years and the occurrence of breakfast consumption declines with age. The frequency of breakfast consumption is predictive of lower BMI levels in children and adolescents.

Snacking Patterns

An examination of food intakes from NFCS and CSFII revealed an increase in snacking prevalence across all age groups of children and adolescents ages 2–18 years—from 77 percent in 1977–1978 to 91 percent in 1994–1996 (Jahns et al., 2001; Figure 2-5). Most of the increase occurred between 1989–1991 and 1994–1996. In 1994–1996, younger children (ages 2–5 years) and older children (ages 6–11 years), except for Hispanics/Latinos, were the highest proportion who snacked; slightly more boys than girls snacked; and more Hispanics/Latinos and whites snacked than African Americans.

The average size (in grams) or calorie content per snack remained relatively constant over time from 1977–1978 to 1994–1996, but the number of snacking occasions increased significantly, thereby increasing the average daily calories from snacks. The size of snacks increased with age during each time period (e.g., from 153 g for ages 2–5 years to 195 g for ages 6–11 years to 307 g for ages 12–18 years in 1994–1996). The average daily calorie intake from snacks increased over time for all age groups because the number of snacking occasions increased by about 0.4 snacking events per day overall. In 1994–1996, snacks contributed 378 calories per day for younger children ages 2–5 years, 462 calories for older children ages 6–11 years, and 612 calories for adolescents ages 12–

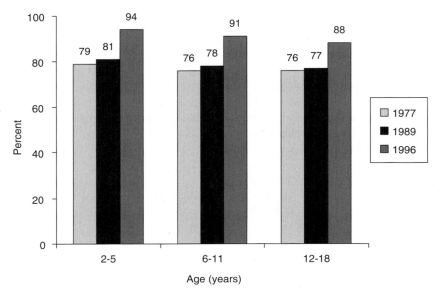

FIGURE 2-5 Trends in prevalence of snacking among U.S. children and adolescents, ages 2–18 years.
SOURCE: Jahns et al. (2001). Reprinted from Journal of Pediatrics, Jahns L, Siega-Riz AM, Popkin BM, The increasing prevalence of snacking among US children from 1977 to 1996, Pages 493–498, 2001, with permission from Elsevier.

18 years, representing an estimated 25 percent of total calorie intake (compared to an estimated 20 percent in 1977–1978). The calcium density (mg/1,000 calories) of both meals and snacks decreased over 20 years, with the magnitude of decline greater for snacks.

Finding: The prevalence of snacking and number of snacking occasions by children and youth have increased steadily over the past 25 years.

Portion Sizes

Although the size of each snack consumed by children and adolescents over the past 20 years has remained relatively constant (Jahns et al., 2001), the portion size and calorie contribution of selected foods per eating occasion did increase based on an analysis of data for all individuals (ages 2 years and older) who participated in NFCS 1977–1978, CSFII 1989–1991, and CSFII 1994–1996 and 1998 (Nielsen and Popkin, 2003). The quantity of salty snacks consumed per eating occasion increased by 0.6 oz

(93 calories), desserts by 0.6 oz (41 calories), carbonated soft drinks by 6.8 oz (49 calories), fruit drinks by 3.8 oz (50 calories), hamburgers by 1.3 oz (97 calories), cheeseburgers by 1.5 oz (138 calories), french fries by 0.5 oz (68 calories), and Mexican dishes by 1.7 oz (133 calories). According to these investigators, the portion size or calorie content of pizza did not change during the time frame examined. There were no statistically significant different trends between age groups, and in most but not all cases, portion sizes increased for these foods whether obtained at home or away from home, with the largest portion sizes in 1994–1998 found in QSRs and the smallest in full serve restaurants (Chapter 3).

When data from CSFII 1989–1991 and CSFII 1994–1996 for foods commonly consumed (e.g., by 7 percent or more of the population ages 2 years and older) were compared, larger portions were reported in 1994–1996 for several foods, including spaghetti with tomato sauce (16 percent increase in portion size), carbonated soft drinks (16 percent increase), fruit drinks (16 percent increase), orange juice (12 percent increase), and RTE cereals (9.6 percent increase) (Smiciklas-Wright et al., 2003). Smaller portions were reported for a few foods such as margarine (18 percent decrease), mayonnaise (10 percent decrease), chicken (11 percent decrease), pizza (14 percent decrease), and macaroni and cheese (17 percent decrease). An increase in portion size was significant for RTE cereals consumed by older children ages 6–11 years and adolescent boys ages 12–19 years, fruit drinks and spaghetti with tomato sauce consumed by adolescent boys, and carbonated soft drinks consumed by adolescent girls. A decrease in portion size was significant for chicken consumed by younger children ages 2–5 years and older children ages 6–11 years, french fries by younger children, and pizza by older children.

Eating Locations and Food Sources

Adolescents ages 12–18 years consumed most of their calorie intake from food prepared or obtained at home, but the percentage decreased between 1977–1978 and 1994–1996 (74 versus 60 percent, respectively) (Nielsen et al., 2002b). A higher percentage of calories was consumed from foods obtained at full serve restaurants and QSRs (6.5 versus 19 percent) and less at school (11 versus 8 percent). Less than 1 percent of calorie intake was from foods obtained from vending machines at both time periods (0.5 versus 0.9 percent) (Nielsen et al., 2002b). Children ages 2–12 years in 1994–1996 consumed more than two-thirds of their calories from food obtained or prepared at home (68 percent) (Lin et al., 1999). However, total calorie intake obtained from away-from-home food sources increased for children from 20 percent to 32 percent between 1977–1978 and 1994–1996 (Lin et al., 1999). Food obtained by children from schools,

QSRs, and full serve restaurants accounted for 9 percent, 10 percent, and 4 percent of total calorie intake, respectively. Similar trends have been reported overall for children and adolescents ages 2–18 years (Nielsen et al., 2002a,b; Figure 2-6; Chapter 3).

Finding: There has been a steady increase in the proportion of calories that children and youth have received from away-from-home foods over the past 20 years. Approximately one-third or more of their calories are derived from foods purchased outside of the home, nearly one-half of which is obtained at full serve restaurants and quick serve restaurants that contain higher fat content than food consumed at home.

In 1994–1996, food consumed by children and adolescents ages 2–17 years that was prepared away from home, compared to food prepared at home, contained more total fat (36.1 versus 31.6 percent of calories) and saturated fat (13.2 versus 11.5 percent of calories), and less cholesterol (106 versus 118 mg/1,000 calories), dietary fiber (6.2 versus 6.9 g/1,000 calories), calcium (437 versus 474 mg/1,000 calories), and iron (6 versus 8.3 g/1,000 calories) (Guthrie et al., 2002). There was no difference in the sodium content (per 1,000 calories) between food consumed at home and food prepared away from home.

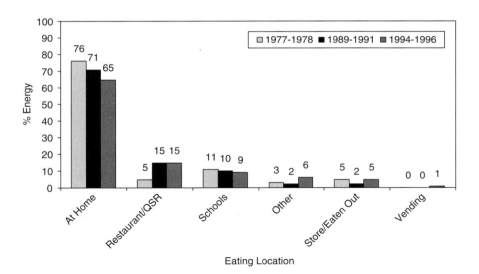

FIGURE 2-6 Trends in energy intake of U.S. children and adolescents, ages 2–18 years, by selected eating location, 1977–1978 to 1994–1996.
SOURCE: Nielsen et al. (2002a).

Infants and Toddlers

Reports from the national dietary surveys usually provide limited details of the food and nutrient intakes of infants (ages <12 months) and toddlers (ages 12–24 months). Yet the first 2 years of life are associated with a transition from a largely milk-based diet to an increasingly complex diet that includes a variety of common foods.

As discussed in Chapter 3, food preferences develop early in life and have been shown to predict consumption habits. Thus, it is important to understand the overall nutritional adequacy and nature of the diets consumed by infants and toddlers. The 2002 Feeding Infants and Toddlers Study has provided important information about the nutrient intakes, food group consumption, and meal and snack patterns for a large, nationally representative, random sample of 3,022 infants and toddlers ages 4 to 24 months (Devaney et al., 2004; Fox et al., 2004; Skinner et al., 2004a,b). FITS intake data are based on multiple-pass 24-hour dietary recalls conducted with a parent or caregiver.

Nutrient and Calorie Intakes

The usual nutrient intakes, from both foods and dietary supplements, of young (4–6 months) and older (7–11 months) infants exceeded the AI, often with the 10th percentile of usual intake either equaling or exceeding the AI (Devaney et al., 2004). The estimated prevalence of nutrient inadequacy for older infants was relatively low for iron (7.5 percent) and zinc (4.2 percent). For toddlers, the prevalence of inadequacy was low (<1 percent) for most nutrients, except for vitamin E. More than half (58 percent) of toddlers had vitamin E intakes below the EAR. The mean intakes for calcium and vitamin D exceeded the AI. The percentages of usual intakes that exceeded the UL were less than 1 percent for most nutrients. However, a relatively high percentage of toddlers had usual intakes for vitamin A (35 percent) and zinc (43 percent) that exceeded the UL. Overall the data suggest that the diets of infants and toddlers are nutritionally adequate, with less than 1 percent of total nutrient intakes coming from supplements. The mean, median, and estimated percentiles of the usual calorie intake distribution all exceeded the comparable EER. The mean usual calorie intake was higher than the mean EER by 10 percent for young infants, 23 percent for older infants, and 31 percent by toddlers. Maternal employment status did not influence calorie intake. The mean intakes of fat, carbohydrates, and protein of young infants exceeded the AI, as did the mean intakes of fat and carbohydrates for older infants. Thirty-eight percent of toddlers had fat intakes outside the AMDR: 29 percent had fat intake below 30 percent of calories and 9 percent had intakes above 40 percent of calories. Mean fiber intake for toddlers was 8 g/day, far below the AI of 19 g.

Finding: Calorie intake by infants and toddlers substantially exceeds their estimated requirements, although validation is needed on the reliability of food intake reporting by parents and caregivers, as well as on body weight estimates.

Food and Beverage Intakes

Food and beverage consumption patterns—reported as the percentage of infants and toddlers who consumed an item at least once in a day—from FITS have been described (Fox et al., 2004; Skinner et al., 2004b). Patterns that have been observed in older children and adults were observed in infants as young as 7 months. Up to one-third of infants and toddlers ages 7–24 months did not consume a discrete serving of a vegetable (18–33 percent) (Fox et al., 2004). In virtually all age groups, fewer than 10 percent consumed dark green leafy vegetables. Potato, starchy vegetable, and other vegetable consumption increased with age, with french fries or other fried potatoes being the third most consumed vegetable at 9–11 months (8.6 percent), second most consumed at 12–14 months (12.9 percent), and most consumed at ages 15–18 months (19.8 percent) and 19–24 months (25.5 percent) (Fox et al., 2004). Similar to vegetable consumption, up to one-third of infants and toddlers ages 7–24 months did not consume a discrete serving of a fruit (23–33 percent) and 46–62 percent consumed fruit juice (primarily apple juice). Most toddlers consumed cereals that were not presweetened, but 18–26 percent of toddlers, depending on age, consumed presweetened cereal (defined as 21.2 g of sugar/100 g). The percentage of infants and toddlers who consumed desserts, sweets, or sweetened beverages increased sharply after the age 6 months (from about 10 percent at age 6 months to 91 percent by ages 19–24 months). Among older toddlers ages 19–24 months, 60 percent consumed a baked dessert (e.g., cake, cookie, pie, or pastry) and 20 percent consumed candy.

Older toddlers primarily drank milk (93 percent), water (77 percent), 100 percent fruit juices (62 percent), and fruit drinks (43 percent), and to a lesser extent carbonated soft drinks (12 percent) and other beverages (11 percent) (Skinner et al., 2004b). Many infants and toddlers consumed at least one sweetened beverage each day, infants ages 7–8 months (7.5 percent), toddlers ages 12–14 months (28.2 percent), and older toddlers ages 19–24 months (44.3 percent) (Fox et al., 2004). Toddlers, ages 12–14 months and 15–18 months, who were in the upper quartile of total calorie intake, showed a higher consumption of sweetened beverages when compared to toddlers in the lower quartile (Briefel et al., 2004).

Beverages, including milks and fruit juices, provided 36 percent of total calorie intake for older toddlers, with less than 25 percent of calories coming from milks. The calcium density of the diet was negatively associated with intake of 100 percent juice, fruit drinks, and carbonated soft drinks. The AAP recommendations for limiting 100 percent juice consumption— age of introduction and amount consumed (to 4–6 oz/day)—were not followed by a majority of parents.

Finding: Infants and toddlers are consuming diets disproportionately high in sweetened foods and beverages and fried potatoes, and disproportionately low in green leafy vegetables.

Meal and Snack Patterns

The median number of daily eating occasions was 7 for infants and toddlers in FITS, regardless of age, and ranged from 3 to 15 (Skinner et al., 2004a). More than 89 percent ate breakfast, lunch, and dinner, and the percentage reported to be eating snacks increased with age. More than 80 percent of toddlers ages 12–24 months ate afternoon snacks, 66 percent consumed a morning snack, and slightly more than 50 percent consumed an evening snack. Among toddlers, snacks provided about 25 percent of daily calorie intake; typical snacks were milk, water, and crackers but also fruit drinks, candy, chips, and cookies. Frequent eating occasions are important for infants and toddlers because of their small stomachs and usually high levels of activity.

Income and Regional-Related Food and Nutrient Patterns

Income and Childhood Obesity

Children who live in poverty experience greater health, social, and nutrition disparities when compared with middle- and high-income children (DHHS, 2000a, 2003; Evans, 2004; Wise, 2004). In 2002, approximately 11.6 million children (17 percent) under the age of 18 years lived in families with incomes below 100 percent of the federal poverty level, and an additional four million children lived in families just above poverty (Federal Interagency Forum on Child and Family Statistics, 2004; Wise, 2004). The poverty rate is much higher for ethnic minority children. In 2000, 32 percent of African American children and 28 percent of Hispanic/Latino children lived in poverty compared to 9 percent of white children (Federal Interagency Forum on Child and Family Statistics, 2004).

Moreover, less than 70 percent of people living at or above the federal poverty level have health insurance (DHHS, 2003). Despite evidence documenting health disparities by income, including nutrition-related health disparities, evidence on the relationship between household income and nutrient intake levels is mixed, and the relationship has varied over time (Devaney et al., 2005).

The prevalence of obesity in children and youth reveals significant disparities by sex and between racial/ethnic groups (Hedley et al., 2004). As seen in Figure 2-7, NHANES data reveal that non-Hispanic black and Mexican-American children and adolescents ages 6–19 years have a greater prevalence of obesity (with a BMI equal to or greater than the 95th percentile of the CDC BMI charts) and are at greater risk of becoming obese (defined as having a BMI between the 85th and the 95th percentile of the CDC BMI charts) than are non-Hispanic whites (Hedley et al., 2004).

Despite the substantial variation in BMI that exists as a function of both socioeconomic status and ethnicity based on NHANES III in girls ages 6–9 years (Winkleby et al., 1999), and the increase in obesity prevalence among African American youth at the lowest income (Strauss and Pollack, 2001), uncertainties remain as to whether these rates can be attributed only to socioeconomic status because these disparities are not the same across ethnic groups and they do not emerge at comparable times during childhood. Also, there is no consensus, albeit many theories, about the mechanisms by which they occur. For example, analysis of the data from the 1988–1994 NHANES shows that the prevalence of obesity in white adolescents is higher among those in low-income families, but there is no clear relationship between family income and obesity in other age or ethnic subgroups (Ogden et al., 2003; Troiano and Flegal, 1998). Two analyses of nationally representative longitudinal data—the National Longitudinal Survey of Youth (Strauss and Knight, 1999; Strauss and Pollack, 2001) and the National Longitudinal Study of Adolescent Health (Goodman, 1999)— have suggested that family socioeconomic status is inversely related to obesity prevalence in children and that the effects of socioeconomic status and race or ethnicity were independent of other variables.

Food insecurity—the limited or uncertain availability of nutritionally adequate and safe foods, or the inability to acquire such foods in a socially acceptable way—is a significant issue for low-income[18] families, especially African American and Hispanic/Latino households that experience this condition at double the national average rate (Food Research Action Center, 2005). In 2004, 38.2 million individuals, including 13.8 million children,

---

[18]Low-income is defined as a household income at or below 130 percent of the poverty level.

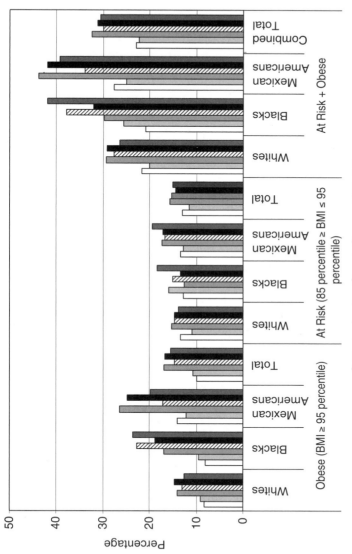

FIGURE 2-7 Percentage of U.S. children and adolescents who are obese or at risk for obesity by age, sex, and ethnicity, 1999–2002.

SOURCE: Hedley et al. (2004).

lived in food-insecure households (an estimated 11.9 percent of all U.S. households), and 3.9 percent (4.4 million) of U.S. households were food insecure with hunger (Nord et al., 2005). An estimated 19 percent of all U.S. children and 38 percent of children living in poverty were classified as living in food-insecure households (Nord et al., 2005).

State-specific prevalence and trends among 2- through 4-year-old children from low-income U.S. families were examined from 1989 to 2000. Results showed significant increases in obesity among low-income children in 30 states and significant decreases in childhood underweight in 26 states (Sherry et al., 2004). Although no geographic predominance was apparent, the number of states reporting obesity prevalence of more than 10 percent increased from 11 in 1989 to 28 in 2000. Reported underweight decreased during the same time frame, as reflected by 9 states in 1989 and 23 states in 2000 that had a prevalence equal to or less than 5 percent (Sherry et al., 2004).

Food insecurity is associated with adverse health outcomes in infants and toddlers younger than 36 months of age (Cook et al., 2004) and with negative academic and psychosocial outcomes including depression in older children (Alaimo et al., 2001a, 2002). When compared with higher income households that were food insufficient, defined as inadequacy in the amount of food intake because of limited money or resources, low-income food insufficient households had more obese children. The available evidence shows that food insufficiency alone has not been associated with obesity except in white girls ages 8 to 16 years (Alaimo et al., 2001b; Casey et al., 2001). Other studies have not been able to show a clear relationship between childhood obesity and food insufficiency or food insecurity after adjusting for other confounding variables (Kaiser et al., 2002; Matheson et al., 2002).

Several states have examined the relationship of federal food assistance policies and programs to obesity in low-income participants. One analysis of the National Longitudinal Survey of Youth has suggested that long-term Food Stamp Program (FSP) participation was positively associated with obesity in young girls, ages 5–11 years; negatively related to obesity in young boys, ages 5–11 years; and not significantly related to obesity in older children (Gibson, 2004). However, the analysis did not control for food insecurity. Another recent analysis, based on the 1997 Child Development Supplement to the Panel Study of Income Dynamics, examined the BMI levels of 1,268 children between the ages of 6 and 12 years, and families and children who participated in the National School Lunch Program (NSLP) or School Breakfast Program (SBP), either for a free, reduced, or subsidized school meal. The sample included children from five family income categories: poor, near poor, working class, moderate income, and high income. Results found that children in the poorest families were less likely to be obese and have lower BMI levels than most other children. Children from high-income families were also less likely to be obese. In contrast, children from families with incomes just above the poverty level—the near poor—are the children at greatest risk for obesity. School meal participation was not a determining factor in a child's risk of obesity (Hofferth and Curtin, 2005). Another published study found that school-aged girls from food-insecure households who participated in the FSP, SBP, and NSLP had a lower risk of becoming obese than their cohorts in food-insecure households who did not participate in food assistance programs (Jones et al., 2003). It cannot yet be concluded whether FSP participation results in obesity. Further research is needed to understand the mechanisms operating among poverty, food insecurity, federal food assistance program participation, and obesity in children and youth (Frongillo, 2003).

Income and Diet Among Younger Children

Dietary intakes of younger children (ages 2–4 years) in NHANES III (1988–1994) who participated in the Special Supplemental Nutrition Program for Women, Infants, and Children have been compared to WIC income-eligible but nonparticipating children and higher income noneligible children (Cole and Fox, 2004). More WIC children consumed fewer than three meals per day than higher income children (16 percent versus 10 percent), with fewer consuming breakfast (88 percent versus 94 percent) (Cole and Fox, 2004). WIC children had higher calorie and calcium intakes compared to the other two groups; however, all three groups appeared to have adequate calcium as well as vitamin C, iron, and zinc intakes when compared to the DRIs. The diets of children participating in WIC generally were similar to the diets of income-eligible, nonparticipants and higher income children. Notable exceptions were higher intakes of calories, total fat, saturated fat, cholesterol, and sodium compared to the higher income children (Cole and Fox, 2004). Also, the WIC children had higher scores for the fruit component of the HEI compared to the income-eligible children, which suggests that eligible but nonparticipating WIC children had lower quality diets.

Income and Diet Among School-Age Children

The diets of school-aged children, ages 5–18 years, who participated in NHANES III (1988–1994) have been analyzed based on income status: income at or below 130 percent of poverty (lowest income), income between 131 and 185 percent of poverty (low income), and income higher than 185 percent of poverty (higher income) (Fox and Cole, 2004). Children in the lowest income group were eligible for participation in the FSP and free meals in the NSLP and SBP; those in the low-income group were eligible for reduced-price meals.

Slightly more children in the lowest income group consumed fewer than three meals per day than those in the higher income group (39 versus 34 percent), and slightly fewer had breakfast (44 versus 48 percent). Only 14 percent of children in the lowest income group met the Dietary Guidelines for total fat (no more than 30 percent of calories) compared to 10 percent in the low-income group and 22 percent in the higher income group. The available evidence reveals that compared with the higher income group, slightly more of the lowest income children consumed less than three meals per day and did not eat breakfast; they had lower intakes of calcium and higher intakes of total fat, saturated fat, and sodium. Few of the children had good diets based on the HEI (Fox and Cole, 2004).

The prevalence of iron deficiency[19] has decreased in the United States (Sherry et al., 2001). This decrease is attributed in part to the widespread use and greater bioavailability of iron-fortified foods and infant formula (IOM, 2005c; Sherry et al., 2001). However, iron deficiency remains a nutritional concern for toddlers and younger children, especially low-income and minority children, and adolescent girls (CDC, 2002; DHHS, 2000a; IOM, 2005c; Looker et al., 1997). Although iron-deficiency anemia is uncommon in the United States, population levels of iron deficiency exceed the Healthy People 2010 objectives of 5 percent for toddlers, 1 percent for younger children, and 7 percent for adolescent girls (DHHS, 2000a). Iron-deficiency anemia is associated with low energy levels, reduced attention span, compromised cognitive performance, developmental delays, and poor educational achievement (IOM, 2001; Pollitt, 1993).

Finding: Certain subgroups, such as low-income and minority children and adolescent girls, have inadequate dietary intakes of specific micronutrients (e.g., vitamins D and B_6, folate, iron, zinc, and magnesium).

Regional Patterns

The NFCS, CSFII, and NHANES provide dietary information for a nationally representative sample of the U.S. civilian, noninstitutionalized population and were not designed to evaluate specific regional differences in dietary habits. Other studies have provided insights into regional differences, especially in selected southern states.

---

[19]Iron deficiency is defined as an abnormal value for at least two of three indicators (e.g., serum ferritin, transferrin saturation, and free erythrocyte protoporphyrin) (CDC, 2002).

The Foods of Our Delta Study was a cross-sectional survey of a culturally diverse population residing in the Lower Mississippi Delta region of Arkansas, Louisiana, and Mississippi (Champagne et al., 2004). Calorie intake did not differ between the children ages 3–18 years in the Delta and CSFII 1994–1996 and 1998.[20] Average intakes of folate were consistently higher in the Delta children due to the mandatory fortification of enriched grain products that occurred between the time of the national survey and the Delta Study. The average food and nutrient intakes of African American children in the Delta region were similar to those of African American children in the U.S. population, with the only difference being fewer servings of RTE cereals in the Delta region.

However, intakes for white children in the Delta Study were significantly lower for dietary fiber, vitamin A, carotene, riboflavin, vitamin B_6, vitamin C, calcium, and iron than for the white U.S. population, and more similar to intakes for African American children both in the Delta region and nationally—except for vitamin C, which was lower, and calcium, which was higher, for whites. Lower intakes of RTE breakfast cereals, fruit, vegetables, and dairy foods accounted for the lower nutrient intakes of the white Delta children. White Delta children had higher added sugar intakes than those in the U.S. population. Overall the intake of fruits, vegetables, and dairy products was poor for the children in the Delta region—similar to children in the U.S. population in general.

Data from the Bogalusa Heart Study[21] provide additional insight into dietary patterns of children (ages 10 years) residing in the South, including trends from 1973 to 1994. The trends in general are consistent with national trends, with a few notable exceptions. For example, the percentage of Bogalusa children consuming desserts and candy and the mean gram amount consumed, decreased significantly, although they have increased nationally (Nicklas et al., 2004a). Similar to national trends, however, the mean amount consumed increased for cheese, salty snacks, and sweetened beverages, and decreased for milk. Unlike the national population, though, the increase in overall sweetened beverage intake in Bogalusa was due to an increase in the amount of tea with sugar consumed, as the amount of fruit drinks and carbonated soft drinks did not change significantly (Rajeshwari et al., 2005).

Examination of the sweetened beverage data from Bogalusa by tertiles of consumption revealed no significant change in mean consumption be-

---

[20]Dietary information in the Foods of Our Delta Study was obtained by methods similar to those used in CSFII 1994–1996 and 1998 (Champagne et al., 2004).

[21]A total of 1,548 10-year-old children, attending fifth grade in the Bogalusa, LA, school system, participated in one of seven cross-sectional surveys from 1973 to 1994 (Nicklas et al., 2004a). Dietary information was collected by a single 24-hour recall.

tween 1973 and 1994 by children in the low tertile (68 g versus 77 g), but an increase for those in the middle (325 g versus 408 g) and high (770 g versus 868 g) tertiles. The total amount of milk consumption was significantly lower (~20 percent) in the middle and high sweetened beverage consumption groups compared to the low or no sweetened beverage consumption groups (Rajeshwari et al., 2005).

The percentage of Bogalusa children who skipped breakfast increased from 8 percent in 1973 to 30 percent in 1978, but decreased to 13 percent after the introduction of the SBP in 1981 (Nicklas et al., 2004b), a level lower than that observed nationally. Also unlike national trends, the percentage of children consuming snacks as well as total eating episodes decreased. On the other hand, similar to national trends, the percentage of Bogalusa children consuming a dinner at home decreased and those consuming a dinner prepared outside the home or a meal at a restaurant increased.

SUMMARY

The committee's review of the health, diet, and eating patterns of children and youth finds several issues and trends relevant to its consideration of the potential for marketing practices to influence these patterns. Children and youth today face new diet-related health problems that were unexpected just a generation ago. The increased prevalence of obesity and type 2 diabetes and the growing incidence of the metabolic syndrome in children and adolescents of all ages and across all ethnic groups have the potential to affect health gains that children have experienced in other dimensions over the past 30–40 years. Children and adolescents today have higher than recommended intakes of saturated fatty acids, *trans* fatty acids, and sodium. Moreover, dietary intakes of calcium, potassium, fiber, magnesium, and vitamin E are sufficiently low to warrant concern. Adolescent girls of childbearing age and low-income toddlers are especially at risk of inadequate intake of iron. Furthermore, recent trends in child health disparities reveal that social disparities persist despite significant improvements in absolute levels of child health. Children who live in poverty experience greater health, social, and nutrition disparities when compared with middle- and high-income children.

The nutrient intakes of children and adolescents reflect their food and beverage choices, which have changed substantially over time. A healthful diet provides recommended amounts of nutrients and other food components within estimated calorie needs to promote normal growth and development, a healthy weight trajectory, and caloric balance. Yet, current consumption patterns suggest disproportionately low intakes of fruits, vegetables, legumes, whole grains, and dairy products, and disproportionately high intakes of high-calorie and low-nutrient foods and beverages.

REFERENCES

AAP (American Academy of Pediatrics). 2001. The use and misuse of fruit juice in pediatrics. *Pediatrics* 107(5):1210–1213.

AAP. 2004. Soft drinks in schools. *Pediatrics* 113(1):152–154.

Affenito SG, Thompson DR, Barton BA, Franko DL, Daniels SR, Obarzanek E, Schreiber GB, Striegel-Moore RH. 2005. Breakfast consumption by African-American and white adolescent girls correlates positively with calcium and fiber intake and negatively with body mass index. *J Am Diet Assoc* 105(6):938–945.

AHA (American Heart Association). 2005. *Heart Disease and Stroke Statistics—2005 Update*. Dallas, TX: AHA. [Online]. Available: http://www.americanheart.org/ downloadable/heart/1105390918119HDSStats2005Update.pdf [accessed April 23, 2005].

Alaimo K, Olson CM, Frongillo EA Jr. 2001a. Food insufficiency and American school-aged children's cognitive, academic, and psychosocial development. *Pediatrics* 108(1):44–53.

Alaimo K, Olson CM, Frongillo EA Jr. 2001b. Low family income and food insufficiency in relation to overweight in US children: Is there a paradox? *Arch Pediatr Adolesc Med* 155(10):1161–1167.

Alaimo K, Olson CM, Frongillo EA. 2002. Family food insufficiency, but not low family income, is positively associated with dysthymia and suicide symptoms in adolescents. *J Nutr* 132(4):719–725.

Albertson AM, Anderson GH, Crockett SJ, Goebel MT. 2003. Ready-to-eat cereal consumption: Its relationship with BMI and nutrient intake of children ages 4 to 12 years. *J Am Diet Assoc* 103(12):1613–1619.

Allison DB, Egan K, Barra LM, Caughman C, Infante M, Heimbach JT. 1999. Estimated intakes of trans fatty and other fatty acids in the US population. *J Am Diet Assoc* 99(2):166–174.

Bandini LG, Must A, Cyr H, Anderson SE, Spadano JL, Dietz WH. 2003. Longitudinal changes in the accuracy of reported energy intake in girls 10–15 y of age. *Am J Clin Nutr* 78(3):480–484.

Barton BA, Eldridge AL, Thompson D, Affenito SG, Striegel-Moore RH, Franko DL, Albertson AM, Crockett SJ. 2005. The relationship of breakfast and cereal consumption to nutrient intake and body mass index: The National Heart, Lung, and Blood Institute Growth and Health Study. *J Am Diet Assoc* 105(9):1383–1389.

Basiotis PP, Carlson A, Gerrior SA, Juan WY, Lino M. 2002. *The Healthy Eating Index: 1999–2000*. U.S. Department of Agriculture, Center for Nutrition Policy and Promotion. Report No. CNPP-12. [Online]. Available: http://www.usda.gov/cnpp/Pubs/HEI/ HEI99-00report.pdf [accessed March 15, 2005].

Beck BR, Shoemaker MR. 2000. Osteoporosis: Understanding key risk factors and therapeutic options. *The Physician and Sports Medicine* 28(2).

Berenson GS, Srinivasan SR, Bao W, Newman WP III, Tracy RE, Wattigney WA. 1998. Association between multiple cardiovascular risk factors and atherosclerosis in children and young adults: The Bogalusa Heart Study. *N Engl J Med* 338(23):1650–1656.

Block G. 2004. Foods contributing to energy intake in the US: Data from NHANES III and NHANES 1999–2000. *J Food Comp Analysis* 17(3-4):439–447.

Briefel RR, Johnson CL. 2004. Secular trends in dietary intake in the United States. *Annu Rev Nutr* 24:401–431.

Briefel R, Reidy K, Karwe V, Jankowski L, Hendricks K. 2004. Toddlers' transition to table foods: Impact on nutrient intakes and food patterns. *J Am Diet Assoc* 104(1 Suppl): S38–S44.

Capps O Jr, Clauson A, Guthrie J, Pittman G, Stockton M. 2005. *Contributions of Nonalcoholic Beverages to the U.S. Diet.* U.S. Department of Agriculture. Economic Research Service. Economic Research Report No. 1. [Online]. Available: http://www.ers.usda.gov/publications/err1/err1.pdf [accessed April 26, 2005].

Carriquiry AL, Kodd KW, Nusser SM. 1997. *Estimating Adjusted Intake and Biochemical Measurement Distributions for NHANES III.* Hyattsville, MD: National Center for Health Statistics.

Casey PH, Szeto K, Lensing S, Bogle M, Weber J. 2001. Children in food-insufficient, low-income families: Prevalence, health, and nutrition status. *Arch Pediatr Adolesc Med* 155(4):508–514.

Cavadini C, Siega-Riz AM, Popkin BM. 2000. US adolescent food intake trends from 1965 to 1996. *Arch Dis Child* 83(1):18–24.

CDC (Centers for Disease Control and Prevention). 1999. Ten great public health achievements—United States, 1990–1999. *MMWR* 48(12):241–243.

CDC. 2002. Iron deficiency—United States, 1999–2000. *MMWR* 51(40):897–899. [Online]. Available: http://www.cdc.gov/mmwr/preview/mmwrhtml/mm5140a1.htm [accessed April 24, 2005].

CDC. 2004. *Obesity Still a Major Problem, New Data Show.* National Center for Health Statistics. [Online]. Available: http://www.cdc.gov/nchs/pressroom/04facts/obesity.htm [accessed November 3, 2004].

CDC. 2005. QuickStats: Prevalence of overweight among children and teenagers, by age group and selected period—United States, 1963–2002. *MMWR* 54(8):203. [Online]. Available: http://www.cdc.gov/mmwr/preview/mmwrhtml/mm5408a6.htm [accessed March 9, 2005].

Champagne CM, Baker NB, DeLany JP, Harsha DW, Bray GA. 1998. Assessment of energy intake underreporting by doubly labeled water and observations on reported nutrient intakes in children. *J Am Diet Assoc* 98(4):426–433.

Champagne CM, Bogle ML, McGee BB, Yadrick K, Allen HR, Kramer TR, Simpson P, Gossett J, Weber J. 2004. Dietary intake in the lower Mississippi delta region: Results from the Foods of Our Delta Study. *J Am Diet Assoc* 104(2):199–207.

Cohen RA, Bloom B. 2005. Trends in health insurance and access to medical care for children under age 19 years: United States, 1998–2003. *Advance Data from Vital and Health Statistics*, No. 355. Hyattsville, MD: National Center for Health Statistics. [Online]. Available: http://www.cdc.gov/nchs/data/ad/ad355.pdf [accessed April 18, 2005].

Cole N, Fox MK. 2004. *Nutrition and Health Characteristics of Low-Income Participants. Volume II, WIC Program Participants and Nonparticipants.* Report No. E-FAN-04-014-2. Washington, DC: U.S. Department of Agriculture, Economic Research Service.

Cook JT, Frank DA, Berkowitz C, Black MM, Casey PH, Cutts DB, Meyers AF, Zaldivar N, Skalicky A, Levenson S, Heeren T, Nord M. 2004. Food insecurity is associated with adverse health outcomes among human infants and toddlers. *J Nutr* 134(6):1432–1438.

Cook S, Weitzman M, Auinger P, Nguyen M, Dietz WH. 2003. Prevalence of a metabolic syndrome phenotype in adolescents: Findings from the third National Health and Nutrition Examination Survey, 1988–1994. *Arch Pediatr Adolesc Med* 157(8):821–827.

Devaney B, Ziegler P, Pac S, Karwe V, Barr SI. 2004. Nutrient intakes of infants and toddlers. *J Am Diet Assoc* 104(1 Suppl):S14–S21.

Devaney B, Kim M, Carriquiry A, Camano-Garcia G. 2005. *Assessing the Nutrient Intakes of Vulnerable Subgroups.* Washington, DC: Economic Research Service, U.S. Department of Agriculture.

DHHS (U.S. Department of Health and Human Services). 2000a. *Healthy People 2010: Understanding and Improving Health.* Washington, DC: DHHS.

DHHS. 2000b. *Oral Health in America: A Report of the Surgeon General.* Rockville, MD: DHHS, National Institute of Dental and Craniofacial Research, National Institutes of Health.

DHHS. 2003. *National Healthcare Disparities Report.* Rockville, MD: DHHS, Agency for Healthcare Research and Quality.

DHHS and USDA (U.S. Department of Agriculture). 2004. *Nutrition and Your Health: Dietary Guidelines for Americans. 2005 Dietary Guidelines Advisory Committee Report.* [Online]. Available: http://www.health.gov/dietaryguidelines/dga2005/report/ [accessed August 10, 2004].

DHHS and USDA. 2005. *Dietary Guidelines for Americans 2005.* [Online]. Available: http://www.healthierus.gov/dietaryguidelines [accessed January 12, 2005].

Dye BA, Shenkin JD, Ogden CL, Marshall TA, Levy SM, Kanellis MJ. 2004. The relationship between healthful eating practices and dental caries in children ages 2–5 years in the United States, 1988–1994. *J Am Dent Assoc* 135(1):55–66.

Enns CW, Mickle SJ, Goldman JD. 2002. Trends in food and nutrient intakes by children in the United States. *Fam Econ Nutr Rev* 14(2):56–68.

Enns CW, Mickle SJ, Goldman JD. 2003. Trends in food and nutrient intakes by adolescents in the United States. *Fam Econ Nutr Rev* 15(2):15–27.

Ervin RB, Wright JD, Reed-Gillette D. 2004. Prevalence of leading types of dietary supplements used in the Third National Health and Nutrition Examination Survey, 1988–94. *Advance Data from Vital and Health Statistics*, No. 349. Hyattsville, MD: National Center for Health Statistics.

Evans GW. 2004. The environment of child poverty. *American Psychologist* 59(2):77–92.

Federal Interagency Forum on Child and Family Statistics. 2004. *America's Children in Brief: Key National Indicators of Well-Being, 2004.* Washington, DC: U.S. Government Printing Office. [Online]. Available: http://childstats.gov [accessed March 8, 2005].

Fisher JO, Mitchell DC, Smiciklas-Wright H, Mannino ML, Birch LL. 2004. Meeting calcium recommendations during middle childhood reflects mother–daughter beverage choices and predicts bone mineral status. *Am J Clin Nutr* 79(4):698–706.

Flegal KM, Troiano RP. 2000. Changes in the distribution of body mass index of adults and children in the US population. *Int J Obes* 24(7):807–818.

Food Research Action Center. 2005. *State of the States: 2005. A Profile of Food and Nutrition Programs Across the Nation.* [Online]. Available: http://www.frac.org/State_Of_States/2005/Report.pdf [accessed March 9, 2005].

Fox MK, Cole N. 2004. *Nutrition and Health Characteristics of Low-Income Populations. Vol III, School-age Children.* Report No. E-FAN-04-014-3. Washington, DC: Economic Research Service, U.S. Department of Agriculture.

Fox MK, Pac S, Devaney B, Jankowski L. 2004. Feeding Intakes and Toddlers Study: What foods are infants and toddlers eating? *J Am Diet Assoc* 104(1 Suppl):S22–S30.

French SA, Lin BL, Guthrie JF. 2003. National trends in soft drink consumption among children and adolescents age 6 to 17 years: Prevalence, amounts, and sources, 1977/1978 to 1994/1998. *J Am Diet Assoc* 103(10):1326–1331.

Frongillo EA. 2003. Understanding obesity and program participation in the context of poverty and food insecurity. *J Nutr* 133(7):2117–2118.

Ganji V, Hampl JS, Betts NM. 2003. Race-, gender- and age-specific differences in dietary micronutrient intakes of US children. *Int J Food Sci and Nutr* 54(6):485–490.

Gartner LM, Greer FR, Section on Breastfeeding and Committee on Nutrition, American Academy of Pediatrics. 2003. Prevention of rickets and vitamin D deficiency: New guidelines for vitamin D intake. *Pediatrics* 111(4):908–910.

Gibson D. 2004. Long-term food stamp program participation is differentially related to overweight in young girls and boys. *J Nutr* 134(2):372–379.

Gift HC, Drury TF, Nowjack-Raymer RE, Selwitz RH. 1996. The state of the nation's oral health: Mid-decade assessment of Healthy People 2000. *J Public Health Dent* 56(2): 84–91.

Gleason P, Suitor C. 2001. *Children's Diets in the Mid-1990s: Dietary Intake and Its Relationship with School Meal Participation.* Report No. CN-01-CD1. Alexandria, VA: U.S. Department of Agriculture.

Goodman E. 1999. The role of socioeconomic status gradients in explaining differences in US adolescents' health. *Am J Public Health* 89(10):1522–1528.

Guthrie JF, Morton JF. 2000. Food sources of added sweeteners in the diets of Americans. *J Am Diet Assoc* 100(1):43–48, 51.

Guthrie JF, Lin B, Frazão E. 2002. Role of food prepared away from home in the American diet, 1977–78 versus 1994–96: Changes and consequences. *J Nutr Educ Behav* 34(3): 140–150.

Haffner SM, Valdez RA, Hazuda HP, Mitchell BD, Morales PA, Stern MP. 1992. Prospective analysis of the insulin-resistance syndrome (syndrome X). *Diabetes* 41(6):715–722.

Haley S, Reed J, Lin B-H, Cook A. 2005. *Sweetener Consumption in the United States.* Report No. SSS-243-01. Washington, DC: Economic Research Service, U.S. Department of Agriculture.

Hedley AA, Ogden CL, Johnson CL, Carroll MD, Curtin LR, Flegal KM. 2004. Prevalence of overweight and obesity among US children, adolescents, and adults, 1999–2002. *J Am Med Assoc* 291(23):2847–2850.

Hetzel BS, Clugston GA. 1999. Iodine. In: Shils ME, Olson JA, Shike M, Ross AC, eds. *Modern Nutrition in Health and Disease.* 9th ed. Baltimore, MD: Williams and Wilkins. Pp. 253–263.

Hofferth S, Curtin S. 2005. Poverty, food programs, and childhood obesity. *J Policy Analysis Management* 24(4):703–726.

Honein MA, Paulozzi LJ, Mathews TJ, Erickson JD, Wong LY. 2001. Impact of folic acid fortification of the US food supply on the occurrence of neural tube defects. *J Am Med Assoc* 285(23):2981–2986.

Huang TT, McCrory MA. 2005. Dairy intake, obesity, and metabolic health in children and adolescents: Knowledge and gaps. *Nutr Rev* 63(3):71–80.

Huang TT, Howarth NC, Lin BH, Roberts SB, McCrory MA. 2004. Energy intake and meal portions: Associations with BMI percentile in U.S. children. *Obes Res* 12(11):1875–1885.

IOM (Institute of Medicine). 1997. *Dietary Reference Intakes for Calcium, Phosphorus, Magnesium, Vitamin D, and Fluoride.* Washington, DC: National Academy Press.

IOM. 1998. *Dietary Reference Intakes for Thiamin, Riboflavin, Niacin, Vitamin B_6, Folate, Vitamin B_{12}, Pantothenic Acid, Biotin, and Choline.* Washington, DC: National Academy Press.

IOM. 2001. *Dietary Reference Intakes for Vitamin A, Vitamin K, Arsenic, Boron, Chromium, Copper, Iodine, Iron, Manganese, Molybdenum, Nickel, Silicon, Vanadium, and Zinc.* Washington, DC: National Academy Press.

IOM. 2002–2005. *Dietary Reference Intakes for Energy, Carbohydrate, Fiber, Fat, Fatty Acids, Cholesterol, Protein, and Amino Acids (Macronutrients).* Washington, DC: The National Academies Press.

IOM. 2003. *Dietary Reference Intakes: Guiding Principles for Nutrition Labeling and Fortification.* Washington, DC: The National Academies Press.

IOM. 2005a. *Dietary Reference Intakes for Water, Potassium, Sodium, Chloride, and Sulfate.* Washington, DC: The National Academies Press.

IOM. 2005b. *Preventing Childhood Obesity: Health in the Balance.* Washington, DC: The National Academies Press.

IOM. 2005c. *The WIC Food Package: Time for a Change.* Washington, DC: The National Academies Press.

Isomaa B, Almgren P, Tuomi T, Forsen B, Lahti K, Nissen M, Taskinen MR, Groop L. 2001. Cardiovascular morbidity and mortality associated with the metabolic syndrome. *Diabetes Care* 24(4):683–689.

Jahns L, Siega-Riz AM, Popkin BM. 2001. The increasing prevalence of snacking among US children from 1977 to 1996. *J Pediatr* 138(4):493–498.

Jones SJ, Jahns L, Laraia BA, Haughton B. 2003. Lower risk of overweight in school-aged food insecure girls who participate in food assistance. Results from the panel study of income dynamics child development supplement. *Arch Pediatr Adolesc Med* 157(8): 780–784.

Kaiser LL, Melgar-Quinonez HR, Lamp CL, Johns MC, Sutherlin JM, Harwood JO. 2002. Food security and nutritional outcomes of preschool-age Mexican-American children. *J Am Diet Assoc* 102(7):924–929.

Kant AK. 2004. Reported consumption of low-nutrient-density foods by American children and adolescents. National and health correlates, NHANES III, 1988 to 1994. *Arch Pediatr Adolesc Med* 157(8):789–796.

Kant AK, Graubard BI. 2003. Predictors of reported consumption of low-nutrient-density foods in a 24-h recall by 8–16 year old US children and adolescents. *Appetite* 41(2): 175–180.

Kenney GM, McFeeters JR, Yee JY. 2005. Preventive dental care and unmet dental needs among low-income children. *Am J Public Health* 95(8):1360–1366.

Kranz S, Siega-Riz AM, Herring AH. 2004. Changes in diet quality of American preschoolers between 1977 and 1998. *Am J Public Health* 94(9):1525–1530.

Kranz S, Mitchell DC, Siega-Riz AM, Smiciklas-Wright H. 2005a. Dietary fiber intake by American preschoolers is associated with more nutrient-dense diets. *J Am Diet Assoc* 105(2):221–225.

Kranz S, Smiciklas-Wright H, Siega-Riz AM, Mitchell D. 2005b. Adverse effect of high added sugar consumption on dietary intake in American preschoolers. *J Pediatr* 146(1): 105–111.

Lakka HM, Laaksonen DE, Lakka TA, Niskanen LK, Kumpusalo E, Tuomilehto J, Salonen JT. 2002. The metabolic syndrome and total and cardiovascular disease mortality in middle-aged men. *J Am Med Assoc* 288(21):2709–2716.

Land KC. 2005. *The Foundation for Child Development Index of Child Well-Being (CWI), 1975–2003, with Projections for 2004.* Durham, NC: Duke University.

Ledikwe JH, Blanck HM, Khan LK, Serdula MK, Seymour JD, Tohill BC, Rolls BJ. 2005. Dietary energy density determined by eight calculation methods in a nationally representative United States population. *J Nutr* 135(2):273–278.

Lin B. 2005. *Nutrition and Health Characteristics of Low-Income Populations: Healthy Eating Index.* Agriculture Information Bulletin 796-1. Washington, DC: Economic Research Service, U.S. Department of Agriculture.

Lin B, Guthrie J, Frazao E. 1999. Quality of children's diets at and away from home: 1994–96. *Food Review* 22(1):2–10.

Livingstone MBE, Robson PJ. 2000. Measurement of dietary intake in children. *Proc Nutr Soc* 59(2):279–293.

Looker AC, Dallman PR, Carroll MD, Gunter EW, Johnson CL. 1997. Prevalence of iron deficiency in the United States. *J Am Med Assoc* 277(12):973–976.

Mahoney LT, Burns TL, Stanford W, Thompson BH, Witt JD, Rost CA, Lauer RM. 1996. Coronary risk factors measured in childhood and young adult life are associated with coronary artery calcification in young adults: The Muscatine Study. *J Am Coll Cardiol* 27(2):277–284.

Matheson DM, Varady J, Varady A, Killen JD. 2002. Household food security and nutritional status of Hispanic children in the fifth grade. *Am J Clin Nutr* 76(1):210–217.

McGill HC Jr, McMahan CA, Herderick EE, Zieske AW, Malcom GT, Tracy RE, Strong JP. 2002. Obesity accelerates the progression of coronary atherosclerosis in young men. *Circulation* 105(23):2712–2718.

Moshfegh A, Goldman J, Cleveland L. 2005. *What We Eat in America, NHANES 2001–2002: Usual Nutrient Intakes from Food Compared to Dietary Reference Intakes.* USDA Agricultural Research Service. [Online]. Available: http://www.ars.usda.gov/SP2User Files/Place/12355000/pdf/usualintaketables2001-02.pdf [accessed October 4, 2005].

Mrdjenovic G, Levitsky DA. 2003. Nutritional and energetic consequences of sweetened drink consumption in 6- to 13-year-old children. *J Pediatr* 142(6):604–610.

Murphy M, Douglass J, Latulippe M, Barr S, Johnson R, Frye C. 2005. Beverages as a source of energy and nutrients in diets of children and adolescents. Experimental Biology Meeting, San Diego, April 1–5. Abstract 275.4. *FASEB J* 19(4):A434.

National SAFE KIDS Campaign. 2003, May. *Report to the Nation: Trends in Unintentional Childhood Injury Mortality, 1987–2000.* [Online]. Available: http://www.usa.safekids. org/content_documents/nskw03_report.pdf [accessed July 22, 2005].

Nicklas TA, Demory-Luce D, Yang SJ, Baranowski T, Zakeri I, Berenson G. 2004a. Children's food consumption patterns have changed over two decades (1973–1994): The Bogalusa Heart Study. *J Am Diet Assoc* 104(7):1127–1140.

Nicklas TA, Morales M, Linares A, Yang SJ, Baranowski T, De Moor C, Berenson G. 2004b. Children's meal patterns have changed over a 21-year period: The Bogalusa Heart Study. *J Am Diet Assoc* 104(5):753–761.

Nielsen SJ, Popkin BM. 2003. Patterns and trends in food portion sizes, 1977–1998. *J Am Med Assoc* 289(4):450–453.

Nielsen SJ, Popkin BM. 2004. Changes in beverage intake between 1997 and 2001. *Am J Prev Med* 27(3):205–210.

Nielsen SJ, Siega-Riz AM, Popkin BM. 2002a. Trends in energy intake in U.S. between 1977 and 1996: Similar shifts seen across age groups. *Obes Res* 10(5):370–378.

Nielsen SJ, Siega-Riz AM, Popkin BM. 2002b. Trends in food locations and sources among adolescents and young adults. *Prev Med* 35(2):107–113.

NIH (National Institutes of Health). 2001. Osteoporosis: Prevention, diagnosis, and therapy. *J Am Med Assoc* 285(6):785–795.

Nord M, Andrews M, Carlson S. 2005. *Household Food Security in the United States, 2004.* Economic Research Report Number 11. Washington, DC: U.S. Department of Agriculture, Economic Research Service.

NRC (National Research Council). 1989. *Recommended Dietary Allowances.* 10th ed. Washington, DC: National Academy Press.

NRC and IOM. 2004. *Children's Health, the Nation's Wealth.* Washington, DC: The National Academies Press.

Ogden CL, Carroll MD, Flegal KM. 2003. Epidemiologic trends in overweight and obesity. *Endocrinol Metab Clin North Am* 32(4):741–760, vii.

Ogden CL, Fryar CD, Carroll MD, Flegal KM. 2004. Mean body weight, height and body mass index, United States, 1960–2002. *Advance Data from Vital and Health Statistics,* No. 347. Hyattsville, MD: National Center for Health Statistics. [Online]. Available: http://www.cdc.gov/nchs/data/ad/ad347.pdf [accessed March 20, 2005].

Park YK, Sempos CT, Barton CN, Vanderveen JE, Yetley EA. 2000. Effectiveness of food fortification in the United States: The case of pellagra. *Am J Public Health* 90(5): 727–738.

Park YK, Meier ER, Bianchi P, Song WO. 2002. Trends in children's consumption of beverages: 1987 to 1998. *Fam Econ Nutr Rev* 14(2):69–79.

Pfeiffer CM, Caudill SP, Gunter EW, Osterloh J, Sampson EJ. 2005. Biochemical indicators of B vitamin status in the US population after folic acid fortification: Results from the National Health and Nutrition Examination Survey 1999–2000. *Am J Clin Nutr* 82(2): 442–450.

Pollitt E. 1993. Iron deficiency and cognitive function. *Annu Rev Nutr* 13:521–537.

Rajeshwari R, Yang SJ, Nicklas TA, Berenson GS. 2005. Secular trends in children's sweetened-beverage consumption (1973 to 1994): The Bogalusa Heart Study. *J Am Diet Assoc* 105(2):208–214.

Rolls BJ, Ello-Martin JA, Tohill BC. 2004. What can intervention studies tell us about the relationship between fruit and vegetable consumption and weight management? *Nutr Rev* 62(1):1–17.

Sherry B, Mei Z, Yip R. 2001. Continuation of the decline in prevalence of anemia in low-income infants and children in five states. *Pediatrics* 107(4):677–682.

Sherry B, Mei Z, Scanlon KS, Mokdad AH, Grummer-Strawn LM. 2004. Trends in state-specific prevalence of overweight and underweight in 2- through 4-year-old children from low-income families from 1989 through 2000. *Arch Pediatr Adolesc Med* 158(12): 1116–1124.

Shils M, Shike M, Olson J, Ross AC. 1999. *Modern Nutrition in Health and Disease*. Baltimore, MD: Williams & Wilkins.

Siega-Riz AM, Popkin BM, Carson T. 1998. Trends in breakfast consumption for children in the United States from 1965 to 1991. *Am J Clin Nutr* 67(4S):748S–756S.

Skinner JD, Ziegler P, Pac S, Devaney B. 2004a. Meal and snack patterns of infants and toddlers. *J Am Diet Assoc* 104(1 Suppl 1):S65–S70.

Skinner JD, Ziegler P, Ponza M. 2004b. Transitions in infants' and toddlers' beverage patterns. *J Am Diet Assoc* 104(1 Suppl 1):S45–S50.

Smiciklas-Wright H, Mitchell DC, Mickle SJ, Goldman JD, Cook A. 2003. Foods commonly eaten in the United States, 1989–1991 and 1994–1996: Are portion sizes changing? *J Am Diet Assoc* 103(1)41–47.

Storey ML, Forshee RA, Anderson PA. 2004. Associations of adequate intake of calcium with diet, beverage consumption, and demographic characteristics among children and adolescents. *J Am Coll Nutr* 23(1):18–33.

Story M, Holt K, Sofka D, eds. 2003. *Bright Futures in Practice: Nutrition*. 2nd ed. Arlington, VA: National Center for Education in Maternal and Child Health. [Online]. Available: http://www.brightfutures.org/nutrition/index.html [accessed August 22, 2005].

Strauss RS, Knight J. 1999. Influence of the home environment on the development of obesity in children. *Pediatrics* 103(6):E85.

Strauss RS, Pollack HA. 2001. Epidemic increase in childhood overweight, 1986–1998. *J Am Med Assoc* 286(22):2845–2848.

Subar AF, Krebs-Smith SM, Cook A, Kahle LL. 1998. Dietary sources of nutrients among US children, 1989–1991. *Pediatrics* 102(4 Pt 1):913–923.

Suitor CW, Gleason PM. 2002. Using Dietary Reference Intake-based methods to estimate the prevalence of inadequate nutrient intake among school-aged children. *J Am Diet Assoc* 102(4):530–536.

Templeton S. 2005. Sugar intake from combined school lunch and competitive food consumption. *J Am Diet Assoc* 105(7):1066–1067.

Templeton SB, Marlette MA, Panemangalore M. 2005. Competitive foods increase the intake of energy and decrease the intake of certain nutrients by adolescents consuming school lunch. *J Am Diet Assoc* 105(2):215–220.

Troiano RP, Flegal KM. 1998. Overweight children and adolescents: Description, epidemiology, and demographics. *Pediatrics* 101(3 Pt 2):497–504.

Troiano RP, Briefel RR, Carroll MD, Bialostosky K. 2000. Energy and fat intakes of children and adolescents in the United States: Data from the National Health and Nutrition Examination Surveys. *Am J Clin Nutr* 72(5 Suppl):1343S–1353S.

USDA (U.S. Department of Agriculture). 1992. *The Food Guide Pyramid. A Guide to Daily Food Choice.* Home and Garden Bulletin 252. Washington, DC: USDA Human Nutrition Information Service.

USDA. 1996. *The Food Guide Pyramid.* Center for Nutrition Policy and Promotion. Washington, DC: U.S. Government Printing Office.

USDA. 1999. *Food and Nutrient Intakes by Children, 1994–96, 1998, Table Set 17.* Food Surveys Research Group, Agricultural Research Service. [Online]. Available: http://www.barc.usda.gov/bhnrc/foodsurvey/home.htm [accessed January 4, 2005].

USDA. 2003a. *Federal Register Notice on Technical Revisions to the Food Guide Pyramid.* Table 2: Energy Levels for Proposed Food Intake Patterns. Center for Nutrition Policy and Promotion. [Online]. Available: http://www.cnpp.usda.gov/pyramid-update/FGP%20docs/TABLE%202.pdf [accessed March 28, 2005].

USDA. 2003b. *The Food Guide Pyramid for Young Children.* Center for Nutrition Policy and Promotion. [Online]. Available: http://www.usda.gov/cnpp/KidsPyra/LittlePyr.pdf [accessed February 24, 2005].

USDA. 2005a. *Interactive Healthy Eating Index.* [Online]. Available: http://209.48.219.53/Default.asp [accessed July 6, 2005].

USDA. 2005b. *MyPyramid: Steps to a Healthier You.* [Online]. Available: http://www.mypyramid.gov/ [accessed April 25, 2005].

USDA. 2005c. *The Food Assistance Landscape.* Food Assistance and Nutrition Research Report No. 28-6. [Online]. Available: http://www.ers.usda.gov/publications/fanrr28-6/fanrr28-6.pdf [accessed April 24, 2005].

USDA. 2005d. *USDA Healthy Eating Index.* [Online]. Available: http://www.cnpp.usda.gov/healthyeating.html [accessed July 6, 2005].

Wang G, Dietz WH. 2002. Economic burden of obesity in youths aged 6 to 17 years: 1979–1999. *Pediatrics* 109(5):e81.

Weinberg, LG, Berner LA, Groves JE. 2004. Nutrient contributions of dairy foods in the United States, continuing survey of food intakes by individuals, 1994–1996, 1998. *J Am Diet Assoc* 104(6):895–902.

Weisberg P, Scanlon KS, Li R, Cogswell ME. 2004. Nutritional rickets among children in the United States: Review of cases reported between 1986 and 2003. *Am J Clin Nutr* 80(6 Suppl):1697S–1705S.

Williams J, Wake M, Hesketh K, Maher E, Waters E. 2005. Health-related quality of life of overweight and obese children. *J Am Med Assoc* 293(1):70–76.

Winkleby MA, Robinson TN, Sundquist J, Kraemer HC. 1999. Ethnic variation in cardiovascular disease risk factors among children and young adults: Findings from the Third National Health and Nutrition Examination Survey, 1988–1994. *J Am Med Assoc* 281(11):1006–1013.

Wise PH. 2004. The transformation of child health in the United States. *Health Affairs* 23(5):9–25.

Wyshak G. 2000. Teenaged girls, carbonated beverage consumption, and bone fractures. *Arch Pediatr Adolesc Med* 154(6):610–613.

3

Factors Shaping Food and Beverage Consumption of Children and Youth

INTRODUCTION

Eating behaviors cannot be understood, explained, or changed without considering the context in which an individual lives (e.g., individual characteristics, home, and family). This context is nested within a broader community context, such as the neighborhood and schools, and societal factors (e.g., marketing, economics, culture). Interactions within and among these contexts affect behavior. A multidimensional approach to understanding the processes and context of the influences shaping children's and youths' eating behaviors can help explain relationships among factors in different domains.

This chapter presents an ecological perspective for understanding factors that influence child and adolescent eating behaviors and food and beverage choices. From this perspective, child and adolescent eating behaviors are conceptualized as a function of individual and environmental influences, or spheres of influence. These include biological factors, familial and social relationships, neighborhood, community, and institutional settings, culture and values, and broader social and economic trends. This chapter describes the following spheres of influence:

- Individual and developmental factors (e.g., developmental, biological, psychological/psychosocial);
- Family and social influences;
- Institutional, neighborhood, and community environments; and
- Macrosystem influences (e.g., marketing, culture and values, food systems).

All of these factors may directly or indirectly influence eating behaviors. If the diets of children and youth are to improve, attention must be given not only to the behavior of individuals but also to the environmental context and conditions in which people live and eat.

Current studies are inadequate to explain with certainty how individual and environmental influences interact to influence dietary behaviors and health outcomes of children and youth. Simultaneous analyses of sociodemographic, psychological, developmental, and environmental factors and their interactions with food choices are rare in the literature. The few cases that do exist are often focused on a specific age group or a single food group, such as fruits and vegetables. The following sections present both empirical evidence and theoretical links to eating behaviors.

INDIVIDUAL AND DEVELOPMENTAL FACTORS

Individual influences on children's eating behaviors include biological and genetic factors, sensory characteristics, psychological and psychosocial factors, developmental stages, consumer socialization, and lifestyle factors.

Biological and Genetic Factors

Biological Factors

Eating is a behavior influenced by physiological factors. It involves many organs and the central nervous system. Hunger, appetite, and satiety are all under neural regulatory control. Physiological factors influence food intake through sensory stimulation (e.g., smell, sight, taste of food), gastrointestinal signals, and circulating factors and chemical signals (e.g., glucose, insulin, peptides). Environmental and cognitive factors can interfere with or override physiological controls of eating and calorie intake. In fact, food intake in humans may depend more on external factors rather than physiological factors (Bell and Rolls, 2001).

Recent advances in the field of behavioral neuroscience have begun to increase the scientific understanding of the neurobiology of eating and food intake, including when and how much food is consumed and when eating is terminated. Gut–brain signals appear to be a critical neural network in the regulation of calorie intake and meal size. The discovery of bioactive food-stimulated gut peptides, adipocyte hormones, and hypothalamic neuropeptides all appear to affect food intake (Schwartz, 2004). It has been suggested that central regulatory mechanisms may contribute to the preference of sugars and fats over other macronutrients and tastes (Drewnowski and Levine, 2003). Much of the neurobiological mechanism research has been done in animal models, or human neuroimaging studies with patterns of brain activation produced by the thought, sight, smell, or taste of food. Thus, the effect of the neurobiology of eating and food intake on human behavior has not been fully elucidated.

Some universal biological food predispositions may exist, including preferences for sweetness and fat texture, avoidance of irritation, avoidance of bitter and strong tastes, a tendency to be suspicious of new foods, and a set of genetic learning predispositions (Rozin, 2002). These predispositions may have served an adaptive function in human history when food was relatively scarce, modest in fat or sugar content, and limited in variety (Rozin, 2002). However, food today is abundant and widely available and thousands of new food products are introduced every year, including those high in sugar, fat, and salt, which appeal to our taste predispositions (Chapter 4). In today's food environment, children's predispositions and adults' responses to them can promote food preferences and intake patterns that foster less healthful eating patterns that can contribute to the development of obesity (Birch, 1999).

Genetic Factors

Although the influences of genes on weight status and obesity are well documented, genetic influences on eating patterns and behaviors have received much less attention. While there is strong support from animal models for a genetic basis to food intake, a limited number of human studies suggest that food selection and intake, specifically for macronutrients (e.g., fats, carbohydrates) and total calories, may be genetically influenced to some extent (Keller et al., 2002). Research from family and twin studies suggests a modest to moderate genetic contribution to eating behaviors (de Castro and Plunkett, 2002; Keller et al., 2002; Klump et al., 2000; Reed et al., 1997). Selected adult twin studies show that heredity accounts for 11–65 percent of the variance in the average overall calorie intake (Keller et al., 2002). These studies also show the importance of nongenetic environmental effects. Studies among family members suggest that genetic influences on nutrient intake among first degree relatives is weak and that nongenetic effects associated with a shared environment are the major contributors to energy intake (Perusse et al., 1988). Studies assessing food preferences in both families and twins have found that the heritable component for individual foods is very low (Reed et al., 1997; Rozin and Millman, 1987). This suggests the important influential role of the environment on dietary patterns. Reported heritability of macronutrient intakes (e.g., fats, carbohydrates) tends to be somewhat stronger. A better understanding is needed to elucidate the complex interplay between human genes and the environment.

Individual variation in taste and food preferences may be genetically influenced (Birch, 1999; Keller and Tepper, 2004). Sensitivity to bitter taste is a heritable trait. Compounds such as 6-n-propylthiouracil (PROP) taste bitter to some people and are tasteless to others. Some, but not all studies have shown that PROP tasters show lower acceptance of cruciferous and other bitter vegetables (e.g., broccoli, cabbage, brussel sprouts), have more food dislikes, and are more sensitive to sweet tastes and the texture of fat (Birch, 1999; Keller and Tepper, 2004). These studies suggest that genetic taste factors may play an important role in the development of food preferences and dietary intake in children (Keller et al., 2002). A better understanding of the genetic basis of taste may lead to the design of better dietary prevention strategies for children (Keller et al., 2002). More research is needed to identify genetic markers that will facilitate our understanding of genetic predispositions and how they interact with feeding and dietary experiences and social and environmental contexts.

Sensory Characteristics and Taste

Sensory Characteristics

Perceptions and responses to the sensory properties of food—taste, smell, and texture—affect food preferences and eating habits (Drewnowski, 1997). Sensory responses are influenced by genetic, physiological, and metabolic variables. Preferences for sweet tastes, saltiness, and fatty textures may be an innate human trait or acquired early in life. By about 4 months, for example, infants begin to show a preference for salt (Birch, 1999). On the other hand, bitter and strong tasting foods are often rejected early in life. From an evolutionary basis, these responses may have served biological functions needed for survival. In nature, sweetness is associated with readily available calories from carbohydrates, and salt is needed for survival. However, bitterness may be associated with natural toxins signaling dietary danger (Mennella et al., 2004, 2005; Rozin, 2002). The tendency to learn to prefer calorie-dense foods may have been adaptive at times in our history when food was scarce (Rozin, 2002).

Innate taste responses are observed immediately after birth. Facial expressions on human newborns show a positive hedonic response to sweet tastes and a negative response to bitter and sour tastes (Drewnowski, 1997). The sensory pleasure response to sweetness and dietary fat may be mediated by the brain through neurotransmitters or endogenous opiate peptides (Benton, 2004).

Studies of young children have shown that their food preferences are influenced primarily by two factors: sweetness and familiarity (Birch, 1999; Drewnowski, 1997). Preferences for fat also may be acquired in early life, as children learn to prefer those flavors of foods that are associated with high-calorie and fat content (Drewnowski, 1997). However, the predisposition to prefer a sweet taste is readily modified by experiences with food and eating (Birch, 1999). One study showed that at birth all infants preferred sweet solutions to water, but by 6 months, preference for sweetened water was linked to the infant's food experience; those infants routinely given sweetened water by their mothers showed a greater preference for it than infants who had been given water that was not sweetened (Beauchamp and Moran, 1982). Substantial evidence shows that predispositions to prefer sweet, fatty, and salty foods and reject bitter ones can be readily altered through experience with food and eating (Birch, 1999).

Flavor is another primary dimension by which young children determine food acceptance (Mennella et al., 2005). Some relatively new evidence has hypothesized that experience with a flavor in amniotic fluid or breast milk may modify an infant's acceptance and enjoyment of similarly flavored foods at weaning, and that this may underlie individual differences in food acceptability and possibly serve as the foundation for lifelong food habits (Mennella et al., 2004). Mennella et al. (2001) found that weaning infants who had exposure to the flavor of carrots in either amniotic fluid or breast milk were perceived to respond more positively to that flavor in a food base than did nonexposed infants. Thus, preliminary research suggests that prenatal and early postnatal exposure to flavors may predispose the young infant to have a favorable response to those flavors in foods.

Taste

One of the most important individual influences on food choice is taste, which also is influenced by the aroma and texture of food. Research has consistently shown that children, adolescents, and adults all report that taste is the most important influence on their food choices (Barr, 1994; French et al., 1999; Glanz et al., 1998; Horacek and Betts, 1998; Neumark-Sztainer et al., 1999). Taste preference has also been found to be directly related to children's fruit and vegetable consumption (Neumark-Sztainer et al., 2003), calcium intake (Barr, 1994), and carbonated soft drink consumption (Grimm et al., 2004). In studies assessing motivation for vending snack choices and food choices at school, adolescents rated taste as the most important factor to consider, followed by hunger and price (French et al., 1999; Shannon et al., 2002). Those who placed greater emphasis on snack taste were less likely to report low-fat vending snacks as current or intended choices. "Healthfulness" and "tastiness" tend to be seen as opposites by children (Wardle and Huon, 2000).

There appears to be widespread belief among children and adolescents that "if a food tastes good, it must not be good for me" and "if a food tastes bad, it is probably good for me" (Baranowski et al., 1993). In one study of teenagers, only one-fourth thought low-fat foods taste good (Shannon et al., 2002). In an experimental study with 9- to 11-year-old children, Wardle and Huon (2000) tested the idea that a "healthy" label would reduce the appeal of a novel drink. Children were asked to taste and rate one or two drinks—one was described and labeled as "a new health drink" and the other as a "new drink." The results showed children rated the drink labeled healthful as tasting less pleasant and said they would be less likely to ask their parents to buy it than the same drink presented just as a "new drink" (Wardle and Huon, 2000).

Developmental Stages

Early childhood lays the foundation for food behaviors and food preferences. The developmental stage[1] of a child has a central influence on eating behaviors. During infancy (ages 0–12 months), feeding is central to the parent–child relationship and for the infant developing a sense of security and trust. Early childhood (ages 1–5 years) is characterized by rapid growth and change in the child's physical, cognitive, communicative, and social development (NRC and IOM, 2000). Eating behaviors move from complete dependence on the caregiver to more self-directed control. During early childhood, parents and primary caretakers largely determine what foods are provided and when eating occurs. Developmental characteristics of young children influence their eating behavior and include dislike for new foods (neophobia), food jags (favoring only one or two foods), and picky eating (e.g., refusal to eat certain foods and not wanting foods to touch each other on the plate) (Story et al., 2002a). These are normative behaviors in young children (Birch, 1999).

Middle childhood (ages 6–11 years) is a time of major cognitive development and mastery of cognitive, physical, and social skills. Children in this age group progress from dependence on their parents to increasing independence, with a growing interest on the development of friendships and the world around them. Their eating behaviors reflect these changes and become more influenced by outside sources.

The dramatic physical, developmental, and social changes that occur during adolescence (ages 12–19 years) can markedly affect eating behaviors and dietary intake. Growing independence and eating away from home, concern with appearance and body weight, the need for peer acceptance, and busy schedules all can impact eating patterns and food choices.

---

[1]In this report, the committee characterized infants and toddlers as under age 2 years, younger children as ages 2–5 years, older children as ages 6–11 years, and teens as ages 12–18 (Chapter 1). These age categories and terms differ slightly from what is presented from the research described in this chapter.

Age-associated declines in diet quality are evident as children move from childhood through adolescence. For example, a recent longitudinal study with girls found that dietary quality declined between ages 5 and 9 years (Mannino et al., 2004). Girls at 9 years of age tended to have inadequate intakes of dairy foods, fruits and vegetables, and several nutrients more often than the younger girls. Other longitudinal studies have shown that dietary decline continues during middle childhood into adolescence; intakes of fruits, vegetables, and milk decreases, and carbonated soft drinks increase (Lytle et al., 2000).

Psychological and Psychosocial Factors

Food Preferences

The complex interactions of many factors shape food preferences, including a child's early experiences with food and eating, positive or negative conditioning, exposure, and genetics (Birch, 1999). Self-reported food preferences are one of the strongest predictors of food choices and dietary intake (Baranowski et al., 2002; Birch and Fisher, 1998; Drewnowski and Hann, 1999; Woodward et al., 1996). Repeated exposures increase children's preference for a food or flavor (Birch, 1999). A longitudinal study of children from ages 2–3 years to 8 years reported that a high percentage of children's food preferences are formed as early as ages 2–3 years, and few changes in preferences occurred over the 5-year period (Skinner et al., 2002). The strongest predictors of the number of foods liked at age 8 years were the number of foods liked at age 4 years (Skinner et al., 2002).

When food is plentiful, food likes and dislikes play an important role in influencing food choices. Among children, sweet foods and high-fat foods tend to be the most preferred foods (Drewnowski, 1997; Rozin, 2002), while vegetables are the least preferred foods (Skinner et al., 2002). Parents often cite dislike as the primary reason for children's low vegetable intakes (Wardle et al., 2003a). It is not clear why vegetables are disliked by children, but it may be because of the sensitivity to the bitter taste of cruciferous vegetables, bland preparation of vegetables, the negative context in which vegetables may be presented—if you want dessert, you have to eat your peas, poor parental modeling, or low exposure. Skinner et al. (2002) found that foods disliked by mothers tended not to be offered to children. A growing body of research suggests that a dislike of foods can be transformed into liking with experience of repeated tasting or exposures (Wardle et al., 2003a). In one study with children, 10 daily exposures to the taste of an unfamiliar vegetable (e.g., raw red pepper) significantly increased children's liking and consumption of the vegetable (Wardle et al., 2003b). Another recent study found that daily exposure for 14 days to the taste of a previously disliked vegetable increased children's (ages 2–6 years) liking and consumption of that vegetable (Wardle et al., 2003a). These results suggest that repeated exposure through frequent tasting may be effective in increasing children's acceptance of vegetables and other healthful, but not necessarily well-liked foods (e.g., whole grains, unsweetened cereals). In homes, schools, and child-care settings, repeated exposure to initially disliked foods in an emotionally positive atmosphere could increase preference and consumption of those foods.

Social factors and the context in which the food is offered are important in shaping children's preferences. Preschool children's preferences for and consumption of disliked vegetables increased when children observed peers choosing and eating the vegetables that the target child disliked (Birch, 1999). Child feeding practices may also impact children's preferences and intake patterns. When children are given foods as rewards for approved behaviors, enhanced preference for those foods results (Birch, 1999). In contrast, when children are rewarded for eating a disliked food such as vegetables, this leads to a decline in the preference for that food (Birch, 1999).

Finding: Food preferences develop as early as 2–3 years of age and are shaped by a child's early experiences, positive or negative conditioning, exposure to foods, and a biological predisposition to prefer sweet, high-fat, and salty foods.

Gender

Gender differences in food choices and dietary intakes emerge as children move into adolescence. During childhood food intakes are similar between girls and boys. U.S. Department of Agriculture (USDA) data from the 1989–1991 Continuing Surveys of Food Intakes by Individuals (CSFII) showed little differences in mean daily intakes of the Food Guide Pyramid groups for grains, vegetables, fruit, dairy, and meat among boys and girls ages 2–5 years and ages 6–11 years (Munoz et al., 1997). Among adolescents, boys ate more servings of grains, more vegetables (including french fries), dairy, and meat servings compared to girls (Chapter 2).

Studies have shown that as a group, adolescent girls are more likely than adolescent boys to have lower intakes of essential vitamins and minerals, and fewer servings of fruits, vegetables, and dairy foods (Gleason and Suitor, 2001; Story et al., 2002b). Boys are more likely to have diets higher in total fat and saturated fat compared to girls (Gleason and Suitor, 2001; Troiano et al., 2000) and to consume larger amounts of carbonated soft drinks (French et al., 2003a). On average, adolescent boys eat larger quantities of food than adolescent girls, so they are more likely to meet daily recommended intakes for vitamins and minerals. Adolescent girls are also more likely to skip meals, especially breakfast, than are adolescent males (Gleason and Suitor, 2001; Chapter 2).

Gender differences in attitudes towards food are also evident during adolescence. Adolescent girls are more likely than adolescent boys to be concerned about health and weight, and this concern is associated with more positive attitudes and behaviors regarding healthful foods. In one study of 1,083 adolescent high school students, girls were more likely than boys to report that low-fat foods are beneficial for future health and maintaining weight (Fulkerson et al., 2004a). Boys were more likely than girls to report that healthful eating is not important to them. Girls' weight concerns may predispose them to have more favorable attitudes toward healthful eating. These results suggest the importance of segmented nutrition education interventions for adolescents.

Concern About Health and Nutrition

Health and nutrition are not a primary influence on the food choices among the majority of children, adolescents, and adults. In a study of 289 adolescents, while nearly two-thirds (61 percent) of the students reported that eating healthful foods was important to them, only 27 percent were motivated by health in making food choices (Shannon et al., 2002). Gender differences are also evident; one-third (36 percent) of girls report being motivated by health concerns compared to only 18 percent of adolescent boys (Shannon et al., 2002). Studies have also shown that students with higher health concerns have lower intakes of fat and higher nutrient intakes compared to those less concerned about health (Horacek and Betts, 1998). Conversely, those least motivated by health concerns had the highest fat intakes. Other studies have shown that children who value health for the foods they choose have better dietary quality (Gibson et al., 1998). Research has demonstrated that age positively predicts the perceived importance of nutrition and the health effects of food; it becomes more important as people age and is most valued by older adults (Glanz et al., 1998).

From a developmental perspective, it is not surprising that health and nutrition are low-priority concerns for adolescents, that adolescents are the most inclined toward eating behaviors that are incompatible with a healthful diet, and that they are less concerned about nutrition compared to their parents or grandparents (Rozin, 2002). Qualitative research has shown that many adolescents do not perceive a need or urgency to change their eating behavior when the future seems so far away (Neumark-Sztainer et al., 1999; Story and Resnick, 1986). For many, the long-term benefits of good health may not outweigh the short-term advantages of convenience and immediate gratification.

Nutrition Knowledge

Although knowing how and why to eat healthfully is important, nutrition knowledge alone does not ensure that children or adolescents will adopt healthful eating behaviors. A meta-analysis of the literature with adults, adolescents, and children found the association of nutrition knowledge with dietary behavior to be very weak ($r = 0.10$) (Axelson et al., 1985). Another more recent study with adults using CSFII data found that adults with more nutrition knowledge consumed more fruit and vegetables (Guthrie et al., 2005). Another study with mothers and children ages 9–11 years found that mothers' nutrition knowledge was strongly correlated to their children's fruit intake, but not to their intake of vegetables or sweets (Gibson et al., 1998). Children's own nutrition knowledge did not correlate with their fruit or vegetable intake (Gibson et al., 1998). Clearly, nutrition knowledge alone is not sufficient to change dietary behaviors.

Stress and Depression

Stress and depression can affect appetite through either an increase or decrease in eating. However, relatively little research has been done with children or adolescents. Cartwright et al. (2003) examined associations between psychological stress and dietary practices in a socioeconomically and ethnically diverse sample of 4,320 children ages 11–12 years. Children completed a Perceived Stress Scale and food frequency questionnaires. Greater stress was associated with eating higher-fat foods, less fruit and vegetable intake, more frequent snacking, and skipping breakfast. These effects were independent of gender, weight, socioeconomic status, and ethnicity.

An extensive body of research supports a strong relationship between depression and eating disorders among adolescents, as well as depression and weight dissatisfaction, negative body image, and disordered eating behaviors (Fulkerson et al., 2004b). Less is known about childhood depression and dietary practices. In a survey of 4,734 ethnically diverse middle and high school students, Fulkerson et al. (2004b) found that depressive symptoms were positively associated with perceived barriers to healthful eating and weight concerns. Adolescents who reported more depressive symptoms were less likely to eat breakfast, lunch, and dinner. No association was seen between depressive symptoms and calorie or nutrient intakes.

Dieting

Dieting is a widespread practice among preadolescents and adolescents, especially girls. Nationwide in 2003, 59 percent of high school girls and 29 percent of high school boys reported trying to lose weight during the 30 days preceding a survey conducted by Grunbaum et al. (2004). Nearly 20 percent of girls had gone without eating for 24 hours or more to lose weight, 11 percent had taken diet pills to lose weight, and 8 percent had vomited or taken laxatives to lose weight during the past 30 days (Grunbaum et al., 2004). The few studies that have examined adolescent weight control behaviors and associations with dietary intakes have had inconsistent results (Barr, 1995; French et al., 1995; Neumark-Sztainer et al., 2000; Story et al., 1998). Studies have shown that adolescents who engage in less healthful weight control behaviors (e.g., vomiting, laxatives, or diet pills) are at increased risk for dietary inadequacy and weight gain (Neumark-Sztainer et al., 2004; Story et al., 1998). Among 4,144 adolescents, girls using less healthful weight control behaviors had significantly lower intakes of fruits and vegetables, grains, calcium, iron, and other micronutrients compared to girls using healthy weight control methods or not dieting (Neumark-Sztainer et al., 2004). No such relationship was found among boys.

Portion Size

Several controlled laboratory and naturalistic studies show that in the short-term, older children and adults eat more with increasing portion sizes and larger package sizes (Rolls, 2003). In a laboratory study (Rolls et al., 2000), 5-year-old children varied their intake at meals directly with changes in portion sizes. When offered larger portions, children ate substantially more. In the same study, young children (about 3.5 years old) did not vary intake in relation to changes in portion size, suggesting that the ability to respond to internal cues of hunger is stronger at younger ages and diminishes with age as external factors become increasingly influential.

Food packaging and portion sizes have increased steadily over the past 30 years (Wansink, 2004; Young and Nestle, 2002). Data suggest that the trend toward larger portion sizes began in the 1970s, increased sharply in the 1980s, and has continued to increase (Young and Nestle, 2002). Package size influences the volume of food consumed. When food packages are doubled in size, consumption in adults generally increases by 18–25 percent for meal-related foods and 30–45 percent for snack-related foods (Wansink, 2004). Data indicate that away-from-home portions sizes have increased over time (Nielsen and Popkin, 2003; Young and Nestle, 2002; Chapter 2). Larger portions not only contain more calories but also encourage people to eat more. Research suggests that individuals tend to overconsume high energy-dense foods beyond physiological satiety (Kral et al., 2004), especially when they are unaware that the portion sizes served to them have been substantially increased (Rolls et al., 2004). Satiety signals are not triggered as effectively with high energy-dense foods (Drewnowski, 1998), and large portions of them consumed on a regular basis are particularly problematic for achieving energy balance and weight management in older children and adults.

In contrast to 15–25 years ago, quick serve restaurants and full serve restaurants use larger portion sizes in their marketing promotions. Restaurants are using larger dinner plates and quick serve restaurants are using larger containers for drinks and french fries (Young and Nestle, 2002). In an analysis, Young and Nestle (2002) found that the containers for virtually all foods and beverages prepared for immediate consumption have increased over time and now appear to be typical and the norm. Given these findings, there is a need for greater attention to food portion size and consuming recommended serving sizes, such as those in the Dietary Guidelines for Americans (DHHS and USDA, 2005).

Finding: The availability and marketing of foods and beverages of larger portion sizes has increased steadily over the past three decades in many venues.

Consumer Socialization and Behavior

Consumer socialization refers to the "processes by which children and adolescents acquire skills, knowledge, and attitudes relevant to their functioning as consumers in the marketplace" (Ward, 1974). Consumer socialization occurs in the context of cognitive, social and developmental changes as children progress through childhood and adolescence and become socialized into their roles as consumers. Over the past 25 years, a large body of consumer research has accumulated on children's knowledge of products, brands, advertising, pricing, shopping skills, decision-making skills and abilities, parental influence and negotiation approaches, and social aspects of the child consumer role. American children are avid consumers and become socialized into this role from an early age (John, 1999). Children's consumer socialization and behavior influences food choices, both by direct purchases and by the substantial influence children have on family purchases.

A child's first request for a product occurs at about 24 months, and 75 percent of the time, this request occurs in a supermarket. McNeal (1999) found that the most common first in-store request is ready-to-eat breakfast cereal (47 percent), followed by snacks (30 percent), and toys (21 percent). Requests are often made for a branded product. Isler et al. (1987) examined the location, types, and frequency of products that children ages 3–11 years requested of their mothers over 30 days. Food accounted for more than half (55 percent) of total requests made by children and included snack and dessert foods (24 percent), candy (17 percent), cereal (7 percent), quick serve restaurant foods (4 percent), and fruit and vegetables (3 percent) (Isler et al., 1987). Nearly two-thirds (65 percent) of all cereal requests were for presweetened breakfast cereals. Research indicates that parents honor children's requests for food about half of the time: carbonated soft drinks (60 percent), cookies (50 percent), and candy (45 percent) (McNeal, 1999). Dual-income families may be more likely to accommodate children's purchase requests (McNeal, 1999).

Adolescents also have a strong influence on grocery store purchases. In one national market research study, more than 60 percent of adolescents reported that they influence their parents' purchase of fast foods (65 percent), pizza (63 percent), and carbonated soft drinks (60 percent) (Zollo, 1999; Chapter 4). Adolescents also shop for the family groceries. A recent study with 4,746 youth found that more than half (52 percent) of adolescent girls and boys do some food shopping each week for their family (Hanson et al., 2006). Girls, younger adolescents, youth from low-income families, and ethnic minority youth were more likely to report assisting their parents with food shopping.

Parents acknowledge the influence that children have on their food purchases. In a national market survey of 930 adult family meal planners, 38 percent of parents reported that children always or often dominate dinner grocery decisions, 52 percent said they sometimes influence dinner grocery decisions, and only 10 percent reported that their children never have an influence (National Pork Producers Council, 2000). Parents reported that their children always or often influenced grocery purchase decisions for snacks (75 percent), breakfast foods (72 percent), desserts (47 percent), and dinner (38 percent) (Chapter 4). Another market study on consumer decision-making found that parents are two to three times more likely to name a child rather than themselves, as the family expert for selection of fast foods, snack foods, and new breakfast cereals (USA Weekend and The Roper Organization, 1989).

Children's consumer socialization research has also examined brand awareness. Children as young as ages 2–3 years can recognize familiar packages in the stores and familiar spokescharacters on products such as food, toys, and clothing (John, 1999). By preschool, children begin to recall brand names from seeing them advertised on television or featured on product packages, especially if the brand names are associated with salient cues such as cartoon spokescharacters, colors (e.g., packages), or pictures (John, 1999). Brand awareness develops first for child-oriented product categories such as cereals, snacks, and toys. By the time they enter the first grade children are familiar with roughly 200 brands, the average 10-year-old recognizes 300–400 brands, and an adult recognizes about 1,500 brands (McNeal, 1999). When children make requests for foods at the supermarket, more than 90 percent are by brand name and of these, 82 percent are for national brands (McNeal, 1999).

Although brand choice can be important to teenagers, they are likely to experiment with numerous brands. Teens are much more brand loyal when buying personal-hygiene products than when buying food or apparel. Of food products, carbonated soft drinks and quick serve restaurants have the highest brand loyalty among teenagers (Zollo, 1999). Because of this fact, many food and beverage marketers have intensified their efforts to develop brand relationships with young consumers (Zollo, 1999; Chapter 4). The marketing literature clearly emphasizes that in order to develop brand loyalty, marketing must start with young children (McNeal, 1999; Chapter 4).

Finding: Children are aware of food brands as young as 2–3 years of age and preschoolers demonstrate brand recognition when cued by spokes- characters and colored packages. The majority of children's food requests are for branded products. Brand loyalty is highest in teens for carbonated soft drinks and quick serve restaurants.

Lifestyle Characteristics

Time and Convenience

Perceived time constraints and convenience strongly influence the food choices of children, adolescents, and adults (Glanz et al., 1998; Neumark-Sztainer et al., 1999). In focus groups with adolescents from low-income families in California, convenience was a major driving factor in determining food choices (California Project LEAN and Food on the Run Campaign, 1998). In another study using focus groups, adolescents discussed wanting to sleep longer in the morning instead of taking the time to eat or prepare breakfast, not wanting to wait in a long lunch line, eating at quick serve restaurants because the food is served quickly, and choosing foods at home that can be prepared quickly (Neumark-Sztainer et al., 1999). Lack of time is also perceived as a major barrier to eating more healthfully. Adolescents often believe they are too busy to worry about food and eating well. Common remarks were "People our age are so busy that we don't have enough time to change bad habits" and "We don't have the time . . . too many pressures" (Story and Resnick, 1986).

Cost of Food

Studies of adults have found that taste is considered to be the most important influence on food selection, followed by cost (Glanz et al., 1998). Adolescents also appear to be price sensitive (California Project LEAN and

Food on the Run Campaign, 1998; French et al., 1997a,b, 1999, 2001a; Neumark-Sztainer et al., 1999). In one study, adolescents rated cost as the third most important reason in selecting vending snacks after taste and hunger (French et al., 1999).

Several studies have empirically demonstrated large effects of price reduction on sales of fresh fruits and vegetables and lower fat vending snacks in high school settings (French et al., 1997a,b, 2001a). A 50 percent price reduction on fresh fruit and vegetables increased weekly sales two- to four-fold during a 3-week period in two high school cafeteria a la carte areas (French et al., 1997b). In a large study involving 12 high schools and 12 worksites, price reductions on low-fat vending machine snacks of 10, 25, and 50 percent, increased sales of these items by 9 percent, 39 percent, and 93 percent, respectively (French et al., 2001a). The results of these studies clearly show the powerful effect of price on adolescent's food choices.

FAMILY AND SOCIAL INFLUENCES

Children's and adolescents' eating behaviors are strongly influenced by their social environments, especially the home and family environment. Interpersonal influences can affect eating behaviors through mechanisms such as food availability, modeling, reinforcement, social support, and perceived norms.

Family

The family is a major influence on children's and adolescents' eating behavior and dietary intake. The family mediates dietary patterns in three primary ways: (1) the family is a provider of the foods that are available and accessible in the home; (2) the family provides the meal structure, when meals occur, and what is offered; and (3) the family transmits food attitudes, food preferences, brand preferences, and values that may affect lifetime eating habits. The home is where the majority of eating occasions and calorie intake occur for both children and adolescents. National CSFII 1994–1996 data indicate that children and adolescents ages 2–19 years consumed 70 percent of their meals and 80 percent of their snacks at home and obtained 68 percent of total calories from home (Lin et al., 1999). Younger children were more likely to eat meals and snacks at home and obtain a greater proportion of calories at home compared to adolescents; for children ages 2–5 years, 76 percent of total daily calories were eaten at home compared to 67 percent for youth ages 6–11 years and 65 percent for adolescents ages 12–19 years (Lin et al., 1999; Chapter 2).

Maternal Employment

American families have undergone profound social changes in family structure and maternal employment over the past 40 years. In 1960, only 9 percent of children lived in single-parent households. In 2004, 28 percent of children lived in single-parent households, and the majority of those parents were mothers (U.S. Census Bureau, 2005). Also, maternal employment has grown significantly in the past 30 years. From 1970 to 2000, the overall maternal labor-force participation rate rose from 38 to 68 percent (NRC and IOM, 2003). A 2003 study showed that 60 percent of mothers with preschool children (younger than age 6 years) and 75 percent of mothers with children ages 6–17 years were employed in the U.S. labor force (DHHS, 2003). Of these employed mothers, 70 and 78 percent work full-time and part-time, respectively (DHHS, 2003). Trends of fewer family meals, the increasing popularity of fast food and eating out, and the increased demand for convenience and prepared foods are likely related to shifts in family composition and work schedules. Family food preparation traditionally has been largely the work of women, and although more of them are working outside of the home, they continue to have the greatest responsibility for home food production (Harnack et al., 1998).

Few studies have investigated the relationship between mothers' work status and children's diets. Studies using data from the late 1980s found that maternal employment had no significant effect on the quality of the diets of preschool children (Johnson et al., 1992, 1993). A recent study explored the effects of mothers' work on their children's nutritional status using CSFII data from 1994–1996 and 1998 (Crepinsek and Burstein, 2004). Children ages 1–17 years with full-time working mothers had lower overall Healthy Eating Index (HEI) scores (indicative of poorer diet quality), lower intakes of iron and fiber, and higher intakes of carbonated soft drinks and fried potatoes, and were more likely to skip morning meals than children of nonworking mothers. Working mothers were also more likely to rely on away-from-home food sources. These differences remained after controlling for family household characteristics, such as income and the number of adults in the household. Children whose mothers worked part-time had more positive eating patterns than those whose mothers worked full-time (Crepinsek and Burstein, 2004).

A recent study assessed the effect of maternal employment on childhood obesity using matched mother–child data from the National Longitudinal Survey of Youth (Anderson et al., 2003). The results indicate that the more hours the mother worked per week, the more likely a child was to be obese. Analyses by subgroups showed that higher socioeconomic status mothers who worked more hours per week over the child's life were the most likely to have an obese child. Potential mechanisms through which children's eating patterns and physical activity may be affected by working parents include less time to prepare family meals, more reliance on eating out or buying fast foods for consumption at home, and less supervision, which may lead to children preparing high-calorie and low-nutrient foods and beverages after school or spending more time indoors (Anderson et al., 2003).

Household Socioeconomic Status

In 2003, 11.6 million, or 16 percent, of children under the age of 18 years lived in families with incomes below the federal poverty level (Federal Interagency Forum on Child and Family Statistics, 2004). Evidence shows that dietary intakes and dietary patterns in families vary depending on economic circumstances. A recent study analyzed 24-hour recall data from the National Health and Nutrition Examination Survey III (1988–1994) (Fox and Cole, 2004). Three groups of children (ages 5–18 years) were compared based on household income: income at or below 130 percent of poverty (lowest income), income between 131 and 185 percent of poverty (low income), and income above 185 percent of poverty (higher income). Children in the lowest income group were more likely than children in the higher income group to have consumed fewer than three meals in the preceding 2 days (39 percent versus 34 percent) and were less likely to eat breakfast every day (44 percent versus 48 percent). Overall, there were no differences between income groups in mean usual calorie intake. However, children in the lowest income group obtained a greater percentage of calories from fat compared to the higher income group. There were no significant differences among income groups on mean HEI scores; the diets of 78 percent of all children showed a need for improvement, and only 6 percent of children had "good" diets (Cole and Fox, 2004; Chapter 2).

Other studies have found socioeconomic status effects. National data from the CSFII 1989–1991 data found that lower calorie intakes were found among children from less affluent households. In addition, children from lower income households were less likely to meet the recommendations for fruit and dairy intakes (Munoz et al., 1997). Other studies have also shown socioeconomic status differences. Adolescents in lower income households were more likely to consume insufficient fruits and vegetables (Lowry et al., 1996; Neumark-Sztainer et al., 1996). The National Growth and Health Study with 9- to 10-year-old girls found that percentage of calories from fat was inversely related to family income and parental education levels (Crawford et al., 1995). However, food insecurity has not been clearly associated with obesity in children or adolescents with the exception of white adolescent girls (Chapter 2).

Food costs may be one barrier to the adoption of healthier diets, especially by low-income households. Calorie-dense foods, some of which are high in refined grains, added sugars and added fat, provide calories at a far lower cost than do lean meats, fish, and fresh vegetables and fruits (Drewnowski, 2004). Surprisingly, there are little data on what it costs to eat a healthful diet in the United States. A recent USDA analysis estimated an annual retail price per pound for 69 types of fruits and 85 types of vegetables (Reed et al., 2004). More than half of the fruits and vegetables were estimated to cost 25 cents or less per serving. It was estimated that three servings of fruits and four servings of vegetables would cost only 64 cents per day. After adjusting for waste and serving size, 63 percent of fruits and 57 percent of vegetables were least expensive in their fresh form (Reed et al., 2004). Based on this study, it appears that consuming fresh fruits and vegetables may be very affordable. More studies need to be conducted on the costs and perceived trade-offs of eating a healthful diet.

Food Availability

Household food availability and accessibility have been identified as strong correlates of food intake in children and adolescents. Availability refers to whether foods are present in the home, and accessibility refers to whether these are available in a form, location, or time that facilitates their consumption, such as precut vegetables in a plastic bag on a front shelf in the refrigerator or a bowl of fruit on a table (Cullen et al., 2003). Using structural equation modeling, Neumark-Sztainer et al. (2003) found that the strongest correlates of fruit and vegetable intake among adolescents were home availability of fruits and vegetables and taste preferences. Home availability was mediated by parental social support for healthful eating, family meal patterns, and household food security (access to an affordable food supply). Even when taste preferences for fruits and vegetables were low, if fruits and vegetables were available in a household, intakes increased. Availability of carbonated soft drinks in the home has also been found to be strongly associated with carbonated soft drink consumption among 8- to 13-year-olds (Grimm et al., 2004).

Family Meals

Recent studies suggest that family meals exert a strong influence on the dietary intake of children and adolescents. Three large population-based studies have all found that increasing the frequency of family meals is associated with more healthful dietary intake patterns in children (Gillman et al., 2000; Neumark-Sztainer et al., 2003; Videon and Manning, 2003).

Increasing the frequency of family dinner has been associated among children ages 9–14 years with consumption of more fruits and vegetables;

less fried foods and carbonated soft drinks; less saturated fats and *trans* fat; more fiber, calcium, folate, and iron; and more vitamins B_6, B_{12}, C, and E (Gillman et al., 2000). The frequency of family meals and associations with dietary intake were also examined in 4,746 middle and high school students (Videon and Manning, 2003). Frequency of family meals was associated positively with intakes of several vitamins and minerals, fruits, vegetables, grains, and calcium-rich foods.

Parental Intakes

Parental diet has been shown to be a strong predictor of children's intake in several studies. The strongest predictor of 2- to 6-year-old children's fruit and vegetable consumption was parental fruit and vegetable consumption (Cooke et al., 2003; Wardle et al., 2005). In another study, 8- to 13-year-old youth whose parents regularly consumed carbonated soft drinks were nearly three times more likely to consume carbonated soft drinks five or more times a week compared with those whose parents did not regularly consume carbonated soft drinks (Grimm et al., 2004). One study found mother–daughter similarities in milk and carbonated soft drinks consumption (Fisher et al., 2000) and in fruit and vegetable intake (Fisher et al., 2002). In another study of adolescents, parental intakes were positively associated with intake of fruits, vegetables, and dairy products in girls and dairy products in boys (Hanson et al., 2005).

The relationship between parent and child intake may be due to a combination of factors including role modeling effects, food availability in the home, or genetic influences (Birch, 1999; Cooke et al., 2003; Neumark-Sztainer et al., 2003). As mentioned earlier, genetic influences on food preferences and intakes among family members are weak. There is evidence that supports the influence of parental role modeling on children's eating behaviors (Brown and Ogden, 2004). This influence may be direct through what parents actually eat or indirect through transmission of eating-related attitudes. The influence of parental role modeling on children's eating is consistent with Social Learning Theory (Bandura, 1977) and the importance of observational learning and modeling (Brown and Ogden, 2004). These findings suggest the importance of making parents and caregivers aware of the critical role they play in children developing healthful eating behaviors. Parents and caregivers can act as role models to encourage the tasting of new foods and model healthful eating behaviors.

Child Feeding Practices

Another factor that may influence a child's food preference and dietary intake is child feeding practices used by parents. In a series of experimental studies with young children, feeding practices commonly used by parents—such as restricting foods considered to be less nutritious, pressuring children to eat, or using foods as rewards—have been shown to inadvertently promote behaviors counter to their intentions (Birch, 1999; Birch and Fisher, 1998). For example, restricting access to palatable foods promotes children's preference for and intake of these "forbidden foods" (Birch, 1999). Forcing or pressuring children to eat certain foods decreases the preference for that food (Birch, 1999). Rewarding children for eating a disliked food (e.g., vegetables) led to a decline in the preference of that food. On the other hand, if children are given both sweet and nonsweet foods as rewards for approved behavior, the preference for those foods is enhanced. In American society, high-fat and sweet food items are used repeatedly in positive child contexts for rewards, treats, and celebrations, thus further reinforcing the preference for these foods. Birch (1999) also found that when children were offered food items that were initially neither liked nor disliked, but were then used as rewards or associated with positive parental attention, the preference for these foods increased. This has implications for child feeding strategies; for example, using vegetables such as carrots as rewards for young children.

Peers

Children and adolescents spend a substantial amount of time with their peers and friends through child-care or school settings, after-school programs, sports activities, or recreation time. The social influence of the peer group affecting food preferences and food choices is not well explored, and the few studies done have not found consistent results. Birch (1999) found that preschool children began to like and eat certain vegetables they previously disliked when they saw their peers eating those foods. This reinforces the importance of peer modeling and observational learning.

Feunekes et al. (1998) examined resemblances in high-fat foods and food intakes within social networks of adolescents, their closest friends, and their parents. Although there were significant associations between parent and adolescent intakes (76–87 percent of the items on the food frequency), only 19 percent of the foods were correlated for adolescents and their friends. These tended to be for snack foods. A recent study examined the resemblances in food preferences between good friends in three third-grade classrooms (Rozin et al., 2004). They found that friendship had no effect on food preferences. It may be that preferences are mediated through role modeling and that a major social influence on food preferences is the preferences of an admired child who is older or media role models (Rozin et al., 2004). Social influences on food intake and the modeling of eating behaviors of admired peers, older youth, and media or celebrity role models need to be explored. Such effects would have implications for designing interventions to improve eating behaviors of children and adolescents.

INSTITUTIONAL, NEIGHBORHOOD, AND COMMUNITY INFLUENCES

Child-Care Facilities

Child care is now the norm for American children. Approximately 80 percent of children ages 5 years and younger with employed mothers are in a child-care arrangement for an average of almost 40 hours per week, and 63 percent of children ages 6–14 years spend an average of 21 hours per week in the care of someone other than a parent before and after school (NRC and IOM, 2003). Nationwide, 32 percent of young children receive center-based care, 16 percent are in family child care, and 6 percent are cared for by a nanny or babysitter in the child's home (Capizzano et al., 2000). Children in full-time child care can receive up to two meals and snacks per day through federal meal programs.

The Child and Adult Care Food Program (CACFP) is a federal program providing meals and snacks to lower income children in child-care centers, the Head Start Program, family child-care homes, and after-school programs. The program serves an average of 2.9 million children per day and provides roughly 1.7 billion meals and snacks to children annually (FRAC, 2005). Child- and adult-care providers who participate in CACFP are reimbursed at fixed rates for each meal and snack served. Given that children in full-time child care could receive up to two meals and snacks per day through these programs, child-care settings could have a substantial impact on children's dietary intakes. However, there is little research that has assessed the nutritional quality of foods in child-care settings. Few data are available about the types and quantities of foods and snacks served to children in child-care settings and their impact on dietary intake. The USDA has established minimum requirements for the meals and snacks offered by participating child-care providers, but they are not required to meet specific nutrient-based standards such as those required for the National School Lunch Program (NSLP) and School Breakfast Program (SBP). Research is also scarce on the impact that the CACFP program has on participants' dietary intakes, and the limited amount of research that is available is not descriptive. A national study on CACFP-participating child-care sites found that the meals and snacks provided 61–71 percent of children's daily energy needs and more than two-thirds of the Recommended Dietary Allowance (RDA) for key nutrients. Meals and snacks exceeded the Dietary Guidelines for Americans for saturated fat (Fox et al., 1997).

Furthermore, there is a child-care system that extends beyond CACFP and includes formal and informal care of children outside of the home. All of these child-care settings have the potential to influence the diets of children but, as with CACFP, there is limited research on the dietary intake of children in these settings.

Schools

The school food environment can have a large impact on children's and adolescents' dietary intake. National data show that foods eaten from the school cafeteria comprise 19–50 percent of students' total daily calorie intake during a school day (Burghardt et al., 1993; Gleason and Suitor, 2001).

Nearly all public schools and 83 percent of all public and private schools combined participate in the NSLP (Burghardt et al., 1993; Fox et al., 2004). About three-quarters of these schools also provide breakfast through the SBP, which is offered in approximately 78 percent of the schools that offer the NSLP (Fox et al., 2004). On an average school day, about 60 percent of children in eligible schools participate in the NSLP program and about 37 percent in the SBP (Fox et al., 2004). NSLP meals are planned to provide approximately one-third of the RDA for specific nutrients and SBP meals are planned to provide a quarter of the RDA for key nutrients. Since 1995, schools participating in the NSLP and SBP have been required by the USDA to offer meals that meet the standards established by the Dietary Guidelines for Americans. Based on national CSFII 1994–1996 data, school meal programs make an important contribution to school-aged children's diets (Gleason and Suitor, 2001). Children who participated in the NSLP showed higher mean intakes of food calories and many micro-nutrients, both at lunch and over 24 hours, compared to nonparticipants. SBP participation was also associated with higher intakes of calories and several key nutrients (Gleason and Suitor, 2001). Although schools have made progress in improving meals through the NSLP and SBP, especially in decreasing fat content, they still have improvements to make to enhance the quality of the food served (Chapter 6).

Just over a decade ago, the NSLP was the primary provider of food during the school day to middle and high school students (Gleason and Suitor, 2001). Today, it represents a much smaller part of the food environment. Students, especially in middle and high schools are faced with a vast array of high-calorie (e.g., high-fat, high-sugar) food and beverage choices. These competitive foods include those sold a la carte in a cafeteria, vending machines, or school stores. Presently, there are no federal nutrition guidelines for competitive foods, unlike the USDA nutrition standards for federally funded school meals (Chapter 6). Over the last five years the availability of competitive foods in middle schools has increased from 83 percent to 97 percent (GAO, 2005). A recent national study found that most high schools offered high-fat cookies or cakes (80 percent) or fried potatoes (62 percent) in a la carte areas, and that 95 percent had vending machines offering carbonated soft drinks, candy, or snacks. Twenty percent of middle and high schools had contracts with quick serve restaurants (Wechsler et al., 2001). In addition, the GAO (2005) recently reported that salty snacks, sweet-baked foods, carbonated soft drinks, and candy were available in at least one-third of high schools and middle schools with competitive foods, although alternative foods were commonly available in all of these schools (e.g., water, milk, juice, fruit, yogurt).

The majority of a la carte foods offered in cafeterias or vending machines are relatively high in fat and sugar and low in nutrients (French et al., 2003b). Kubik et al. (2003) examined the associations between 598 young adolescents' dietary behaviors and school vending machines and a la carte programs. The availability of a la carte items was inversely associated with fruit and vegetable consumption and positively associated with total fat and saturated fat intake. Snack vending machines were negatively associated with fruit consumption (Kubik et al., 2003). In a longitudinal study, Cullen and Zakeri (2004) found that middle school students who had access to school snack bars consumed fewer fruits and nonstarchy vegetables, less milk, and more sweetened beverages compared to the previous school year when they were in elementary school and only had access to lunch meals served at school. These studies demonstrate that the widespread availability of high-calorie (e.g., high-fat, high-sugar) and low-nutrient foods and beverages in schools negatively impacts the diets of children and adolescents. A combination of interventions and policies are needed to reduce access to high-calorie and low-nutrient foods and beverages in schools and to promote more healthful options.

Quick Serve and Full Serve Restaurants

One of the most important food-related lifestyle changes of the past two decades is the increase of consumption of food prepared away from home. Data from the CSFII indicate that Americans consume about a third of calories from food prepared away from home, up from less than a fifth in 1977–1978 (Guthrie et al., 2002). Americans now spend 47 percent of their food dollars on meals and snacks obtained away from home (Stewart et al., 2004). Total away-from-home food expenditures amounted to $415 billion in 2002; accounting for inflation, this is a 23 percent increase since 1992 (Stewart et al., 2004). In 2002, full serve restaurants and quick serve restaurants captured the majority of the away-from-home food dollars, with 40 percent and 38 percent of total sales, respectively in 2002 (Stewart et al., 2004). Consumer spending at full serve restaurants and quick serve restaurants is expected to increase even more over the next decade, with the larger increase at full serve restaurants (Stewart et al., 2004). Meals and snacks consumed away from home contain more calories and total fat and saturated fat than at-home foods (Guthrie et al., 2002; Lin et al., 1996; Chapter 2).

Quick serve restaurants are especially popular among families with children and adolescents because they offer convenience and relatively low cost for the meals purchased. Children and adolescents consume the largest proportion of calories away from home at quick serve restaurants (Guthrie et al., 2002). Consumption of fast food by children ages 2–17 years increased five-fold from the late-1970s to the mid-1990s, from 2 percent of total calorie intake to 10 percent (Guthrie et al., 2002). CSFII (1994–1996 and 1998) data using 24-hour diet recalls indicate that on a typical day, 30 percent of children ages 4–19 years reported consuming fast food (Bowman et al., 2004). Consumption was prevalent in both sexes, all racial/ethnic groups, and all regions of the country; increased consumption was independently associated with male gender, older age, higher household incomes, non-Hispanic/Latino black individuals, and residing in the southern region of the United States. In a recent study, Austin et al. (2005) examined the median distance of quick serve restaurants around schools in the Chicago area. They reported that these restaurants were clustered around schools, 3 to 4 times as many quick serve restaurants were within walking distance of the school than would be expected if the restaurants were distributed evenly throughout the city.

Fast food consumption can have a negative impact on the nutritional quality of children's and adolescents' diets. CSFII data show that children who consumed fast food, compared with those who did not, consumed more total calories (187 additional calories) and total fat, more carbonated soft drinks, less milk, and fewer fruits and nonstarchy vegetables. In a survey of 4,746 multiethnic adolescents, French et al. (2001b) found that the frequency of quick serve restaurants use was positively associated with total calories, percentage of calories from fat, and daily servings of carbonated soft drinks and french fries, and negatively associated with daily servings of fruit, vegetables, and milk. Another study (Zoumas-Morse et al., 2001) found that while restaurant meals accounted for only 6 percent of all reported eating occasions, the calorie content of those meals was 55 percent higher than the average calorie intake of meals eaten at home.

Limited research has examined the relationships among income, race/ethnicity, and quick serve restaurants relative to neighborhood socio-demographic characteristics. Morland et al. (2002b) examined this relationship in a four-state multiethnic study and found no consistent relationship between wealth (as measured by median home values) and eating at quick serve restaurants. They also found no difference between the numbers of quick serve restaurants in African American and white neighborhoods. Block et al. (2004) reported contrasting results in a study using geocoding in New Orleans, Louisiana. They found that predominantly African American neighborhoods have 2.4 quick serve restaurants per square mile compared to 1.5 restaurants in predominantly white neighborhoods. However, population density was not controlled for in the analysis. More studies are needed to examine the geographic association between neighborhood quick serve restaurants density and low-income and ethnic and racial neighborhoods.

A recent study by Lewis et al. (2005) examined availability and food options at 659 restaurants in less affluent and more affluent areas in Los Angeles County to compare residents' access to healthful meals prepared and purchased away from home. Poorer neighborhoods with a higher population of African American residents had fewer healthful options available, both in food selection and in food preparation, and the neighborhood restaurants heavily promoted the less healthful food options. The results indicate that the food environment in poorer neighborhoods makes it difficult for residents to eat healthful foods away from home.

Because Americans are eating out more frequently, eating more fruits and vegetables is a challenge. Food eaten away from home accounts for less than a half a serving of fruit, and one-and-a-quarter servings of vegetables. Fried potatoes make up approximately 35 percent of vegetables eaten away from home, compared with 10 percent of at-home vegetable consumption (Guthrie et al., 2005).

Neighborhood Characteristics and Food Retail Outlets

Neighborhood grocery stores or supermarkets are important contributors to the eating patterns and nutrient intakes of residents. Studies show that more affluent neighborhoods have greater access to supermarkets and healthful foods than low-income neighborhoods. Direct links have been observed between access to supermarkets and healthier dietary intake (Cheadle et al., 1991; Glanz and Yaroch, 2004; Laraia et al., 2004). However, nearly all of this research has been conducted with adults, not with children or adolescents. A recent study found that adult fruit and vegetable intake increased with each additional supermarket in a census tract; African Americans' fruit and vegetable intake increased by 32 percent for each additional supermarket and whites' intake increased by 11 percent (Morland et al., 2002a).

Supermarkets offer the greatest variety of food at the lowest cost. However, supermarkets are less prevalent in low-income neighborhoods (Horowitz et al., 2004; Morland et al., 2002b). In a multiethnic study using census tract data across four states in different regions of the United States, Morland et al. (2002b) found that low-income neighborhoods had three times fewer supermarkets but comparable numbers of small grocers and convenience stores as middle- and upper-income neighborhoods. Zenk et al. (2005) evaluated the spatial accessibility of large chain supermarkets in relation to neighborhood racial composition and poverty in metropolitan Detroit using a geographic information system. Distance to the nearest supermarket was similar among the least impoverished neighborhoods, regardless of racial composition. However, the most impoverished neighborhoods in which African Americans lived were an average of 1.1 miles farther from the nearest supermarket than were white neighborhoods. Laraia et al. (2004) found that pregnant women living greater than 4 miles from a supermarket were more than twice as likely to have poorer quality diets compared to women living within 2 miles of a supermarket, even after controlling for individual socioeconomic status characteristics and the availability of grocery and convenience stores. In a much smaller study, child fruit and vegetable consumption was not significantly associated with availability in grocery stores (Edmonds et al., 2001).

Food retail stores in low-income neighborhoods may also offer a different mix of food. Horowitz et al. (2004) compared the selections in food stores in two adjacent New York City neighborhoods; a low-income minority neighborhood in East Harlem and an affluent, predominantly white neighborhood on the Upper East Side. Five types of products were assessed: fresh fruits, fresh green vegetables or tomatoes, high-fiber bread, low-fat milk, and diet carbonated soft drinks. Only 18 percent of East Harlem stores stocked these foods, compared with 58 percent of stores on the Upper East Side. Only 9 percent of East Harlem bodegas (small stores serving Hispanics/Latinos) carried all items versus 48 percent of Upper East Side bodegas. Collectively, these studies suggest the importance of the local neighborhood food environment for influencing diet quality.

MACROSYSTEM INFLUENCES

Individual food choices depend greatly on sociocultural, marketing, and economic systems that govern food production, distribution, and consumption. The federal nutrition assistance programs and government policies can also impact the diets of participants.

Culture and Values

Cultural factors influence food behavior. Values and beliefs are core aspects of any culture and shape perceptions of food, health, and well-being. In addition to shared belief and value systems, hallmarks of culture include language, social relationships, institutions, clothing, music, and foods. Culture embodies a socially grounded way of learning that shapes the way an individual thinks, feels, and acts (IOM, 2002). Cultural behaviors, values, and beliefs are learned in childhood, are transmitted from one generation to the next, and are often deeply held. Individuals learn to make sense of the outside world within a cultural framework and cultural processes. Within every culture, intracultural variation exists that cuts across ethnic, regional, geographic, gender, and generational domains. There is also much shared across seemingly diverse cultures. For example, media exposure (e.g., television) increases similarity across cultures. Likewise, there are examples of large quick serve restaurants and food and beverage companies that have restaurants and distribute their products in many countries around the world today and therefore may promote common food preferences among people worldwide. The growing ethnic diversity in the United States and the continuous influx of new immigrants has also contributed to exposure to new foods and preparation methods and to shifts in food preferences, as well as an expansion of the American food repertoire.

Food behaviors are learned through enculturation, which is the process by which culture is transmitted from one generation to the next. Culture influences a child's eating behaviors both directly and indirectly. Direct influence occurs through parents, care providers, siblings, or peers. Indirect acquisition occurs through observed social norms or through marketing and the media (e.g., advertising, television, videos, movies, Internet) (Chapter 4).

Cultural values and traditions can also mediate or moderate body image and how obesity is perceived. Physical appearance and how one looks is an important issue in the lives of children and adolescents. Perception of overall appearance including body image is an important component of global self-esteem among children and adolescents (Levine and Smolak, 2002; Smolak and Levine, 2001). How much one weighs, usually an outcome of eating patterns, strongly influences physical appearance and self-image, especially for girls. Girls' concern about physical appearance is often linked to their weight or body shape, and weight concerns and the desire to be thin appear to be developing at earlier ages. Research suggests that about 20 percent of 5-year-old girls (Davison et al., 2000), 30–45 percent of 8- to 13-year-old girls (Field et al., 1999a; Schreiber et al., 1996), and roughly 40–70 percent of adolescent girls (Levine and Smolak, 2002; Story et al., 1995) report concerns about their weight and a desire to be thinner. The widespread nature of weight and body shape dissatisfaction in adolescent girls is characterized as "normative discontent" (Levine and Smolak, 2002).

In a study of multiethnic girls in middle and high school, only a quarter (27 percent) had high body satisfaction (Kelly et al., 2005). High body satisfaction was most common among African American girls (47 percent) and underweight girls (39 percent). Hispanic/Latina, Asian, and American Indian girls report body dissatisfaction as frequently as or more frequently than white girls (Robinson et al., 1996; Story et al., 1995).

Children and adolescents who have higher levels of body dissatisfaction and body image concerns report lower global self-worth and poorer self-esteem (Ricciardelli and McCabe, 2001; Smolak and Levine, 2001). Dissatisfaction with weight and shape and a poor body image is linked to dieting, less healthful weight control methods, depression, anxiety and eating disorders (Davison et al., 2003; Ohring et al., 2002; Stice and Whitenton, 2002). Body dissatisfaction tends to be higher in boys and girls who are heavier, although it is not restricted to those who are obese (Davison et al., 2003; Levine and Smolak, 2002; Ricciardelli and McCabe, 2001).

Gender differences in body satisfaction become apparent in late childhood. Girls have a higher prevalence of body dissatisfaction than boys and choose thinner "ideal" images for themselves (Cohane and Pope, 2001). Few studies have been conducted with boys, but recent studies report substantial numbers of adolescent boys who have weight concerns and are dissatisfied with their bodies (Labre, 2002; McCabe and Riccariardelli, 2004; Story et al., 1995). Preadolescent boys are largely satisfied with their bodies, with about one-third wanting to be thinner (McCabe and Ricciardelli, 2004). Adolescent boys tend to be equally divided between wanting to lose weight and gain weight (Cohane and Pope, 2001; McCabe and Ricciardelli, 2004). Recent reviews suggest that as the male body ideal has become increasingly muscular, body dissatisfaction has increased among adolescent males (Labre, 2002).

A major source of body dissatisfaction among girls and boys are the perceived societal pressures for them to conform to the sociocultural ideal for beauty and attractiveness (Levine and Smolak, 2002; McCabe and Ricciardelli, 2004). Sociocultural standards for males emphasize strength and muscularity and this standard appears to be consistent across a broad range of cultural groups (McCabe and Ricciardelli, 2004). Sociocultural ideals of beauty for girls emphasize thinness, although this is less pronounced for African American girls (Levine and Smolak, 2002). African American girls are more satisfied with their bodies than white, Hispanic/Latina or American Indian girls (Kelly et al., 2005). Nichter (2000) conducted serial in-depth interviews with middle school and high school girls and found that African American girls were much more likely to be satisfied with their bodies than were the white girls. African American girls expressed that beauty was a matter of projecting attitude and moving with confidence and style rather than being thin (Nichter, 2000).

Cross-sectional surveys find that greater exposure to teen media is associated with higher weight concern (Field et al., 1999b; McCabe et al., 2002). It is hypothesized that mass media—with the pervasive emphasis on an ideal body shape that is often unrealistically thin—is associated with internalization of the slender beauty ideal, and resulting increases in body dissatisfaction among girls (Levine and Smolak, 2002). However, superimposed on the backdrop of a "thin-ideal" for girls is the wide range of other influences on girls' lives, including cultural factors and the subculture of her family and friends, her personal attitudes and related experiences. These factors may serve to reinforce sociocultural pressures or may act as a protective buffer and promote high body satisfaction.

The eating behaviors and physical inactivity associated with obesity have become the social norm in many communities across the United States (IOM, 2005a). Understanding the audience and the cultural and social context is the first step in designing successful health-promotion interventions (IOM, 2002). In order to be effective, nutrition and health-promotion and disease-prevention interventions need to be sensitive to salient cultural values. As individuals, families, institutions, and organizations across the United States make behavioral changes, social norms are also likely to change, so that healthful eating and regular physical activity will be the accepted and encouraged standard (IOM, 2005a).

Food Production, Processing, and Distribution Systems

The U.S. food system is a vital part of the American economy. In 2000, the food marketing system accounted for 7.7 percent of the U.S. gross domestic product and employed more than 12 percent of the U.S. labor force (Martinez, 2002). An increasing share of what consumers spend on food goes to marketing services added after the product leaves the farm. In 2000, more than 80 percent of the U.S. food dollar went toward value-added services and materials—processing, distribution, labor, packaging, and transportation. An efficient food system has resulted in an abundant and affordable food supply. Income growth has outpaced increases in food expenditures, leading to continuous reductions in the share of income spent on food (Martinez, 2002). Americans now spend less of their income on food than ever before. In 2003, expenditures for food accounted for 13.1 percent of disposable income, with 7.7 percent spent for foods at home and 5.4 percent for foods acquired away from home (U.S. Department of Labor and U.S. Bureau of Labor Statistics, 2005; Chapter 4).

The American food supply arises from a combination of domestic agricultural production and imported foodstuffs. What is actually produced and imported depends on business practices in purchasing, processing, distributing, and marketing food, and these practices are influenced by government policy and regulation. Consumer and institutional food purchases, in turn, create the markets to which businesses respond.

An analysis of the American food supply as it existed in 1996 did not match dietary recommendations according to the Food Guide Pyramid. The American food supply contained more grains, fats, and sugars than recommended, and less fruit, vegetables, dairy, and meat (Kantor, 1998). It is not clear that this imbalance between the actual food supply and healthful diets can be largely attributed to consumer demand because American agriculture is not purely market-driven. Government policies provide selective subsidies for some types of agriculture, make public lands available for activities such as cattle grazing, impose selective import restrictions and tariffs, and constrain agricultural practices for environmental and health purposes (Chapter 6). Consequently, some foods are relatively inexpensive and available in great supply, whereas others are more expensive and not widely available.

Many foods do not require intense processing and preparation. These include vegetables, fruits, nuts, meats, and dairy. These foods often have short shelf lives and require refrigeration. Branding is a marketing feature that provides a name or symbol that legally identifies a company or its product and serves as a differentiation in the marketplace (Roberts, 2004). Traditionally, these foods are not strongly associated with particular brands. More recently, branding has emerged as an important differentiation for these product categories in the marketplace. As generic foodstuffs, they are also not heavily advertised and marketed when compared to company-specific product brands.

In contrast, many manufactured foods require considerable processing before they are distributed. These foods include prepared entrees, baked goods, salty snacks, confectioneries, and carbonated soft drinks. Many of these foods are processed and manufactured to have long shelf lives and frequently do not require refrigeration. These processed foods are more likely to be strongly branded and heavily marketed and advertised. The imbalance between the food supply and the USDA food guidance system roughly approximates the differences between generic unprocessed foods and branded processed foods. The latter are much more likely to contain added sugars, sodium, fats, and oils and are also most heavily promoted through marketing communication efforts (Chapter 4). Branding does not determine the healthfulness of a food. Rather, the degree of processing, added sugar, fat, or salt, and nutrient content will determine the healthfulness of foods and beverages.

Food Marketing, Media, and Advertising

One socializing force that potentially impacts children's eating behavior is the media. Today's youth live in a media-saturated environment

(Rideout et al., 1999; Roberts et al., 2005). Advertising and other forms of marketing permeate nearly all media platforms to which youth are exposed (Brown and Witherspoon, 2002). Children and adolescents are currently exposed to an increasing and unprecedented amount of advertising, marketing, and commercialism through a wide range of vehicles and venues (Chapter 4). Over the past 35 years, there has been growth in a marketing research enterprise specifically focused on catering to the preferences and desires of children and youth.

Federal Food Assistance Programs

The nation's domestic federal nutrition assistance programs provide an important source of food for many low-income children and adults. One in five Americans receive food assistance from at least one of the 15 nutrition assistance programs over the course of a year (USDA, 2005; Chapter 6). The USDA administers these programs that are designed to provide children and low-income households with access to food and a more nutritious diet, to provide nutrition education, and to assist America's farmers by giving them an outlet for distributing foods purchased under farmer assistance programs (Levedahl and Oliveira, 1999). Even with these programs, some low-income households may still not get adequate amounts of high-quality food (Levedahl and Oliveira, 1999).

Expenditures for USDA's 15 nutrition assistance programs totaled $46 billion in 2004. Five programs accounted for 94 percent of USDA's total expenditures for food assistance—the Food Stamp Program (FSP); NSLP; SBP; Special Supplemental Nutrition Program for Women, Infants and Children (WIC); and CACFP. The FSP is the principal food assistance program, serving 1 in 12 Americans, or nearly 24 million low-income people per month, more than half of whom are children (USDA, 2005). The FSP provides recipients with a monthly allotment of coupons that can be redeemed for food at authorized food retail stores. Few restrictions are placed on what foods recipients can purchase. Recently, there have been targeted efforts to strengthen and reshape nutrition education in the FSP to help motivate consumers to choose healthful foods.

The WIC program provides 8 million participants with supplemental food packages each month. Participants include at-risk, low-income pregnant, breastfeeding, and postpartum women, as well as children up to age 5 years, who constitute 76 percent of all WIC participants (IOM, 2005b). Half of U.S. infants and one in four young children participate in WIC. An IOM committee recently reviewed the WIC food packages and provided comprehensive recommendations to improve its contents, such as adding more fruits and vegetables; adding more high-calcium food choices such as yogurt, soymilk, and tofu; and expanding culturally acceptable food options (IOM, 2005b).

The Child Nutrition Programs, which include the NSLP, SBP, CACFP, and the Summer Food Programs, target children enrolled in public and nonprofit private schools, child-care institutions, and summer recreation programs. The NSLP discussed earlier is the largest of these programs, serving almost 29 million children every school day. Nearly half (49 percent) of the school lunches served are provided free to students and another 10 percent are provided at a reduced price (USDA, 2005). In recent years, there has been an increased emphasis on providing more nutritious food through these programs (Levedahl and Oliveira, 1999). Concern has centered on improving the quality of foods served in these programs, increasing the availability of fruits and vegetables, and improving the nutritional quality of commodity foods. Recently, efforts have been made to pilot programs to promote fresh fruits and vegetables in schools. The 2002 Farm Bill provided funds for the Fruit and Vegetable Pilot Program (FVPP) in 25 schools in four states and one Indian reservation (ERS, 2002). The recent Child Nutrition and WIC Reauthorization Act expanded the program to four more states and two more Indian reservations (Committee on Education and the Workforce, 2004).

Although the USDA's nutrition assistance programs vary greatly in size, target populations, and delivery mechanisms, they all provide children of low-income households with food, the means to purchase food, and nutrition education. Although the food assistance programs have been shown to increase the quantity of food consumed by participants, the effect of these programs on improving the quality of their diets has been more difficult to ascertain (Levedahl and Oliveira, 1999). Although a number of studies have attempted to quantify the effects of the nutrition assistance programs, there has been no comprehensive assessment of the effects of the programs on the diet and health outcomes of participants. A recent USDA-funded study reviewed research on the impact of the USDA's nutrition assistance programs on participants' health and diet outcomes. The main conclusion is that findings must be interpreted with caution due to the limitations of the studies (Fox et al., 2004). For targeted programs such as WIC, the NSLP, and SBP, nutrient intake is generally increased. The FSP increases household food intake, although whether nutritional quality is higher is unclear (Fox et al., 2004). There is a need for a well-designed comprehensive study on how nutrition and health status are impacted by participation in nutrition assistance programs.

Nutrition assistance programs serve a large proportion of low-income children who need these programs to meet their daily calorie and nutritional needs. These children should have access to nutrient-rich foods that are ethnically and culturally appropriate. The USDA could explore innovative pilot programs to increase access to healthful foods or provide incentives for the purchase of these items. Examples include further expanding the FVPP to more schools; supporting farm-to-school programs, school gardens, and WIC gardens, ensuring that food stamp recipients have access to supermarkets, farmers' markets, and other venues to provide fresh, high-quality, and affordable produce, and other healthful foods, fruit and vegetable vouchers, or bonus coupons for food stamp users (IOM, 2005a; Chapter 6).

Government Regulations and Policies

Government policies and regulations related to food and agriculture can directly and indirectly affect the supply or prices of food, the nutritional composition of foods, food safety, the information consumers receive about food, and consumer confidence in the food supply, all of which can influence consumer food choices (Ralston, 1999). As discussed in more depth in Chapter 6, the effects of policies and regulations, such as subsidies and taxation, on food choices depends on how the policy affects the cost of producing commodities, how those costs relate to final retail prices, how responsive consumers are to price changes, and how the policy directly influences consumer preference for the product (Ralston, 1999).

A highly productive and efficient agriculture production system contributes to an ample supply of food in the United States. However, there has been little examination of how agricultural and economic public policies and the resulting food and agricultural environment affect food choice or obesity (Tillotson, 2004), including how the types and quantities of foods available through the federal food and nutrition assistance programs influence healthy diets for children and youth.

SUMMARY

The committee's review of the elements shaping the food and beverage consumption of children and adolescents underscores the importance of using an ecological perspective to understand the interactions among factors that influence food preferences and eating behaviors. Multiple influences—individual and developmental factors, family and social elements, institutions, communities, and macrosystems—interact to shape the food and beverage consumption patterns of children and youth. This ecological perspective can be used to develop more effective strategies and programs to improve dietary behaviors.

Nutrition knowledge of children and youth by itself does not necessarily motivate their food choices and dietary behaviors. Food preferences develop as early as ages 2–3 years and are shaped by a child's early experiences, positive or negative conditioning, exposure to foods, and a biological predisposition to prefer sweet, high-fat, and salty foods. Thus, the challenge of helping young people adopt healthful eating behaviors will require multifaceted and coordinated efforts aimed at the individual and family, the physical environment such as schools and neighborhoods, the macrosystem such as the food marketing system, and government policies and regulations. These efforts need to focus on changing individual behaviors, the social environment, and social norms around eating behaviors. Individual change is more likely to be facilitated and sustained in an environment that supports healthful food choices. Special attention needs to be focused on ensuring that low-income and ethnic minority children and youth have access to healthful and nutritious foods and beverages.

REFERENCES

Anderson PM, Butcher KF, Levine PB. 2003. Maternal employment and overweight children. *J Health Econ* 22(3):477–504.

Austin SB, Melly SJ, Sanchez BN, Patel A, Buka S, Gortmaker SL. 2005. Clustering of fast-food restaurants around schools: A novel application of spatial statistics to the study of food environments. *Am J Public Health* 95(9):1575–1581.

Axelson ML, Federline TL, Brinberg D. 1985. A meta-analysis of food- and nutrition-related research. *J Nutr Ed* 17(2):51–54.

Bandura A. 1977. *Social Learning Theory*. Englewood Cliffs, NJ: Prentice-Hall, Inc.

Baranowski T, Domel S, Gould R, Baranowski J, Leonard S, Treiber F, Mullis R. 1993. Increasing fruit and vegetable consumption among 4th and 5th grade students: Results from focus groups using reciprocal determinism. *J Nutr Ed* 25(3):114–120.

Baranowski T, Pery CL, Parcel GS. 2002. How individuals, environments, and health behavior interact. In: Glanz K, Rimer BK, Lewis FM, eds. *Health Behavior and Health Education. Theory, Research, and Practice*. 3rd ed. San Francisco, CA: Jossey-Bass. Pp. 165–184.

Barr SI. 1994. Associations of social and demographic variables with calcium intakes of high school students. *J Am Diet Assoc* 94(3):260–269.

Barr SI. 1995. Dieting attitudes and behavior in urban high school students: Implications for calcium intake. *J Adolesc Health* 16(6):458–464.

Beauchamp GK, Moran M. 1982. Dietary experience and sweet taste preference in human infants. *Appetite* 3(2):139–152.

Bell EA, Rolls BJ. 2001. Regulation of energy intake: Factors contributing to obesity. In: Bowman BA, Russell RM, eds. *Present Knowledge in Nutrition*. 8th ed. Washington, DC: International Life Sciences Institute Press. Pp. 31–40.

Benton D. 2004. Role of parents in the determination of the food preferences of children and the development of obesity. *Int J Obes Relat Metab Disord* 28(7):858–869.

Birch LL. 1999. Development of food preferences. *Annu Rev Nutr* 19:41–62.

Birch LL, Fisher JO. 1998. Development of eating behaviors among children and adolescents. *Pediatrics* 101(3 Pt 2):539–549.

Block JP, Scribner RA, DeSalvo KB. 2004. Fast food, race/ethnicity, and income: A geographic analysis. *Am J Prev Med* 27(3):211–217.

Bowman SA, Gortmaker SL, Ebbeling CB, Pereira MA, Ludwig DS. 2004. Effects of fast-food consumption on energy intake and diet quality among children in a national household survey. *Pediatrics* 113(1):112–118.

Brown JD, Witherspoon EM. 2002. The mass media and American adolescents' health. *J Adolesc Health* 31(6 suppl):153–170.

Brown R, Ogden J. 2004. Children's eating attitudes and behaviour: A study of the modelling and control theories of parental influence. *Health Ed Res* 19(3):261–271.

Burghardt J, Gordon A, Chapman N, Gleason P, Fraker T. 1993. *The School Nutrition Dietary Assessment Study: School Food Service, Meals Offered, and Dietary Intakes.* Washington, DC: U.S. Department of Agriculture.

California Project LEAN and Food on the Run Campaign. 1998. *A Focus Group Report on Adolescent Behaviors, Perceptions, Values and Attitudes on Health, Nutrition and Physical Activity. A Qualitative Exploration.* Sacramento, CA: California Department of Health/Public Health Institute.

Capizzano J, Adams G, Sonenstein F. 2000. Child care arrangements for children under five: Variation across states. In: *New Federalism. National Survey of America's Families.* Report No. B-7. Washington, DC: The Urban Institute.

Cartwright M, Wardle J, Steggles N, Simon AE, Croker H, Jarvis MJ. 2003. Stress and dietary practices in adolescents. *Health Psychol* 22(4):362–369.

Cheadle A, Psaty BM, Curry S, Wagner E, Diehr P, Koepsell T, Kristal A. 1991. Community-level comparisons between the grocery store environment and individual dietary practices. *Prev Med* 20(2):250–261.

Cohane GH, Pope HG Jr. 2001. Body image in boys: A review of the literature. *Int J Eat Disord* 29(4):373–379.

Cole N, Fox MK. 2004. *Nutrition and Health Characteristics of Low-Income Participants. Volume II, WIC Program Participants and Nonparticipants.* Report No. E-FAN-04-014-2. Washington, DC: Economic Research Service, U.S. Department of Agriculture.

Committee on Education and the Workforce. 2004. *Child Nutrition and WIC Reauthorization Act Bill Summary.* [Online]. Available at: http://edworkforce.house.gov/issues/108th/education/childnutrition/billsummaryfinal.htm [accessed August 22, 2005].

Cooke LJ, Wardle J, Gibson EL, Saponchnik M, Sheiham A, Lawson M. 2003. Demographic, familial and trait predictors of fruit and vegetable consumption by pre-school children. *Pub Health Nutr* 7(2):295–302.

Crawford PB, Obarzanek E, Schreiber GB, Barrier P, Goldman S, Frederick MM, Sabry ZI. 1995. The effects of race, household income, and parental education on nutrient intakes of 9- and 10-year-old girls. NHLBI Growth and Health Study. *Ann Epidemiol* 5(5):360–368.

Crepinsek MK, Burstein NR. 2004. *Maternal Employment and Children's Nutrition. Volume I, Diet Quality and the Role of the CACFP.* Report No. E-FAN-04-006-1. Washington, DC: Economic Research Service, U.S. Department of Agriculture.

Cullen KW, Zakeri I. 2004. Fruits, vegetables, milk, and sweetened beverages consumption and access to a la carte/snack bar meals at school. *Am J Public Health* 94(3):463–467.

Cullen KW, Baranowski T, Owens E, Marsh T, Rittenberry L, de Moor C. 2003. Availability, accessibility, and preferences for fruit, 100% fruit juice, and vegetables influence children's dietary behavior. *Health Ed Behav* 30(5):615–626.

Davison KK, Markey CN, Birch LL. 2000. Etiology of body dissatisfaction and weight concerns among 5-year-old girls. *Appetite* 35(2):143–151.

Davison KK, Markey CN, Birch LL. 2003. A longitudinal examination of patterns in girls' weight concerns and body dissatisfaction from ages 5 to 9 years. *Int J Eat Disord* 33(3):320–332.

de Castro JM, Plunkett S. 2002. A general model of intake regulation. *Neurosci Biobehav Rev* 26(5):581–595.
DHHS (U.S. Department of Health and Human Services). 2003. *Child Health USA 2002*. Rockville, MD: DHHS.
DHHS and USDA (U.S. Department of Agriculture). 2005. *Dietary Guidelines for Americans 2005*. [Online]. Available: http://www.healthierus.gov/dietaryguidelines [accessed January 12, 2005].
Drewnowski A. 1997. Taste preferences and food intake. *Annu Rev Nutr* 17:237–253.
Drewnowski A. 1998. Energy density, palatability, and satiety: Implications for weight control. *Nutr Rev* 56(12):347–353.
Drewnowski A. 2004. Obesity and the food environment: Dietary energy density and diet costs. *Am J Prev Med* 27(3 suppl):154–162.
Drewnowski A, Hann C. 1999. Food preferences and reported frequencies of food consumption as predictors of current diet in young women. *Am J Clin Nutr* 70(1):28–36.
Drewnowski A, Levine AS. 2003. Sugar and fat—from genes to culture. *J Nutr* 133(3):829S–830S.
Edmonds J, Baranowski T, Baranowski J, Cullen KW, Myres D. 2001. Ecological and socioeconomic correlates of fruit, juice, and vegetable consumption among African-American boys. *Prev Med* 32(6):476–481.
ERS (Economic Research Service). 2002. *Farm Policy. Title IV Nutrition Programs*. [Online]. Available at: http://www.ers.usda.gov/Features/farmbill/titles/titleIVnutritionprograms.htm [accessed August 22, 2005].
Federal Interagency Forum on Child and Family Statistics. 2004. *America's Children in Brief: Key National Indicators of Well-being, 2004*. Washington, DC: U.S. Government Printing Office.
Feunekes GI, de Graaf C, Meyboom S, van Staveren WA. 1998. Food choice and fat intake of adolescents and adults: Associations of intakes within social networks. *Prev Med* 27(5 Pt 1):645–656.
Field AE, Camargo CA Jr, Taylor CB, Berkey CS, Frazier AL, Gillman MW, Colditz GA. 1999a. Overweight, weight concerns, and bulimic behaviors among girls and boys. *J Am Acad Child Adolesc Psychiatry* 38(6):754–760.
Field AE, Cheung L, Wolf AM, Herzog DB, Gortmaker SL, Colditz GA. 1999b. Exposure to the mass media and weight concerns among girls. *Pediatrics* 103(3):E36.
Fisher JO, Mitchell DC, Smiciklas-Wright H, Birch LL. 2000. Maternal milk consumption predicts the tradeoff between milk and soft drinks in young girls' diets. *J Nutr* 131(2):246–250.
Fisher JO, Mitchell DC, Smiciklas-Wright H, Birch LL. 2002. Parental influences on young girls' fruit and vegetable, micronutrient, and fat intakes. *J Am Diet Assoc* 102(1):58–64.
Fox MK, Cole N. 2004. *Nutrition and Health Characteristics of Low-Income Populations Volume III, School Age Children*. Report No. E-FAN-04-014-3. Washington, DC: Economic Research Service, U.S. Department of Agriculture.
Fox MK, Glantz FB, Geitz L, Burstein N. 1997. *Early Childhood and Child Care Study. Nutritional Assessment of the CACFP: Final Report. Volume II*. Cambridge, MA: Abt Associates, Inc.
Fox MK, Hamilton W, Lin BH. 2004. *Effects of Food Assistance and Nutrition Programs on Nutrition and Health. Volume 4*. Food Assistance and Nutrition Research Program Report No 19-4. Washington, DC: U.S. Department of Agriculture.
FRAC (Food Research and Action Center). 2005. *Federal Food Programs. Child and Adult Care Food Program*. [Online] Available: http://www.frac.org/html/federal_food_programs/programs/cacfp.html [accessed August 19, 2005].

French SA, Perry CL, Leon GR, Fulkerson JA. 1995. Dieting behaviors and weight change history in female adolescents. *Health Psychol* 14(6):548–555.

French SA, Jeffery RW, Story M, Hannan P, Snyder MP. 1997a. A pricing strategy to promote low-fat snack choices through vending machines. *Am J Public Health* 87(5): 849–851.

French SA, Story M, Jeffery RW, Snyder P, Eisenberg M, Sidebottom A, Murray D. 1997b. Pricing strategy to promote fruit and vegetable purchase in high school cafeterias. *J Am Diet Assoc* 97(9):1008–1010.

French SA, Story M, Hannan P, Breitlow KK, Jeffery RW, Baxter JS, Snyder MP. 1999. Cognitive and demographic correlates of low-fat vending snack choices among adolescents and adults. *J Am Diet Assoc* 99(4):471–475.

French SA, Jeffery RW, Story M, Breitlow KK, Baxter JS, Hannan P, Snyder MP. 2001a. Pricing and promotion effects on low-fat vending snack purchases: The CHIPS Study. *Am J Public Health* 91(1):112–117.

French SA, Story M, Neumark-Sztainer D, Fulkerson JA, Hannan P. 2001b. Fast food restaurant use among adolescents: Associations with nutrient intake, food choices and behavioral and psychosocial variables. *Int J Obes Relat Metab Disord* 25(12):1823–1833.

French SA, Lin BH, Guthrie JF. 2003a. National trends in soft drink consumption among children and adolescents age 6 to 17 years: Prevalence, amounts, and sources, 1977/1978 to 1994/1998. *J Am Diet Assoc* 103(10):1326–1331.

French SA, Story M, Fulkerson JA, Gerlach AF. 2003b. Food environment in secondary schools: A la carte, vending machines, and food policies and practices. *Am J Public Health* 93(7):1161–1167.

Fulkerson JA, French SA, Story M. 2004a. Adolescents' attitudes about and consumption of low-fat foods: Associations with sex and weight-control behaviors. *J Am Diet Assoc* 104(2):233–237.

Fulkerson JA, Sherwood NE, Perry CL, Neumark-Sztainer D, Story M. 2004b. Depressive symptoms and adolescent eating and health behaviors: A multifaceted view in a population-based sample. *Prev Med* 38(6):865–875.

GAO (U.S. Government Accountability Office). 2005. *School Meal Programs. Competitive Foods are Widely Available and Generate Substantial Revenues for Schools.* Report No. GAO-05-563. Washington, DC: GAO.

Gibson EL, Wardle J, Watts CJ. 1998. Fruit and vegetable consumption, nutritional knowledge and beliefs in mothers and children. *Appetite* 31(2):205–228.

Gillman MW, Rifas-Shiman SL, Frazier AL, Rockett HR, Camargo CA Jr, Field AE, Berkey CS, Colditz GA. 2000. Family dinner and diet quality among older children and adolescents. *Arch Fam Med* 9(3):235–240.

Glanz K, Yaroch AL. 2004. Strategies for increasing fruit and vegetable intake in grocery stores and communities: Policy, pricing, and environmental change. *Prev Med* 39(suppl 2):S75–S80.

Glanz K, Basil M, Maibach E, Goldberg J, Snyder D. 1998. Why Americans eat what they do: Taste, nutrition, cost, convenience, and weight control concerns as influences on food consumption. *J Am Diet Assoc* 98(10):1118–1126.

Gleason P, Suitor C. 2001. *Children's Diets in the Mid-1990s: Dietary Intake and Its Relationship with School Meal Participation.* Report No. CN-01-CD1. Alexandria, VA: U.S. Department of Agriculture, Food and Nutrition Service, Office of Analysis, Nutrition and Evaluation.

Grimm GC, Harnack L, Story M. 2004. Factors associated with soft drink consumption in school-aged children. *J Am Diet Assoc* 104(8):1244–1249.

Grunbaum JA, Kann L, Kinchen S, Ross J, Hawkins J, Lowry R, Harris WA, McManus T, Chyen D, Collins J. 2004. Youth risk behavior surveillance—United States, 2003. *MMWR Surveill Summ* 53(2):1–96.

Guthrie JF, Lin BH, Frazao E. 2002. Role of food prepared away from home in the American diet, 1977–78 versus 1994–96: Changes and consequences. *J Nutr Ed Behav* 34(3): 140–150.

Guthrie JF, Lin BH, Reed J, Stewart H. 2005. Understanding economic and behavioral influences on fruit and vegetable choices. *Amber Waves* 3(2):36–41.

Hanson NI, Neumark-Sztainer D, Eisenberg ME, Story M, Wall M. 2005. Associations between parental report of the home food environment and adolescent intakes of fruits, vegetables and dairy foods. *Public Health Nutr* 8(1):77–85.

Hanson NI, Story M, Eisenberg M, Neumark-Sztainer D. 2006. Food preparation and purchasing roles among adolescents: Associations with sociodemographic characteristics and diet quality. *J Am Diet Assoc* 106(2).

Harnack L, Story M, Martinson B, Neumark-Sztainer D, Stang J. 1998. Guess who's cooking? The role of men in meal planning, shopping, and preparation in US families. *J Am Diet Assoc* 98(9):995–1000.

Horacek TM, Betts NM. 1998. Students cluster into 4 groups according to the factors influencing their dietary intake. *J Am Diet Assoc* 98(12):1464–1467.

Horowitz CR, Colson KA, Hebert PL, Lancaster K. 2004. Barriers to buying healthy foods for people with diabetes: Evidence of environmental disparities. *Am J Public Health* 94(9):1549–1554.

IOM (Institute of Medicine). 2002. *Speaking of Health. Assessing Health Communication Strategies for Diverse Populations.* Washington, DC: The National Academies Press. Pp. 224–254.

IOM. 2005a. *Preventing Childhood Obesity: Health in the Balance.* Washington, DC: The National Academies Press.

IOM. 2005b. The *WIC Food Packages: Time for a Change.* Washington, DC: The National Academies Press.

Isler L, Popper ET, Ward S. 1987. Children's purchase requests and parental responses: Results from a diary study. *J Advertising Res* 27(5):28–39.

John D. 1999. Consumer socialization of children: A retrospective look at twenty-five years of research. *J Consum Res* 26(3):183–213.

Johnson RK, Crouter AC, Smiciklas-Wright H. 1993. Effects of maternal employment on family food consumption patterns and children's diets. *J Nutr Ed* 25(3):130–133.

Johnson RK, Smiciklas-Wright H, Crouter AC, Willits FK. 1992. Maternal employment and the quality of young children's diets: Empirical evidence based on the 1987–1988 Nationwide Food Consumption Survey. *Pediatrics* 90(2 Pt 1):245–249.

Kantor LS. 1998. *A Dietary Assessment of the US Food Supply: Comparing Per Capita Food Consumption with Food Guide Pyramid Serving Recommendations.* Agricultural Economic Report No. 772. Washington, DC: U.S. Department of Agriculture.

Keller KL, Tepper BJ. 2004. Inherited taste sensitivity to 6-n-propylthiouracil in diet and body weight in children. *Obes Res* 12(6):904–912.

Keller KL, Peitrobelli A, Must S, Faith MS. 2002. Genetics of eating and its relation to obesity. *Curr Atheroscler Rpt* 4(3):176–182.

Kelly AM, Wall M, Eisenberg ME, Story M, Neumark-Sztainer D. 2005. Adolescent girls with high body satisfaction: Who are they and what can they teach us. *J Adolesc Health* 37:391–396.

Klump KL, McGue M, Iacono WG. 2000. Age differences in genetic and environmental influences on eating attitudes and behaviors in preadolescent and adolescent female twins. *J Abnorm Psychol* 109(2):239–251.

Kral TV, Roe LS, Rolls BJ. 2004. Combined effects of energy density and portion size on energy intake in women. *Am J Clin Nutr* 79(6):962–968.

Kubik MY, Lytle LA, Hannan PJ, Perry CL, Story M. 2003. The association of the school food environment with dietary behaviors of young adolescents. *Am J Public Health* 93(7):1168–1173.

Labre MP. 2002. Adolescent boys and the muscular male body ideal. *J Adolesc Health* 30(4):233–242.

Laraia BA, Siega-Riz AM, Kaufman JS, Jones SJ. 2004. Proximity of supermarkets is positively associated with diet quality index for pregnancy. *Prev Med* 39(5):869–875.

Levedahl JW, Oliveira V. 1999. Dietary impacts of food assistance programs. In: Frazao E, ed. *America's Eating Habits: Changes and Consequences*. Agriculture Information Bulletin No. 750. Washington, DC: U.S. Department of Agriculture.

Levine MP, Smolak L. 2002. Body image development in adolescence. In: Cash TF, Pruzinsky T, eds. *Body Image: A Handbook of Theory, Research, and Clinical Practice*. New York: Guilford Press. Pp. 74–82.

Lewis LB, Sloane DC, Nascimento LM, Diamant AL, Guinyard JJ, Yancey AK, Flynn G. 2005. African Americans' access to healthy food options in South Los Angeles restaurants. *Am J Public Health* 95(4):668–673.

Lin BH, Guthrie J, Blaylock J. 1996. *The Diets of America's Children: Influences of Dining Out, Household Characteristics, and Nutrition Knowledge*. Agricultural Economic Report No. 746. Washington, DC: U.S. Department of Agriculture.

Lin BH, Guthrie J, Frazao E. 1999. Quality of children's diets at and away from home: 1994–96. *Food Rev* 22(1):2–10.

Lowry R, Kann L, Collins JL, Kolbe LJ. 1996. The effect of socioeconomic status on chronic disease risk behaviors among US adolescents. *J Am Med Assoc* 276(10):792–797.

Lytle LA, Seifert S, Greenstein J, McGovern P. 2000. How do children's eating patterns and food choices change over time? Results from a cohort study. *Am J Health Promot* 14(4):222–228.

Mannino ML, Lee Y, Mitchell DC, Smiciklas-Wright H, Birch LL. 2004. The quality of girls' diets declines and tracks across middle childhood. *Int J Behav Nutr Phys Act* 1(1):5.

Martinez SW. 2002. Introduction. In: Harris JM, Kaufman PR, Martinez SW, Price C. *The U.S. Food Marketing System, 2002. Competition, Coordination, and Technological Innovations into the 21st Century*. Agricultural Economic Report No. 811. Washington, DC: U.S. Department of Agriculture.

McCabe MP, Ricciardelli LA. 2004. Body image dissatisfaction among males across the lifespan: A review of past literature. *J Psychosom Res* 56(6):675–685.

McCabe MP, Ricciardelli LA, Finemore J. 2002. The role of puberty, media and popularity with peers on strategies to increase weight, decrease weight and increase muscle tone among adolescent boys and girls. *J Psychosom Res* 52(3):145–153.

McNeal J. 1999. *The Kids Market: Myth and Realities*. Ithaca, NY: Paramount Market Publishing.

Mennella JA, Jagnow CP, Beauchamp GK. 2001. Prenatal and postnatal flavor learning by human infants. *Pediatrics* 107(6):e88.

Mennella JA, Griffin CE, Beauchamp GK. 2004. Flavor programming during infancy. *Pediatrics* 113(4):840–845.

Mennella JA, Pepino MY, Reed DR. 2005. Genetic and environmental determinants of bitter perception and sweet preferences. *Pediatrics* 115(2):e216–e222.

Morland K, Wing S, Diez Roux A. 2002a. The contextual effect of the local food environment on residents' diets: The atherosclerosis risk in communities study. *Am J Public Health* 92(11):1761–1767.

Morland K, Wing S, Diez Roux A, Poole C. 2002b. Neighborhood characteristics associated with the location of food stores and food service places. *Am J Prev Med* 22(1):23–29.

Munoz KA, Krebs-Smith SM, Ballard-Barbash R, Cleveland LE. 1997. Food intakes of US children and adolescents compared with recommendations. *Pediatrics* 100(3 Pt 1): 323–329.

National Pork Producers Council. 2000. *The Kitchen Report III.* Des Moines, IA: National Pork Producers Council. Pp. 1–10.

Neumark-Sztainer D, Story M, Resnick MD, Blum RW. 1996. Correlates of inadequate fruit and vegetable consumption among adolescents. *Prev Med* 25(5):497–505.

Neumark-Sztainer D, Story M, Perry C, Casey MA. 1999. Factors influencing food choices of adolescents: Findings from focus-group discussions with adolescents. *J Am Diet Assoc* 99(8):929–937.

Neumark-Sztainer D, Rock CL, Thornquist MD, Cheskin LJ, Neuhouser ML, Barnett MJ. 2000. Weight-control behaviors among adults and adolescents: Associations with dietary intake. *Prev Med* 30(5):381–391.

Neumark-Sztainer D, Wall M, Perry C, Story M. 2003. Correlates of fruit and vegetable intake among adolescents. Findings from Project EAT. *Prev Med* 37(3):198–208.

Neumark-Sztainer D, Hannan PJ, Story M, Perry CL. 2004. Weight-control behaviors among adolescent girls and boys: Implications for dietary intake. *J Am Diet Assoc* 104(6): 913–920.

Nichter M. 2000. *Fat Talk: What Girls and Their Parents Say About Dieting.* Cambridge, MA: Harvard University Press.

Nielsen SJ, Popkin BM. 2003. Patterns and trends in food portion sizes, 1977–1998. *J Am Med Assoc* 289(4):450–453.

NRC and IOM (National Research Council and Institute of Medicine). 2000. *From Neurons to Neighborhoods: The Science of Early Childhood Development.* Shonkoff JP, Phillips DA, eds. Washington, DC: National Academy Press.

NRC and IOM. 2003. *Working Families and Growing Kids: Caring for Children and Adolescents.* Washington, DC: The National Academies Press.

Ohring R, Graber JA, Brooks-Gunn J. 2002. Girls' recurrent and concurrent body dissatisfaction: Correlates and consequences over 8 years. *Int J Eat Disord* 31(4):404–415.

Perusse L, Tremblay A, Leblanc C, Cloninger CR, Reich T, Rice J, Bouchard C. 1988. Familial resemblance in energy intake: Contribution of genetic and environmental factors. *Am J Clin Nutr* 47(4):629–635.

Ralston K. 1999. How Government Policies and Regulations Can Affect Dietary Choices. In: Frazao E, ed. *America's Eating Habits: Changes and Consequences.* Agriculture Information Bulletin No. 750. Washington, DC: U.S. Department of Agriculture.

Reed DR, Bachmanov AA, Beauchamp GK, Tordoff MG, Price RA. 1997. Heritable variation in food preferences and their contribution to obesity. *Behav Genet* 27(4):373–387.

Reed J, Frazao E, Itskowitz R. 2004. *How Much Do Americans Pay for Fruits and Vegetables?* Agriculture Information Bulletin 790. Washington, DC: Economic Research Service, U.S. Department of Agriculture.

Ricciardelli LA, McCabe MP. 2001. Children's body image concerns and eating disturbance: A review of the literature. *Clin Psychol Rev* 21(3):325–344.

Rideout V, Foehr UG, Roberts DF, Brodie M. 1999. *Kids and Media at the New Millennium.* Menlo Park, CA: Henry J. Kaiser Family Foundation.

Roberts DF, Foehr UG, Rideout V. 2005. *Generation M: Media in the Lives of 8–18 Year Olds.* Menlo Park, CA: Henry J. Kaiser Family Foundation.

Roberts K. 2004. *The Future Beyond Brands: Lovemarks.* New York: PowerHouse Books.

Robinson TN, Killen JD, Litt IF, Hammer LD, Wilson DM, Haydel KF, Hayward C, Taylor CB. 1996. Ethnicity and body dissatisfaction: Are Hispanic and Asian girls at increased risk for eating disorders? *J Adolesc Health* 19(6):384–393.

Rolls BJ. 2003. The supersizing of America: Portion size and the obesity epidemic. *Nutr Today* 38(2):42–53.

Rolls BJ, Engell D, Birch LL. 2000. Serving portion size influences 5-year-old but not 3-year-old children's food intakes. *J Am Diet Assoc* 100(2):232–234.

Rolls BJ, Roe LS, Kral TV, Meengs JS, Wall DE. 2004. Increasing the portion size of a packaged snack increases energy intake in men and women. *Appetite* 42(1):63–69.

Rozin P. 2002. Human food intake and choice: Biological, psychological and cultural perspectives. In: Anderson H, Blundell J, Chiva M, eds. *Food Selection From Genes to Culture*. Levallois-Perret, France: Danone Institute. Pp. 7–25.

Rozin P, Millman L. 1987. Family environment, not heredity, accounts for family resemblances in food preferences and attitudes: A twin study. *Appetite* 8(2):125–134.

Rozin P, Riklis J, Margolis L. 2004. Mutual exposure or close peer relationships do not seem to foster increased similarity in food, music, or television program preferences. *Appetite* 42(1):41–48.

Schreiber GB, Robins M, Striegel-Moore R, Obarzanek E, Morrison JA, Wright DJ. 1996. Weight modification efforts reported by black and white preadolescent girls: National Heart, Lung, and Blood Institute Growth and Health Study. *Pediatrics* 98(1):63–70.

Schwartz GJ. 2004. Biology of eating behavior in obesity. *Obes Res* 12(suppl 2):102S–106S.

Shannon C, Story M, Fulkerson JA, French SA. 2002. Factors in the school cafeteria influencing food choices by high school students. *J Sch Health* 72(6):229–234.

Skinner JD, Carruth BR, Wendy B, Ziegler PJ. 2002. Children's food preferences: A longitudinal analysis. *J Am Diet Assoc* 102(11):1638–1647.

Smolak L, Levine MP. 2001. Body image in children. In: Thompson JK, Smolak L, eds. *Body Image, Eating Disorders, and Obesity in Youth: Assessment, Prevention, and Treatment*. Washington, DC: American Psychological Association. Pp. 41–66.

Stewart H, Blisard N, Bhuyan S, Nayga RM. 2004. *The Demand for Food Away From Home. Full-Service or Fast Food?* Agricultural Economic Report No. 829. Washington, DC: U.S. Department of Agriculture.

Stice E, Whitenton K. 2002. Risk factors for body dissatisfaction in adolescent girls: A longitudinal investigation. *Dev Psychol* 38(5):669–678.

Story M, Resnick MD. 1986. Adolescents' view on food and nutrition. *J Nutr Ed* 18(4): 188–192.

Story M, French SA, Resnick MD, Blum RW. 1995. Ethnic/racial and socioeconomic differences in dieting behaviors and body image perceptions in adolescents. *Int J Eat Disord* 18(2):173–179.

Story M, Neumark-Sztainer D, Sherwood N, Stang J, Murray D. 1998. Dieting status and its relationship to eating and physical activity behaviors in a representative sample of US adolescents. *J Am Diet Assoc* 98(10):1127–1135, 1255.

Story M, Holt K, Sofka D, eds. 2002a. *Bright Futures in Practice: Nutrition*. Arlington, VA: National Center for Education in Maternal and Child Health.

Story M, Neumark-Sztainer D, French S. 2002b. Individual and environmental influences on adolescent eating behaviors. *J Am Diet Assoc* 102(3):S40–S51.

Tillotson JE. 2004. America's obesity: Conflicting public policies, industrial economic development, and unintended human consequences. *Annu Rev Nutr* 24:617–643.

Troiano RP, Briefel RR, Carroll MD, Bialostosky K. 2000. Energy and fat intakes of children and adolescents in the United States: Data from the National Health and Nutrition Examination surveys. *Am J Clin Nutr* 72(5 suppl):1343S–1353S.

U.S. Census Bureau. 2005. *Living Arrangements of Children Under 18 Years Old: 1960 to Present.* [Online]. Available: http://www.census.gov/population/socdemo/hh-fam/ch1.pdf [accessed August 18, 2005].

U.S. Department of Agriculture (USDA). 2005. *The Food Assistance Landscape, March 2005.* Food Assistance and Nutrition Research Report No. 28-6. Washington, DC: USDA.

U.S. Department of Labor and U.S. Bureau of Labor Statistics. 2005. *Consumer Expenditures in 2003.* Report 986. Washington, DC: U.S. Department of Labor.

USA Weekend and The Roper Organization. 1989. *A USA Weekend/Roper Report on Consumer Decision-Making in American Families.* New York: The Roper Organization.

Videon TM, Manning CK. 2003. Influences on adolescent eating patterns: The importance of family meals. *J Adolesc Health* 32(5):365–373.

Wansink B. 2004. Environmental factors that increase the food intake and consumption volume of unknowing consumers. *Annu Rev Nutr* 24:455–479.

Ward S. 1974. Consumer socialization. *J Consum Res* 1(2):1–14.

Wardle J, Huon G. 2000. An experimental investigation of the influence of health information on children's taste preferences. *Health Ed Res* 15(1):39–44.

Wardle J, Cooke LJ, Gibson EL, Sapochnik M, Sheiham A, Lawson M. 2003a. Increasing children's acceptance of vegetables; a randomized trial of parent-led exposure. *Appetite* 40(2):155–162.

Wardle J, Herrera ML, Cooke L, Gibson EL. 2003b. Modifying children's food preferences: The effects of exposure and reward on acceptance of an unfamiliar vegetable. *Eur J Clin Nutr* 57(2):341–348.

Wardle J, Carnell S, Cooke L. 2005. Parental control over feeding and children's fruit and vegetable intake: How are they related? *J Am Diet Assoc* 105(2):227–232.

Wechsler H, Brener ND, Kuester S, Miller C. 2001. Food service and foods and beverages available at school: Results from the School Health Policies and Programs Study 2000. *J Sch Health* 71(7):313–324.

Woodward DR, Boon JA, Cumming FJ, Ball PJ, Williams HM, Hornsby H. 1996. Adolescents' reported usage of selected foods in relation to their perceptions and social norms for those foods. *Appetite* 27(2):109–117.

Young LR, Nestle M. 2002. The contribution of expanding portion sizes to the US obesity epidemic. *Am J Public Health* 92(2):246–249.

Zenk SN, Schulz AJ, Israel BA, James SA, Bao S, Wilson ML. 2005. Neighborhood racial composition, neighborhood poverty, and the spatial accessibility of supermarkets in metropolitan Detroit. *Am J Public Health* 95(4):660–667.

Zollo P. 1999. *Wise Up to Teens: Insight into Marketing and Advertising to Teenagers.* 2nd ed. Ithaca, NY: New Strategist Publications, Inc.

Zoumas-Morse C, Rock CL, Sobo, EJ, Neuhouser ML. 2001. Children's patterns of macronutrient intake and associations with restaurant and home eating. *J Am Diet Assoc* 101(8):923–925.

4

Food and Beverage Marketing to Children and Youth

INTRODUCTION

This chapter considers how food and beverage products are developed and marketed to appeal to the preferences of children and youth and to stimulate sales. It provides definitions of certain commonly used marketing terms and approaches; provides an overview of various target markets such as tweens, teens, and ethnic minorities; and offers a description of the marketing research enterprise directed at children and youth. An overview is provided of the marketing environment, including a profile of food and beverage companies and retailers, full serve and quick serve restaurants, and trade associations. It discusses food, beverage, and meal product development, the implications of the evolving purchasing power of American children and youth, and the general marketing strategies, tactics, and messaging used by industry. The chapter also reviews children's and adolescents' media use patterns and advertising exposure, and discusses the range of marketing vehicles and venues used by companies to reach them with advertising and marketing messages. A discussion of company and industry guidelines and policies, including self-regulatory programs, health and wellness advisory councils, public–private partnerships, and coalitions concludes the chapter.

To explore this domain, the committee drew from several different types of reviews, reports and materials, including supplementing the peer-reviewed literature with information from industry and marketing sources. Thus, the evidentiary sources cited in this chapter include articles published in marketing, advertising, or industry trade journals; commissioned papers examining the current and future food and beverage marketing trends affecting children and youth; government, company, and trade organization websites; annual reports of companies;[1] foundation or nonprofit organization reports and briefs; popular magazines and books relevant to advertising and marketing; and news releases. Sources also included materials from presentations, testimony, and documents provided during and following the January 2005 public workshop held to consider industry perspectives and activities. To assess the degree to which new food and beverage products have been targeted to children and youth across various product categories, the committee also conducted an analysis of trends in the proliferation of children's products using ProductScan®, a large commercial database of products (Marketing Intelligence Service, 2005) that has tracked new product introductions in the U.S. marketplace since 1980 (Williams, 2005b).

Because marketing research could enhance understanding on the relationships of marketing strategies to children's food and beverage consumption patterns and diets and diet-related health outcomes, as well as the design of strategies to improve the healthfulness of messages, several market research firms were contacted for information. Some—The Geppetto Group, The Strottman Group, KidShop/KidzEyes, and Yankelovich Partners—provided child- and youth-specific data for the committee's consideration and use. Others were unable to provide information, either because of time constraints, economic considerations, or on the basis that the data were proprietary and not intended for public use. A summary of the marketing research information considered by the committee is included in Appendix E, Table E-1.

MARKETING TERMINOLOGY AND APPROACHES

Marketing professionals use a variety of strategies to influence consumer preferences, stimulate consumer demand, promote frequency of purchases, build brand awareness and brand loyalty, encourage potential or existing customers to try new products, and increase sales. From a marketing perspective, businesses engage in a variety of activities that are designed to meet customers' needs and to create the context where consumers perceive value in exchange for their money. Marketing is defined by the American Marketing Association (AMA) as "an organizational function and a set

---

[1]Many companies and marketing firms discussed in this chapter are incorporated (Inc.). For ease of reading, the Inc. has been removed after a company name in the text, tables, and reference citations. The discussion of trade names or commercial products in this report is solely for the purpose of providing specific information or illustrative examples and does not imply endorsement by the Institute of Medicine.

of processes for creating, communicating, and delivering value to customers and for managing customer relationships in ways that benefit an organization and its stakeholders" (AMA, 2005a). Conducting marketing research is a fundamental activity of the marketing process, providing information that helps identify opportunities and problems, refine strategies, and monitor performance (AMA, 2005a).

The four traditional components of marketing are as follows:

- *Product* (e.g., features, quality, quantity, packaging)
- *Place* (e.g., location, outlets, distribution points used to reach target markets)
- *Price* (e.g., strategy, determinants, levels)
- *Promotion* (e.g., advertising, consumer promotion, trade promotion, public relations)

Figure 4-1 shows one approach to a graphic representation of the elements that influence a marketing strategy: defining the target market, determining the marketing mix to meet the needs of that market, and assessing

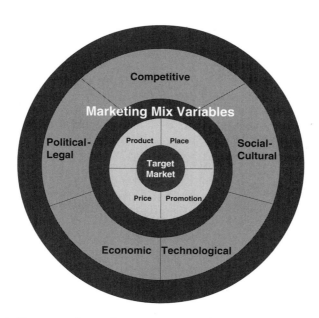

FIGURE 4-1 Elements of a marketing strategy and its environmental framework. SOURCE: Based on Boone and Kurtz (1998). From Contemporary Marketing, 9E 9th edition by Boone. ©1998. Reprinted with permission of South-Western, a division of Thomson Learning: www.thomsonrights.com.

the relevant competitive, social-cultural, technological, economic, political-legal, and environmental factors (Boone and Kurtz, 1998).

Branding

A key aim of marketing is product branding—providing a name or symbol that legally identifies a company, a single product, or a product line to differentiate it from other companies or products in the marketplace (Roberts, 2004). Elements of branding strategy may be characterized on several dimensions: (1) brand differentiation, to distinguish one brand from another in the same product line; (2) building brand image (or *brand presence*) to raise consumers' awareness about a brand and the competition; (3) developing brand equity (also referred to as *brand relevance* and *brand performance*), to build brand familiarity and perceived quality with the intent to meet a customer's expectations and purchase intent, which is the extent to which a consumer intends to continue purchasing a specific brand; (4) assessing brand momentum (or *brand advantage*) to determine whether customers think a brand is improving or whether their interest in a specific brand is declining; and (5) building and sustaining brand loyalty (also referred to as *brand bonding*), which is the degree to which consumers will consistently purchase the same brand within a product category (BrandWeek, 2005; Survey Value, 2005).

In effect, the purpose of branding is to promote product sales by taking a product and identifying it with a lifestyle to which consumers aspire (Roberts, 2004). With food and beverage products, product development can be part of the branding process, as with many prepared entrees, baked goods, savory snacks, confectionery, and carbonated soft drinks (CSDs)[2]. Nonprocessed foods such as vegetables and fruits are more difficult challenges for brand differentiation, and are generally less promoted than processed food brands. This may be beginning to change, however, as there is a developing trend toward branding produce and promoting innovative features such as new shapes or colors, special varieties (e.g., baby or seedless watermelon, champagne grapes) and ethnic fruits and vegetables that help to build consumer awareness, sales, and profits (Pollack Associates, 2004).

Processed foods are highly branded and lend themselves to major advertising (Gallo, 1999). More than 80 percent of U.S. grocery products

---

[2]Carbonated soft drinks is a common marketing term used to refer to a category of cold, nonalcoholic, sweetened beverages that uses the process of carbonation to enhance its taste and texture. The complete term, carbonated soft drinks, is used in other chapters of this report instead of CSDs due to the lack of familiarity of this term among nonmarketing audiences.

are branded whereas only 19 percent of fruits and vegetables are nationally branded (Harris, 2002). Results from a Grocery Manufacturers Association (GMA) survey of 800 consumers found that Americans across all demographic groups consider a product's brand before making a final purchase selection, and consumers will pay a higher price for perceived quality in premium branded products and will go to a different store if a preferred brand is not available (GMA, 2002; Pollack Associates, 2004). Key factors that influenced their brand selection include experience (36 percent indicated that prior family exposure influences brand choice) and peer endorsement (13 percent) (GMA, 2002). Branding has become a normalized part of life for American children and adolescents (Schor, 2004), as marketers seek to develop positive and sustained brand relationships with young consumers and their parents in order to create brand recognition and foster brand loyalty, brand advantage, and brand equity (McDonald's Corporation, 1996; McNeal, 1999; Moore et al., 2002).

Advertising

Advertising is the most visible form of marketing. It is paid public presentation and promotion of ideas, goods, or services by a sponsor (Kotler and Armstrong, 2004), intended to bring a product to the attention of consumers through a variety of media channels such as broadcast and cable television, radio, print, billboards, the Internet, or personal contact (Boone and Kurtz, 1998). Marketers recognize its value by itself, and also view it as contributing to the success of other strategies by (1) building brand awareness and brand loyalty among potential consumers, and (2) creating perceived value by persuading consumers that they are getting more than the product itself (e.g., social esteem, peer respect).

Consumer Promotion

Consumer promotion, also called sales promotion, represents the promotional efforts that are designed to have an immediate impact on sales. Consumer promotion includes media and nonmedia marketing communications targeted directly to the consumer that are used for a predetermined and limited time to increase consumer demand, stimulate market demand, or improve product availability. Examples of sales promotion include coupons, discounts and sales, contests, point-of-purchase displays, rebates, and gifts and incentives (Boone and Kurtz, 1998).

Trade Promotion

Trade promotion is a broad category of marketing that targets intermediaries, such as grocery stores, convenience stores, and other food retail outlets. Trade promotion strategies include provision of in-store displays, agreements for shelf space and positioning, free merchandise, buy-back allowances,[3] and merchandise allowances,[4] as well as sales contests to encourage wholesalers or retailers to give unusual attention to selling more of a specific product or lines (Boone and Kurtz, 1998). Companies usually spend as much of their marketing budgets on trade promotion as on expenditures for advertising and all other consumer-oriented sales promotion, combined (Boone and Kurtz, 1998; GMA Forum, 2005).

Market Segmentation and Target Markets

Identifying and reaching unique target markets is important for businesses to promote sales in a competitive marketplace. Target markets may be segmented by demographic characteristics (e.g., age, gender, income, race or ethnicity), psychographic features (e.g., values, attitudes, beliefs, lifestyles), behavioral patterns (e.g., brand loyalty, usage rates, price sensitivities), and geographic characteristics (e.g., region, population density) (Neal, 2005; QuickMBA, 2004). As the ethnic, racial, and cultural composition of the U.S. population changes and boundaries among groups become less distinct through intermarriage and cultural adaptation, the criteria that marketers have used to target specific groups of consumers may change (Grier and Brumbaugh, 2004).

Companies often alter the types of products and services marketed (marketing mix) for customers in each market segment in order to meet the demand for products and services and to maximize sales. Marketers may change only one element of the marketing mix (e.g., promotional approach), or tailor each element of the marketing mix to a specific population segment—the product and how it is packaged, the pricing strategies, the place(s) or channel(s) through which the product is distributed and made available to consumers in a target market, and the promotional strategies (Neal, 2005; QuickMBA, 2004).

Children and youth represent an important demographic market because they are potential customers, they influence purchases made by parents and households, and they constitute the future adult market (McNeal, 1998; Moore et al., 2002). Table 4-1 summarizes the U.S. Census Bureau

---

[3] A form of sales promotion in which retailers are offered an incentive to restock their store or warehouse with the product to the level in place prior to a count and recount promotion offer.

[4] Introductory offers and periodic discounts offered by a company to promote and introduce the company's line of branded products.

TABLE 4-1 Marketing Categories by Population Sizes

Group	Age Range	Population Size
Infants and Toddlers	0–2 years	
	Girls	5,575,564
	Boys	5,841,112
Children	3–8 years	
	Girls	11,734,700
	Boys	12,306,607
Tweens[a]	9–12 years	
	Girls	8,159,391
	Boys	8,572,920
Teens[b]	13–19 years	
	Girls	13,758,399
	Boys	14,524,572

[a]In this report, the committee characterized infants and toddlers as under age 2 years, younger children as ages 2–5 years, older children as ages 6–11 years, and teens as ages 12–18 (Chapter 1). These age categories and terms differ slightly from what is described in this chapter. Marketers distinguish the tween market segment from children and teens, defining it as young people who have attitudes and behaviors that are "in between" the ages of 8–12 years or 9–14 years (Siegel et al., 2001; The Intelligence Group/Youth Intelligence, 2005).
[b]The U.S. Census Bureau defines teens as young people ages 13–19 years.
SOURCE: U.S. Census Bureau (2000).

age categories that differ from the age categories used in this report (Chapter 1 and Chapter 5) and commonly used by marketers. The Census Bureau age categories include infants and toddlers (ages 0–2 years), younger and older children (ages 3–8 years), tweens (ages 9–12 years), and younger and older teens (ages 13–19 years).

Children and youth under the age of 19 years comprise more than a fourth of the U.S. population. From 1990–2003, this population increased by 14 percent (U.S. Census Bureau, 2001, 2004). Ethnic minorities represent attractive targets for food and beverage marketers due to their size, growth, and purchasing power (Williams, 2005a). Marketers segment target audiences by age, gender, and race/ethnicity to build brand awareness and brand loyalty early in life that will be sustained into adulthood. African American consumers have been targeted by both mainstream and African American-owned marketers, often using very different marketing styles (Williams and Tharp, 2001). Food and beverage companies market to African American family preferences. An analysis of 2004 Nielsen Monitor-Plus data of food and beverage advertising that appeared in African American media showed significant spending by food and beverage companies for high-calorie and low-nutrient foods and beverages.

In six magazines targeted to African Americans (e.g., Jet, Ebony, Black Enterprise, Essence, Vibe, and Savoy), the top three categories advertised were regular CSDs ($1.8 million), cookies and crackers ($1.6 million), and fruit juices and fruit-flavored drinks ($1.5 million). Advertising spending for the top three food and beverage categories on Black Entertainment Television (BET) were regular CSDs ($10.8 million), candy and gum ($8.8 million), and fruit juices and fruit-flavored drinks ($5.3 million) (Williams, 2005a). Magazine Publishers of America estimates that 15 percent of teens ages 12–19 years are African American, and are a major influence on youth culture, spending 6 percent more per month than the average U.S. teen, which is estimated at $428 monthly (MPA, 2004b).

In 2004, the industry advertising and marketing expenditures were estimated at $260.9 million to reach consumers through Hispanic/Latino-oriented broadcast television networks, cable television, and Spanish-language newspapers and magazines (Endicott et al., 2005). Among the food, beverage, and retailer companies, PepsiCo spent $68.5 million, McDonald's Corporation spent $65.8 million, Wal-Mart Stores spent $55.9 million, Yum! Brands spent $30.8 million, The Coca-Cola Company spent $27.7 million, the Kellogg Company spent $25.2 million, and Wendy's International spent $20.4 million to advertise brands to reach Hispanic/Latino consumers (Endicott et al., 2005). An example of an ethnically targeted marketing effort to Hispanics/Latinos is PepsiCo's Frito-Lay™ Flaming Hot Corn Chips advertising campaign (MPA, 2004c).

The Hispanic/Latino teen market is the fastest growing ethnic youth segment in the United States. This market currently represents 4.6 million young consumers, or 20 percent of all U.S. teens. Market researchers forecast that the Hispanic/Latino youth population is expected to grow six times faster than the rest of the teen market by 2020 (MPA, 2004c). Marketers view the Hispanic/Latino youth market as providing a variety of business opportunities across many types of products and services (Valdés, 2000). In 1998, the total annual purchasing power of Hispanic/Latino teens was estimated at $19 billion—4 percent higher than non-Hispanic/Latino teens (MPA, 2004c). This so-called Generation Ñino includes tweens, teens, and young people who are bilingual and bicultural as they retain their Hispanic/Latino identity and navigate comfortably in this culture and American cultures (Valdés, 2000).

Cultural influences among different racial/ethnic groups are also possible. For example, "hip-hop" youth culture originated among African American youth in the inner city, and is now embraced by a generation of African American, white, Hispanic/Latino, and Asian youth (Williams and Tharp, 2001). "Urban culture" is a term used to describe a target market that has a particular lifestyle. Urban culture transcends both racial and ethnic boundaries by bringing together a lifestyle of fashion, attitudes, street language, and music from all backgrounds (Williams and Tharp, 2001). MTV has been a leading entertainment network partnering with PepsiCo and The Coca-Cola Company to launch advertising campaigns featuring hip-hop culture such as break dancing to market CSDs and urban culture to teens (Holt, 2004; PBS Frontline, 2001).

With respect to economic segmentation, there is some descriptive evidence suggesting that ethnic minorities living in poorer neighborhoods have fewer healthier options and neighborhood restaurants heavily promote less healthful foods (Lewis et al., 2005; Chapter 3). Despite concerns expressed that marketers disproportionately target racial/ethnic minorities with high-calorie, low-nutrient foods and beverages, there is a need for greater empirical evidence to support the claim (Grier, 2005; Samuels et al., 2003). The committee was not able to find available evidence to assess whether market segmentation has been a significant influence on children's food and beverage product development.

Embedded Marketing Strategies

Embedded marketing strategies blend commercial content with programming or editorial content, or other lifestyle experiences, to add brand exposure and avoid resistance to direct advertising. Product placement, or brand placement, is an embedded marketing technique that refers to the inclusion of a corporate or brand name, product package, signage, or other trademark either visually or verbally in television programs, films, video games, magazines, books, and music, or across a range of these media simultaneously (Babin and Carder, 1996; Nebenzahl and Secunda, 1993; PQMedia, 2005). Product placement is generally arranged in return for a fee payment, although occasionally other *quid pro quo* accommodations are involved (Balasubramanian, 1994; PQMedia, 2005).

Another form of embedded marketing technique used by marketers is known as viral marketing, representing the "buzz," "word of mouth," or "street marketing" that occurs when individuals talk about a product to one another, either in conversations or virtual communication via an electronic platform such as the Internet (Henry, 2003; Holt, 2004; Kaikati and Kaikati, 2004). Viral branding and marketing focus on the paths of public influence, including diffusion of innovation, word of mouth, and public relations (Holt, 2004).

Measured Media and Unmeasured Media

Marketers pay to advertise and promote branded products through a variety of media channels, termed measured and unmeasured media in the marketing literature. Measured media spending refers to the categories that are tracked by media research companies such as Nielsen, TNSMI/CMR, and Forrester. Commonly tracked measured media spending categories include television (e.g., network, spot, cable, syndicated, Spanish-language network), radio (e.g., network, national spot, local), magazines (e.g., local, Sunday magazine), business publications, newspapers (e.g., local, national), outdoor, the Yellow Pages, and the Internet (Brown et al., 2004, 2005).

Unmeasured media spending refers to the difference between a company's reported or estimated advertising costs and its measured media spending. Unmeasured media spending includes activities such as sales promotions, coupons, direct mail, catalogs, and special events, and it is not systematically tracked (Brown et al., 2004, 2005). Marketers use a variety of techniques to assess the effects of advertising in measured media on consumers. They measure the cost of advertising or promotion, usually expressed in terms of consumer exposure to advertising messages or "impressions," representing a message seen by one viewer. Thus, consumers who report that they remember or recall an advertisement have "retained impressions" of the specific advertisement. Marketers also track consumers' recall, retention, processing of messages, and purchase intent or purchase behavior. A second measure of the impact of an advertisement used by marketers is the increase in sales as a result of the advertising or promotional campaign. Because several factors may influence sales in the marketplace, it may be difficult to isolate the effect of advertising on sales of a particular product during a given time period. Thus, companies and marketers use other measures to guide their decisions, including communications research, an analysis of purchase dynamics (e.g., trial purchase, repeat purchase, frequency of purchase), and tracking consumer awareness and attitudes regarding specific product categories and specific brands (Collier Shannon Scott and Georgetown Economic Services, 2005c).

Once the purchase behavior of the exposed and unexposed groups are evaluated for a pre- and post-period, marketers determine brand penetration (the percentage of households that purchased an advertised product), volume (the average number or weight of an advertised product for every 100 households), dollars spent (the average dollars spent on the advertised product for every 100 households), and the dollar share (the percentage of sales that the advertised brand represents of total category sales) (MPA, 1999).

Marketing Research

Substantial investments have been made in marketing research directed to U.S. children and youth, and this research has grown into a major marketing tool over the past 30 years (Austin and Rich, 2001; McNeal,

1999; Schor, 2004). Its evolution and focus on youth has been rapid. Companies and private marketing research and public relations firms currently conduct marketing research that involves children and adolescents of all ages in the stages of product development, market testing, and the design of messages that are delivered to them (Schor, 2004). Examples of selected marketing research firms and marketing reports that the committee considered through its data-gathering process are listed in Appendix E, Table E-1.

Marketing research firms use a variety of methods, such as convenience surveys, opinion polls, focus groups, participant observation, photography, and ethnographic studies to collect information about their target markets (e.g., age and income of consumers, purchasing power, spending patterns, consumer attitudes and opinions)—including, in some cases, market research focus groups with early- and preschool age children (Austin and Rich, 2001; Buzz Marketing Group, 2004; Friend and Stapylton-Smith, 1999; Nestle, 2002; PBS Frontline, 2001; Peleo-Lazar, 2005; Schor, 2004; Teinowitz and McArthur, 2005; Yankelovich, 2005). Cultural anthropologists and psychologists have become regular resources for marketing research firms to study the culture of children and youth, and to research how children and teens process information and respond to advertising (Montgomery and Pasnik, 1996; Schor, 2004).

Some marketing research is developed for public use but most is proprietary. Public research is conducted primarily by academic institutions and may be financed by public or private funds. Proprietary research is conducted for commercial purposes by private companies, marketing research and public relations firms, or companies that are associated with the marketing industry, and is not publicly available. Appendix E, Table E-1 provides examples of the types of proprietary research focused specifically on the eating habits and lifestyles of children and youth and the companies or marketing research firms that collect and sell these data. Because the majority of nonacademic research conducted by marketing research firms, public relations firms, and companies is proprietary, these data are unavailable to help assess the direct relationship between advertising and sales (Nestle et al., 1998), as well as the impact of advertising and other forms of marketing on children's and adolescents' food choices and diet (Swinburn et al., 2004; Chapter 5).

Finding: Marketing research can provide important insights about how marketing techniques might help improve the diets of children and youth. Yet, much of the relevant marketing research on the profile and impact of food and beverage marketing to children and youth is currently unavailable to the public, including for use in designing and targeting efforts to improve the diets of children and youth.

MARKETING ENVIRONMENT

Companies, Retailers, Restaurants, and Trade Associations

Food and Beverage Companies

Two federal government series reports provide estimates of food expenditures in the United States: The Economic Research Service (ERS) Food Expenditure Series published by the U.S. Department of Agriculture (USDA), which provides actual food sales information obtained from total food sales of retail establishments that sell food items, based on food sales in the Bureau of the Census Retail Trade Reports; and the U.S. Bureau of Labor Statistics (BLS) Consumer Expenditure Survey, which is based on annual household expenditure surveys that measure food purchases of the consuming units or households surveyed (ERS/USDA, 2005a). Food and beverage expenditures have grown at approximately 6.4 percent per year for the past 40 years[5] (ERS/USDA, 2004, 2005b). Sales for total U.S. food and beverage consumption were $895.4 billion in 2004 (ERS/USDA, 2005b). The BLS survey reports the distribution of food expenditures for food categories by selected demographic categories. Consumer expenditures for food in 2002 accounted for 13.2 percent of a household's disposable income, with 7.6 percent spent for foods at home and 5.6 percent for foods acquired away from home (U.S. Department of Labor, 2004; Table 4-2).

Many factors have contributed to the growth of the modern American food industry, including agricultural improvement, new food processing technologies, expanded transportation facilities, and evolving communication systems (Tillotson, 2004). Historically, the growth of the processed-food retail sector in the United States has been important both for supporting economic growth and feeding an evolving, nonagricultural society (Tillotson, 2004).

The majority of the top 25 global food and beverage companies are also leading producers of child- or youth-specific branded food and beverage products (Food Engineering, 2004). These companies include Nestlé S.A., Kraft Foods, Cargill, PepsiCo, The Coca-Cola Company, Cadbury Schweppes, Mars, ConAgra, General Mills, and the Kellogg Company (Williams, 2005b). Worldwide revenues for leading food and beverage companies in 2003 and 2004 are shown in Table 4-3.

---

[5]The USDA differentiates food sales from food expenditures. The latter includes noncash sales in the ERS food expenditure series. The Bureau of Labor Statistics Consumer Price Index for Food grew at a rate of 4.6 percent from 1967 to 2004 so more than half of the growth in food sales was due to higher prices. Total food expenditures for 2004 have not yet been completed.

TABLE 4-2 Average Annual Expenditures of Households and Percent Distribution of Total Food Expenditures, 2002

| Category | Total Expenditure ($) Thousands | | Percent of Total Food-at-Home Expenditures |
	Total	By Category	
Food at home	3,099		
Cereals and bakery products		450	14
Meats, poultry, fish, and eggs		798	26
Dairy products		328	11
Fruits and vegetables		552	18
Other food at home		970	31
Food away from home	2,276	n/a	
Total Food	5,375		

NOTE: Food represents 13.2 percent of total expenditures (made up of 7.6 percent for food at home and 5.6 percent for food away from home).
SOURCE: U.S. Department of Labor (2004).

TABLE 4-3 Selected Leading Food and Beverage Companies' Global Revenues, 2003 and 2004

Company	2003 Revenues ($ billion)	2004 Revenues ($ billion)
Nestlé S.A.	69.0	72.6
Cargill	59.9	62.9
Kraft Foods	31.0	32.2
PepsiCo	27.0	29.3
The Coca-Cola Company	17.3	18.2
Mars	17.0*	18.0*
ConAgra Foods	19.8	14.5
General Mills	10.5	11.1
Kellogg Company	8.8	9.6
The Hershey Company	4.2	4.4
TOTAL	264.5	272.8

NOTE: Cargill primarily provides food ingredients and value-added services to food and beverage manufacturers. *Mars, including Masterfoods, does not publicly release its annual revenues.
SOURCES: Business Wire (2005), DataMonitor (2004, 2005), Kraft Foods (2004), The Hershey Company (2005).

Companies continuously develop new products or reformulate existing products to keep pace with changing consumer tastes and preferences, new technology, and competition. In 2000, a typical supermarket offered an estimated 40,000 products from more than 16,000 food processing companies (Harris, 2002). Selected leading food companies' top brands, total sales, and marketing media expenditures for these brands in 2004 are shown in Table 4-4.

The beverage industry includes the manufacturers, distributors, and franchise companies engaged in the production and sale of many different product brands, including regular, no-calorie, and low-calorie CSDs; ready-to-drink teas and coffees; bottled waters, fruit juices, and nonjuice fruit drinks; sports and energy drinks; and milk-based beverages (ABA, 2004, 2005a). Over the past several years, there has been a significant expansion of diet, low-fat, low-calorie, and caffeine-free varieties of traditional beverage products (FitchRatings, 2004). In 2003, more than 5,200 new ready-to-drink, nonalcoholic beverages were introduced in the United States (ABA, 2004). In the same year, single-serving bottled water sales increased by 21.5 percent and single-serving sports drink sales increased by 17.9 percent.

In 2003, two companies represented 75 percent of the market share for CSDs—The Coca-Cola Company (44 percent) and PepsiCo (31.8 percent) (Beverage Digest, 2004). The leading beverage brands, companies, and marketing media expenditures in 2004 are shown in Table 4-5.

The food and beverage industry attracts large financial investments based on the expectation of continued growth and profitability (Tillotson, 2004). According to an opinion survey of the 10 leading global food companies, the strategies identified as most likely to help the leading food companies grow over the next 3 years were: (1) innovating and launching new products into developed markets; (2) category expansion such as moving from confectionery to frozen foods; and (3) merger and acquisition activities in developed markets and high-growth potential markets (Business Insights, 2005a).

With respect to healthful products, the prospects were viewed as mixed. The heightened public interest in health and wellness and increased concern about obesity presents certain marketing risks—such as increased costs associated with developing, reformulating, packaging, test marketing, and promoting food and beverage products, as well as uncertainty related to creating and sustaining consumer demand for these new products. However, the public interest and concern also presents potentially profitable marketing opportunities not yet fully explored—food and beverage manufacturers can compete for and expand their market share for healthier food and beverage product categories, be role models for the industry by substantially shifting overall product portfolios toward healthier products, and

TABLE 4-4 Selected Leading Companies' Top Food Brands, Total Sales, and Marketing Media Expenditures by Category, 2004

Brand	Company Name	Headquarters	Total Sales ($ millions)	Marketing Media Expenditures ($ millions)
Ready-to-Eat Cereals				
Cheerios	General Mills	Minneapolis, MN	289.7	34.5
Frosted Flakes	Kellogg NA Company	Battle Creek, MI	243.3	10.0
Honey Nut Cheerios	General Mills	Minneapolis, MN	239.6	38.3
Honey Bunches of Oats	Kraft Foods	Tarrytown, NY	222.8	17.8
Cinnamon Toast Crunch	General Mills	Minneapolis, MN	164.9	24.9
Cereal Bars				
Chewy Granola	Quaker Oats	Chicago, IL	125.7	2.8
Nature Valley	Campbell Mithun	Minneapolis, MN	107.6	7.1
Nutri-Grain	Kellogg NA Company	Battle Creek, MI	102.5	23.3
Rice Krispies Treats	Kellogg NA Company	Battle Creek, MI	70.5	n/a
Crackers				
Ritz	Kraft Foods	Glenview, IL	232.4	12.9
Pepperidge Farm Goldfish	Campbell Soup Company	Camden, NJ	167.8	9.1
Premium Saltines	Kraft Foods	East Hanover, NJ	157.5	n/a
Cheez-It Savory	Kellogg NA Company	Battle Creek, MI	139.8	22.2
Wheat Thins	Kraft Foods	East Hanover, NJ	126.2	21.9
Triscuit	Kraft Foods	East Hanover, NJ	108.2	16.3
Salty Snacks				
Lay's	PepsiCo	Purchase, NY	743.1	23.7
Doritos	PepsiCo	Purchase, NY	657.0	9.7
Tostitos	PepsiCo	Purchase, NY	417.0	1.3
Cheetos	PepsiCo	Purchase, NY	380.3	2.4
Wavy Lay's	PepsiCo	Purchase, NY	278.3	n/a

continues

TABLE 4-4 Continued

Brand	Company Name	Headquarters	Total Sales ($ millions)	Marketing Media Expenditures ($ millions)
Refrigerated Orange Juice				
Tropicana Pure Premium	PepsiCo	Purchase, NY	1,149.8	31.9
Minute Maid	The Coca-Cola Company	Atlanta, GA	402.8	28.1
Florida's Natural	Citrus World	Lake Wales, FL	234.2	20.7
Refrigerated Yogurt				
Yoplait	General Mills	Minneapolis, MN	283.5	36.0
Yoplait Light	General Mills	Minneapolis, MN	174.4	n/a
Dannon Light	Dannon Company	Tarrytown, NY	164.1	3.9
Luncheon Meats				
Oscar Mayer	Kraft Foods	Madison, WI	808.8	18.0
Hillshire Farm Deli	Sara Lee Corporation	Chicago, IL	244.0	20.1
Buddig	Carl Buddig & Company	Homewood, IL	138.0	0.1
Meat Alternatives				
Morningstar Farms	Kellogg NA Company	Battle Creek, MI	73.7	8.9
Boca Burger	Kraft Foods	Madison, WI	53.1	1.7
Morningstar Farms Grillers	Kellogg NA Company	Battle Creek, MI	28.2	n/a

SOURCE: Reprinted with permission, from BrandWeek (2005). ©Brandweek Research 2005 / Sources: Information Resources, Inc. (sales); TNS (media). Sales data reflect U.S. supermarkets, drugstores, and mass merchandisers, excluding Wal Mart.

TABLE 4-5 Leading Beverage Brands, Total Sales, and Marketing Media Expenditures by Category, 2004

Brand	Company Name	Headquarters	Total Sales (millions of cases)*	Marketing Media Expenditures ($ millions)
Carbonated Soft Drinks				
Coke Classic	The Coca-Cola Company	Atlanta, GA	1,832.7	123.4
Pepsi	PepsiCo	Purchase, NY	1,179.5	104.0
Diet Coke	The Coca-Cola Company	Atlanta, GA	998.0	22.8
Mountain Dew	PepsiCo	Purchase, NY	648.0	52.5
Diet Pepsi	PepsiCo	Purchase, NY	625.0	32.9
Sprite	The Coca-Cola Company	Atlanta, GA	580.5	43.9
Dr Pepper	Cadbury Schweppes	London, U.K.	574.1	68.8
Caffeine Free Diet Coke	The Coca-Cola Company	Atlanta, GA	170.0	n/a
Diet Dr Pepper	Cadbury Schweppes	London, U.K.	140.1	24.6
Sierra Mist	PepsiCo	Purchase, NY	138.8	41.4

Brand	Company Name	Headquarters	Total Sales ($ millions)	Marketing Media Expenditures ($ millions)
New Age/Sports/Water				
Gatorade	PepsiCo	Purchase, NY	2,648.9	127.6
Aquafina	PepsiCo	Purchase, NY	1,061.1	21.4
Dasani	The Coca-Cola Company	Atlanta, GA	925.1	17.5
Lipton	PepsiCo	Purchase, NY	668.3	0.2
Red Bull	Red Bull NA	Santa Monica, CA	594.5	31.6
Snapple	Cadbury Schweppes	London, U.K.	531.1	10.5
Minute Maid Single Serve	The Coca-Cola Company	Atlanta, GA	503.4	35.7
Powerade	The Coca-Cola Company	Atlanta, GA	460.2	10.5
Poland Spring	Nestlé Waters	Greenwich, CT	450.3	3.1
AriZona	Ferolito	Vultaggio, NY	369.0	n/a

SOURCE: Reprinted with permission, from BrandWeek (2005). ©Brandweek Research 2005 / Sources: Beverage Digest (sales in millions of cases); TNS (media). *Total sales in dollars were not reported.

serve as socially responsible corporate stakeholders in the response to child-hood obesity. In making positive changes that expand consumers' selection of healthier foods and beverages, despite the challenges of market forces and the marketplace, companies may also be seeking to avoid the risk of either stronger government regulation or litigation possibilities that have been identified by industry analysts (FitchRatings, 2004; JP Morgan, 2003; UBS Warburg, 2002).

Food and Beverage Retailers

In 2004, Americans visited supermarkets an average of 2.2 times per week (FMI, 2004). A supermarket is defined as any full-line, self-service grocery store generating a sales volume of $2 million or more annually (FMI, 2004). Supermarket sales in 2004 totaled $457.4 billion (FMI, 2004). Several supermarket designs exist in the United States including conventional, superstore, combination food and drug, warehouse clubs, economy limited-assortment store,[6] and hypermarket[7] (Kaufman, 2002). A variety of principles shape the marketing strategies of food retailers: penetration, to attract the maximum number of households; frequency, to engage shoppers so they will make repeat shopping trips; and spending, to encourage consumers to purchase more during each trip (ACNielsen, 2004). Carbonated beverages, candy, and snack foods were identified as top food categories that drove penetration and frequency in 2003 (ACNielsen, 2004; Kelley et al., 2004).

A recent consumer survey conducted by the Food Marketing Institute found that women are the primary grocery shoppers in two-thirds of households, and only 16 percent have a shared responsibility between women and men. According to the survey, the most common reasons why shoppers report not eating a healthful diet is the desire for convenience foods (which they believe are not as healthful as home-prepared meals), perceived cost, and confusion about what constitutes healthful choices (FMI, 2003). The survey found that younger shoppers are especially interested in prepared foods, partly because they report that food preparation is more difficult for them.

---

[6]Economy limited-assortment stores are lower priced supermarkets that typically sell a limited number of brands and sizes, many of which are private-label brand goods, at lower prices than traditional supermarkets. They are not full-service supermarkets, and they generally require customers to bring their own bags and bag their own purchases.

[7]Hypermarkets combine a supermarket and a department store, resulting in an extremely spacious retail facility that carries an enormous range of products under one roof, including full lines of fresh groceries and apparel.

Shopping frequency in traditional retail outlets, such as grocery stores, declined from 1993 to 2001 (Deutche Bank Securities, 2004) but increased in superstores (e.g., Wal-Mart), warehouse clubs (e.g., B.J's, Costco, Sam's), and nontraditional outlets such as convenience stores and drug stores, which are among the fastest growing venues where shoppers purchase food (ACNielsen, 2004; Deutche Bank Securities, 2004). Food merchandising at drug stores has increased in recent years with the more aisles offering seasonally available, limited assortments of food. In 2003, food and beverages led drug store sales at 27 percent of total sales. Candy was the third largest category of food sold in drug stores, based on total sales, followed by carbonated beverages (ACNielsen, 2004).

Full Serve and Quick Serve Restaurants

People are getting their meals from outside the home more often. In 2002, approximately half (46 percent) of Americans' food dollar was spent on away-from-home foods that were either fully prepared and eaten either outside the home or brought into the home for consumption, up from 27 percent of Americans' food dollar in 1962 (Variyam, 2005b; Table 4-2). With increases in household incomes and the proportion of two-working-parent families, a larger share of food spending is devoted to prepared and out-of-home foods and meals (Jekanowski, 1999; Kaufman, 2002; Variyam, 2005a). The share of Americans' daily caloric intake from away-from-home foods increased from 18 percent in 1977–1978 to 32 percent in 1994–1996 (Variyam, 2005b).

Restaurants have become part of the American lifestyle. The restaurant industry estimates that the full serve restaurant and quick serve restaurant (QSR)[8] or fast food restaurant sector will provide approximately 70 billion meals or snacks to U.S. consumers in 2005 (NRA, 2005). More than 900,000 commercial restaurants are projected to generate an estimated $476 billion in annual sales in 2005, up from $42.8 billion in 1970 (NRA, 2005). Consumer per-capita spending at fast food outlets such as QSRs are expected to rise by 6 percent between 2000 and 2020 (Stewart et al., 2004). In 2004, the leading 10 QSR chains accounted for $73.4 billion in sales (Table 4-6).

---

[8]Quick serve restaurants is a common industry and marketing term used to refer to a category of restaurants characterized by food that is supplied quickly after ordering and with minimal service. Food and beverages purchased may be consumed at the restaurant or served as take-out. The complete term, quick serve restaurants, is used in other chapters of this report instead of QSRs due to the lack of familiarity of this term among nonmarketing audiences.

TABLE 4-6 Leading QSR Chains by Total Sales and Marketing Media Expenditures, 2004

Brand	Segment	Company Name	Headquarters	Total Sales ($ billions)	Marketing Media Expenditures ($ millions)
McDonald's	Burger	McDonald's Corporation	Oak Brook, IL	24.4	528.8
Wendy's	Burger	Wendy's International	Dublin, OH	7.7	331.3
Burger King	Burger	Burger King Corporation	Miami, FL	7.7	287.1
Subway	Sandwich	Doctor's Associates	Milford, CT	6.3	287.1
Taco Bell	Mexican	Yum! Brands, Taco Bell Corporation	Irvine, CA	5.7	194.4
Pizza Hut	Pizza/pasta	Yum! Brands, Pizza Hut	Dallas, TX	5.3	185.2
KFC	Chicken	Yum! Brands, KFC Corporation	Louisville, KY	4.9	212.1
Starbucks	Snack	Starbucks	Seattle, WA	4.8	26.4
Dunkin' Donuts	Snack	Dunkin' Brands	Canton, MA	3.4	61.8
Domino's Pizza	Pizza/pasta	Domino's Pizza	Ann Arbor, MI	3.2	130.8

SOURCE: Reprinted with permission, from BrandWeek (2005). ©Brandweek Research 2005 / Sources: Technomic (sales); TNS (media).

TABLE 4-7 Major Trade Associations Representing U.S. and Global Food and Beverage Manufacturers and Distributors

Association	Segment Represented
American Bakers Association	Wholesale baking industry
American Beverage Association	Beverage manufacturers, marketers, distributors, franchise companies of non-alcoholic beverages
Food Products Association	Food and beverage manufacturers
Grocery Manufacturers Association	Branded food, beverage, and consumer product companies
International Dairy Foods Association	Dairy food manufacturers, marketers, distributors, and industry suppliers
National Confectioners Association	Confectionery and candy manufacturers and suppliers
National Restaurant Association	Full serve restaurants and QSRs
Snack Food Association	Snack manufacturers and suppliers
United Fresh Fruit & Vegetable Association	Growers, shippers, processors, brokers, wholesalers and distributors of produce

Trade Associations

Trade associations represent their industry members in several capacities including government relations, regulatory guidance, media interactions, and nutrition institutions. These organizations often compile data on annual industry sales and consumer trends pertaining to their segments, educate manufacturers on technological advances and retailing practices, offer standards and guidelines for practice, and provide their member companies with technical research and support. A variety of trade associations represent different segments of the food and beverage industry, retail and wholesale sectors, and the restaurant industry (Table 4-7).

Growing Purchasing Power of Children and Youth

Children and youth collectively represent a powerful economic and demographic segment. They are a primary market, spending discretionary income on a variety of products that they acquire from allowances and other sources. Children and youth are also an influence market, determining a large proportion of what is spent by parents and households. Finally, children and youth are the future market, representing tomorrow's adult customers for branded products and services (McNeal, 1999; MPA, 2004a).

With discretionary income from allowances and other sources including gifts from parents, relatives, and friends, household chores, and outside jobs (Doss et al., 1995; McNeal, 1998; Teenage Research Unlimited, 2004), in 2002 children ages 4–12 years spent $30 billion on direct purchases (Schor, 2004), up from $6.1 billion in 1989 and $23.4 billion in 1997 (McNeal, 1999). Of the various spending categories, one-third of children's direct purchases are for sweets, snacks, and beverages followed by toys and apparel (Schor, 2004). Of the top 10 items children ages 8–12 years reported they could select without parental permission, the top 4 were for food categories: candy or snacks (66 percent did not need permission to purchase), soft drinks (63 percent), fast food (54 percent), and breakfast cereals (49 percent) (Chaplin, 1999).

In 2003, 12- to 19-year-olds alone spent an estimated $175 billion (Teenage Research Unlimited, 2004). Income varies greatly within the teen market as the population matures (MPA, 2004a). Adolescents have more discretionary income than their peers a few decades ago. Approximately 37.2 percent of all teens ages 12–17 years have savings or checking accounts in their own name, and 5.3 percent have access to credit cards in their own name or their parents' name (MPA, 2004a). According to Teenage Research Unlimited (2005), which provides a continuous tracking and segmentation of the U.S. teen market to assess trends, lifestyles, attitudes, product and brand usage, the total weekly spending by teens is $98.25, with Hispanic ($107.48) and African American ($100.25) teens' weekly spending being slightly higher than white ($95.72) teen spending. As shown in Table 4-8, food or beverages—particularly candy, soda or soft drinks,

TABLE 4-8 Top 10 Items Teens, Ages 13–17 Years, Purchased with Their Own Money

		Percent (%)	
	Overall Teen Rank/Item	Boys	Girls
1	Clothes	21	43
2	Food	30	31
3	Candy	24	34
3	Soda or soft drinks	26	32
4	Salty snacks	15	22
4	CDs or recorded music	19	18
5	Lunch	13	22
6	Shoes	15	16
7	Video games	18	5
8	Jewelry	7	15
9	Magazines	9	12
10	Ice cream	7	10

SOURCE: Reprinted with permission from the Roper Youth Report (2003).

and salty snacks/chips—were ranked among the top 4 items that teens ages 13–17 years last bought with their own money in 2003 (Roper Youth Report, 2003). Another marketing research study reports that younger and older children purchase candy most frequently with their own money while teens also frequently purchase gum, drinks, and other snacks in addition to candy (Yankelovich, 2003).

Shopping malls represent the most frequent shopping place for adolescents. Boys and girls ages 14–17 years who shop at malls spend a reported $46.80 per visit. They visit malls more frequently than any other age group at a rate of once weekly, and also spend the most time per visit when compared to other places (MPA, 2004a). Teens also shop in many other venues including discount stores, convenience stores, and grocery stores. Girls shop more frequently than boys at almost every shopping venue (MPA, 2004a).

Children and adolescents also influence household purchase decisions. The purchase influence of children and adolescents increases with age and is currently estimated at $500 billion annually for 2- to 14-year-olds (*U.S. Market for Kids' Foods and Beverages*, 2003). In 1993, children and youth together wielded a purchase influence of $295 billion. Of this amount, children ages 3–11 years exerted a purchase influence totaling $125 billion and youth ages 12–17 years represented a purchase influence of $170 billion (Stipp, 1993). In recent years, there has been a substantial increase in the number of children and their parents who report that young consumers ages 8–17 years are playing more prominent roles in household purchasing decisions ranging from food to entertainment to media (Roper Youth Report, 2003).

Both parents and their children report that young people have the highest purchase influence on food, when compared to other nonfood spending categories such as music, electronics, and home decor (Roper Youth Report, 2003). In 2003, 78 percent of children and youth ages 8–17 years reported that they influenced family food purchases and 84 percent of their parents concurred (Roper Youth Report, 2003). Children and youth, ages 6–17 years report that they help their parents select snack foods, breakfast cereal, soft drinks, candy, cookies, and even the QSRs where they eat (Yankelovich, 2003). Marketing research has found that nearly three-quarters (73 percent) of mothers of children and teens ages 6–17 years state that their children have influence over the types of brands and groceries they buy for the family (Yankelovich, 2003). Marketing research also suggests that parents believe that their children's preferences are important in determining where food is purchased, as 21 percent of parents in one survey report that their child's preference for certain snack foods is an important factor in deciding where to shop (Yankelovich, 2003).

New Product Development Targeted to Children and Youth

New product development is a central focus of innovation in the food and beverage industry. A recent survey of 30 U.S. food and beverage companies found that 71 percent had reformulated products and 29 percent had introduced new products across 3,000 product categories since 2002 (GMA, 2004). Many of these were targeted to children. Annual sales of food and beverages to children and youth were more than $27 billion in 2002 (*U.S. Market for Kids' Foods and Beverages*, 2003). In 2004, product introductions targeted to children appeared to account for more than 10 percent of all new food and beverage products according to an analysis of the ProductScan® database (Harris, 2005). Candy was the largest category (46 percent) and others included snacks (8 percent), cookies (6 percent), cereals (5 percent), and beverages (5 percent). Nearly half of the new beverage products were fruit and fruit-flavored drinks. About 15 percent of all new children's foods and beverages between 2000 and 2004 were whole-grain, low-fat, and low-sugar products, up from 9 percent for the previous 5 years (Harris, 2005).

Proliferation of Children's Products

The committee analyzed the 50 food categories and 16 beverage categories contained in the ProductScan® database for trends in new product introductions targeted to children (Williams, 2005b). ProductScan® is an online global database that has tracked new consumer products and packaged goods introductions into the U.S. marketplace since 1980 (Marketing Intelligence Service, 2005). In the ProductScan® database, a new product is defined as a packaged, branded item that constitutes a new brand, line, variety, package type, package size or formulation, introduced to the retail shelf within the previous 90 days (Williams, 2005b).

Since 1994, the ProductScan® database has been structured to allow identification of products specifically targeted to children (ages 4–12 years) and to teens (ages 13–19 years). Searching the full 1980–2004 database using the keyword "children," suggests generally that new products targeted to children during 1980–1994 were significantly fewer than from 1994 to the present (Williams, 2005b). However, the age specificity of the search capacity has been improved for recent years. Figure 4-2a shows the year-by-year new product introductions in the ProductScan® database from 1994 to 2004 for all food products targeted to the total market and Figure 4-2b shows the year-by-year new product introductions in the ProductScan® database from 1994 to 2004 to children and youth. The number of new food and beverage products targeted to children and adolescents by

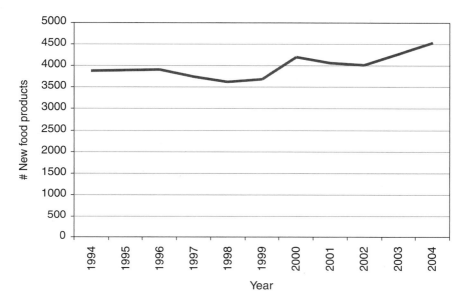

FIGURE 4-2a New food products targeted to the total market, 1994–2004.
SOURCE: Williams (2005b).

company, manufacturer, or distributor from 1994–2004 is shown in Appendix E, Table E-2.

Figure 4-3a shows similar data for all beverage products targeted to the total market, and Figure 4-3b shows data for beverage products targeted specifically to children and adolescents.

For both foods and beverages, the overall trend lines increased upward from 1994 to 2004, but as indicated by the slope of the trend lines, the growth rate in new product introductions for both food and beverage products targeted to children and youth is greater than the growth rate for food and beverage products targeted to the general market. The decline that occurred between 2003 and 2004 for both food and beverage products targeted to children and youth, relative to those targeted to the general market, may be due to recent scrutiny addressed to the introduction of new products targeted to children. It is uncertain whether the recent decline in new products targeted to children is attributed to an overall

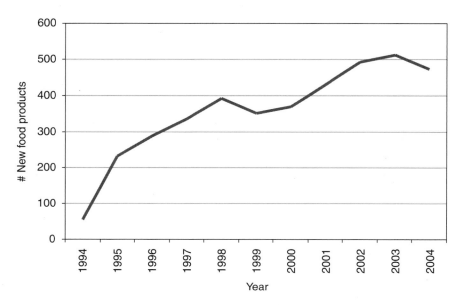

FIGURE 4-2b New food products targeted to children and adolescents, 1994–2004.
SOURCE: Williams (2005b).

decrease in all new products, or whether it represents a selective reduction in certain categories, such as those products deemed to be less healthful for children and youth. Overall, in the period 1994–2004, there were 3,936 new food products and 511 new beverage products targeted to children and youth (Williams, 2005b). Products high in total calories, sugar, or fat and low in nutrients dominated the profile of new foods and beverages targeted to children and youth, as indicated in Tables 4-9 and 4-10.

For example, for food products, the categories of candies, snacks, cookies, and ice cream accounted for 58 percent of all new products targeted to children in 1994–2004, compared to 27 percent of all new products targeted to the general market. For beverage products, the categories of fruit and fruit-flavored drinks accounted for 40 percent of all new products targeted to children, compared to 22 percent of all new products targeted to the general market. These results concur with those reported by Harris (2005). On the other hand, one industry analysis has forecasted that healthful food and beverage products for children will be among the most active and profitable new product categories for industry over the next 5 years from 2005 to 2009 (Business Insights, 2005b).

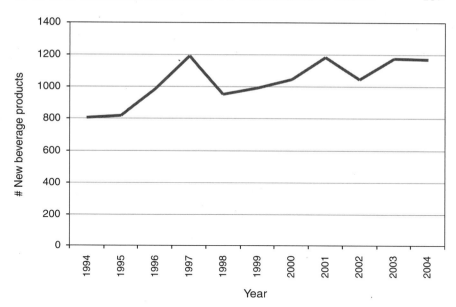

FIGURE 4-3a New beverage products targeted to the total market, 1994–2004.
SOURCE: Williams (2005b).

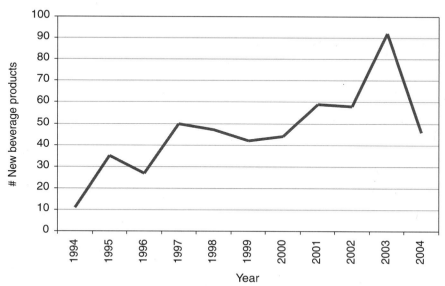

FIGURE 4-3b New beverage products targeted to children and adolescents, 1994–2004.
SOURCE: Williams (2005b).

TABLE 4-9 Top Food Categories for New Products Targeted to Children and Adolescents, 1994–2004

Category	Number of New Products
Candies—nonchocolate	1,407
Chewing gum	354
Snacks	265
Candies—chocolate	236
Cereals	231
Cookies	225
Meals	171
Ice cream & frozen yogurt	168
Pasta	98
Yogurt	77
Crackers	71
Snack bars	70
Pastry	66
Desserts	55
Cheese	50
Mixes	49
Fruits	41
Sweet toppings	27
Cakes	25
Chips	25
Popcorn	25
Soup	21
Bread products	20
Jams	20
Poultry	16
Nut butters	13
Vegetables	11
Meat	11
Sauces & gravies	11
Meat substitutes	10
Catsup	10
Meal replacements	9
Fish	8
Staples	8
Baby food	6
Rice	4
Salad dressings	4
Spices	3
Nuts & seeds	2
Dairycase foods	2
Mustard	2
Sauces	2
Salads	1
Entrée mixes	1

continues

TABLE 4-9 Continued

Category	Number of New Products
Margarine, butter, & spreads	1
Oil, shortening, & cooking sprays	1
Pickles, olives, & condiments	1
Dips & salad toppings	1
Miscellaneous foods	1
Total	3,936

SOURCE: Williams (2005b).

TABLE 4-10 Top Beverage Categories for New Products Targeted to Children, 1994–2004

Category	Number of New Products
Fruit drinks	203
Milk, nondairy milk, & yogurt drinks	96
Beverage mixes & flavorings	60
Carbonated soft drinks	39
Bottled water	34
Sports beverages	34
Health drinks	10
Baby beverages	10
Vegetable drinks	3
Miscellaneous drinks	22
Total	511

SOURCE: Williams (2005b).

Finding: Children and youth ages 4–17 years have increasing discretionary income and purchasing capacity, are being targeted more directly by marketers, and frequently spend their discretionary income on high-calorie and low-nutrient foods and beverages.

Children's Versions of Classic Products

In addition to the development of new products oriented to children and youth, food and beverage companies have devoted considerable attention to enhancing the appeal of existing products to a younger market, using novel package designs, names, and co-branding with recognizable cartoon or fictional characters (Mintel International Group Ltd., 2003). For example, Heinz introduced Heinz EZ Squirt™, a "kid-friendly" ketchup, available in "Blastin' Green" and "Funky Purple" colors, and substantially increased the company's market share in 2003 (McGinn, 2003). However, like many products, they proved to have a short-lived novelty appeal and were withdrawn from the market soon after their introduction.

By contrast, conventional wisdom suggested that children would not like yogurt due to its generally sour flavor. Yogurt has demonstrated an interesting evolution both in product and child taste adaptation. Whole new products have been introduced that appeal to children's preferences for sweet tastes. Dannon pioneered children's yogurt with Dannon Sprinklin's®, a version of its regular yogurt flavors with candy sprinkles encased on the cap that children could add to the yogurt (Dannon, 2005). Dannon later developed a drinkable yogurt called Danimals®, and Frusion® smoothies, a 10-ounce bottle of real fruit and low-fat yogurt within its child product portfolio. Both of these brands offer sweeter yogurt taste and portability for children (Dannon, 2005). General Mills followed with several innovations in the yogurt category that intended to make yogurt appealing to children. The first of these products was a line extending its Trix® cereal into its Yoplait® yogurt line with a mixed fruit and sweetened formulation of traditional yogurt (General Mills, 2005a). General Mills changed the yogurt packaging format with the launch of Go-Gurt®, which comes in long tubes, and Go-Gurt® smoothies that are sold in small plastic bottle-shaped containers (General Mills, 2005b). Other companies that have developed and market dairy-based products for children include Kraft Foods, which developed Twist-ums™ string cheese sticks, and The Coca-Cola Company, which manufactures Swerve™, a milk-based beverage product consisting of 51 percent skim milk (The Coca-Cola Company, 2005a).

Convenience and Portability

Convenience and portability have become guiding principles in the food company business. Swanson & Sons began this trend when the company created the first TV dinner in 1953 (Lauro, 2002). The dinners were marketed as quick meals that required minimal preparation time. The meals came in various forms and generally included meat, a starch, a vegetable, and dessert. In the 1960s, Swanson removed the words "TV dinner" from the packaging and has since introduced lighter meals in microwave-safe trays for consumers. Swanson TV dinners still remain in the public memory as the dinner phenomenon of the 1950s generation that grew up with television (Pinnacle Foods Corporation, 2003).

Easy preparation of meals has allowed children greater flexibility and independence in preparing their own meals. The concept of the TV dinner evolved into child-targeted variations of the dinner meal in the 1980s.

ConAgra Foods launched Kid Cuisine® as a line of frozen food entrées intended especially for children and young teens (ConAgra Foods, 2004). Using various character appeals, first a cartoon chef and later an animated penguin, Kid Cuisine® offered meals similar to Swanson TV dinners. ConAgra Foods markets 11 different varieties of the Kid Cuisine® meal, from chicken breast nuggets to alien invasion pepperoni pizza (ConAgra Foods, 2004).

Marketing research conducted by Nickelodeon suggests that nearly three-quarters of children and youth report that they decide on their own what they eat for breakfast most or all of the time (Smalls, 2005b). Breakfast options have undergone substantial innovations over the past 40 years from ready-to-eat (RTE) sweetened breakfast cereals to breakfast bars and pastries. The breakfast pastry category was pioneered by the Kellogg Company with the introduction of Pop-Tarts® in 1963, allowing children to prepare their own breakfasts by putting a flat pastry into the toaster, an approach since adopted by a number of companies. The company has doubled sales in the United States from 1 billion in the early 1990s to an estimated 2 billion Pop-Tarts® annually (Prichard, 2003). Other breakfast innovations with child appeal include a number of breakfast bars by various companies with ingredients ranging from cereal, fruit, and milk to chocolate and cookies.

A new lunch combination category was specifically designed for children by Kraft Foods in 1988 when the Oscar Mayer Lunchables® was launched (Kraft Foods, 2005a). This line of convenience foods was the first prepackaged, RTE lunch that offered meat, cheese, and crackers, now in three sizes of packages—the largest with 40 percent more food (Kraft Foods, 2005a). Sports drink beverages have also become popular over the past three decades. Gatorade® Thirst Quencher was created in 1965 at the University of Florida to help athletes stay hydrated during active sports (Gatorade, 2004), and now represents a category of products marketed widely as a product for children and youth.

Finding: Child-targeted food and beverage products have steadily increased over the past decade, and are typically high in total calories, sugars, salt, fat, and low in nutrients.

MARKETING STRATEGIES, TACTICS, AND MESSAGING

Advertising and Marketing of Foods and Beverages in the United States

The scope of marketing expenditures in the United States is very large. Gross marketing expenditures in 2004 for all products, including food, beverages, and other manufactured items, totaled $264 billion, including

TABLE 4-11 U.S. Advertising Spending in Selected Food-Related Categories by Purchased Measured Media, 2004

| | | U.S. Measured Media | |
Category	Total Measured Media ($ millions)	Magazine	Newspaper
Food, beverages, candy[a]	6,840	1,743	51
Restaurants and fast food	4,418	179	176

[a]This category includes beverages, confectionery, snacks, dairy, produce, meat, bakery goods, prepared foods or ingredients, and mixes and seasonings (Brown et al., 2005). SOURCE: Brown et al. (2005). Reprinted with permission from the June 27, 2005, issue of Advertising Age. © Crain Communications, Inc. 2005.

$141 billion for advertising in measured media (Brown et al., 2005). Appendix E, Table E-3 lists selected leading advertisers ranked by category, total U.S. revenues, and total advertising spending for 2003 and 2004. The committee does not have a definitive breakout of the portion devoted to food and beverages. As a proxy, Table 4-11 displays total advertising spending in measured media for selected categories: food and beverages including candy, and restaurants and fast food outlets.

An estimated $6.84 billion was spent on advertising in the food, beverage, and candy category, and $4.42 billion was spent on advertising for restaurants and fast food for a total of $11.26 billion in food and beverage advertising (Brown et al., 2005; Table 4-11). In 2003, food marketers spent $1.75 billion to advertise products to children on national cable television alone, which included NICK ($756.5 million), TDSN ($86 million), and TOON ($910 million) (Nielsen Monitor-Plus, 2005). The children's media and entertainment industry are represented by four major companies— Disney, Time Warner, News Corporation, and Viacom—which own several forms of children's media production and distribution systems, including ownership in broadcast networks and children's cable networks (Allen, 2001).

Advertising intensity is one measure of the marketing emphasis given to a product category. It represents the ratio of a food's share of advertising to its share of consumers' disposable income. Although food accounts for approximately 16 percent of total advertising, it accounts for a much smaller percentage of disposable income, suggesting a high level of advertising intensity. This intensity varies significantly across different food categories. In 1999, confectionery and salty snacks (e.g., candy, gum, mints, cookies, crackers, nuts, and chips) accounted for 13.2 percent of total food advertising expenditures, but only 5.4 percent of the household food budget share, which represented an advertising intensity of 2.4, the highest of any food

Outdoor	Television	Cable Network	Radio	Internet
78	3,418	1,331	140	79
204	3,123	567	147	22

category examined (Gallo, 1999). CSDs have an advertising intensity of 1.8, the third highest category. Fruits, vegetables, and grains have the lowest advertising intensity of 0.1—though these products account for 1.9 percent of advertising expenditures, they represent 14.7 percent of food-at-home budget shares (Gallo, 1999). More recent data for advertising intensity of various food and beverage categories are not available.

Changing Composition of Marketing Expenditures

There is evidence that the balance between advertising in measured media and other marketing techniques is changing. Available analyses use different techniques, data, and time frames, complicating precise tracking of trends. One unpublished analysis of estimated inflation-adjusted expenditures for U.S. food and restaurant television advertising from 1993 to 2004, based on Nielsen Media Research data, has suggested that real expenditures on food and restaurant advertising on television viewed by adult, child, and youth audiences have fallen over the past decade, from nearly $6 billion in 1994 to less than $5 billion in 2004 (Collier Shannon Scott and Georgetown Economic Services, 2004; Figure 4-4).

Industry sources have reported several converging trends that are attributed to reducing television's effectiveness in reaching consumers and target markets, including declining brand loyalty across a variety of product categories, audience fragmentation[9] across different channels and di-

---

[9]Audience fragmentation occurs when a target group, such as a television viewing audience, watches a greater diversity of television programming and divides its attention and screen time across many media platforms. The result is a smaller audience, which makes it more challenging for marketing messages to effectively reach target markets.

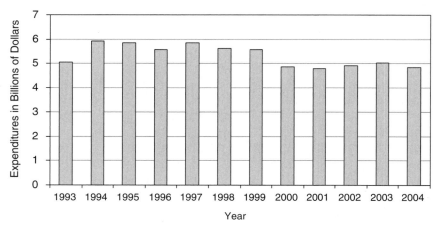

FIGURE 4-4 Estimated inflation-adjusted expenditures on food, beverages, and restaurant advertising on television, 1993–2004.
NOTE: Based on an analysis of Nielsen Media Research data.
SOURCE: Collier Shannon Scott and Georgetown Economic Services (2005b).

verse media platforms, increased advertising costs, rising price elasticity, and increased trade promotion spending by food and beverage manufacturers that is accompanied by decreased spending for advertising and consumer promotion (Deutche Bank Securities, 2004; Smith et al., 2005). Industry and marketing sources suggest that food and beverage companies and restaurants have been progressively reducing their television advertising budgets, reinvesting in other communication channels, and using integrated marketing strategies to reach consumers more effectively (Collier Shannon Scott and Georgetown Economic Services, 2005b; Deutche Bank Securities, 2004). An independent analysis that could confirm these trends was not available to the committee.

A recent trade promotion spending and merchandising study, based on 400 responses from an array of retailers and manufacturers across all connected sectors (Cannondale Associates, 2005), estimated the general distribution of companies' marketing expenditures for trade promotion, account-specific marketing, consumer promotion, and advertising from 1997 to 2004 (GMA Forum, 2005) (Figure 4-5). In general, for all companies, trade promotion was approximately 44 percent of marketing expenditures in 1997 and 48 percent in 2004. Advertising expenditures increased slightly from 23 percent in 1997 to 26 percent in 2004 (GMA Forum, 2005). Marketing budget allocations may differ based on the type of company and the size of the company, with food companies generally allocating more for

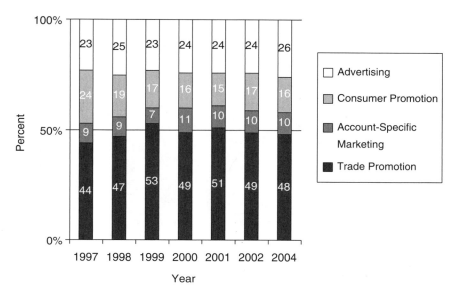

FIGURE 4-5 Allocation of all companies' marketing expenditures (including food companies), 1997–2004.
NOTE: See pages 137-138 for a description of marketing categories.
SOURCE: Reprinted with permission, from GMA Forum (2005).

trade promotion than other types of companies. One analysis indicates that food companies devote 55 percent of their marketing budgets for trade promotion, 25 percent for consumer promotion (including account-specific marketing), and 20 percent for advertising (GMA Forum, 2005).

Although expenditures on traditional television advertising for food and beverage products have slowed over the past decade, television still remains the primary promotional medium when compared to other measured media categories (Brown et al., 2005; Table 4-11). It appears that more food, beverage, and restaurant advertising dollars are shifting from television into unmeasured media sales promotion (e.g., product placement, character licensing, in-school marketing, special event marketing) (Collier Shannon Scott and Georgetown Economic Services, 2004, 2005b; PQMedia, 2005). For example, the investment in the value of all product placement increased from $190 million in 1974 to $3.46 billion in 2004, reflecting a trend away from traditional advertising to alternative marketing strategies (PQMedia, 2005; Figure 4-6). From 1974 to 2004, all product placement (including food and beverages) in television increased from $71 million to $1.88 billion. During the same period, as reported by

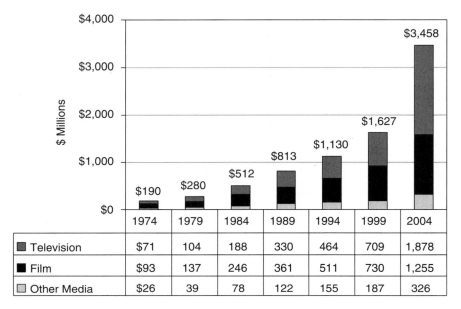

	1974	1979	1984	1989	1994	1999	2004
■ Television	$71	104	188	330	464	709	1,878
■ Film	$93	137	246	361	511	730	1,255
□ Other Media	$26	39	78	122	155	187	326

FIGURE 4-6 Product placement spending in media, 1974–2004.
NOTE: Other media include magazines, newspapers, video games, music, books, radio, and the Internet.
SOURCE: Reprinted with permission, from PQMedia (2005).

PQMedia (2005), product placement expenditures in film increased from $93 million to $1.26 billion, and increased more slowly in other media such as video games, magazines, music, books, and the Internet, from $26 million to $326 million (Figure 4-6).

Finding: Television is the primary promotional medium for measured media marketing of food and beverage products to children and youth, but a notable shift is occurring toward unmeasured sales promotion (e.g., product placement, character licensing, in-school marketing, special event marketing).

Advertising and Marketing to Children and Youth

In 2004, an estimated $15 billion was spent on all advertising and marketing directed at children and youth (Schor, 2004), of which a substantial share was devoted to food and beverage marketing. Advertising food and beverage products to children began to emerge in the United States as early as the 1950s (Guest, 1955), and grew during the 1960s, with the growth of the baby boomers as an untapped consumer market (McNeal, 1964, 1999). Over the decade of the 1990s, there was an estimated 20-fold increase in expenditures on advertisements that targeted children (Strasburger, 2001). Currently, advertising and marketing reach young consumers through many settings (e.g., schools, child care, grocery stores, shopping malls, theaters, sporting events, sponsored events, kids' clubs) and media (e.g., network and digital television, cable television, radio, magazines, books, the Internet, video games, and advergames). Marketing is both direct, targeted to children and youth, and indirect, targeted to mothers who are the gatekeepers of the household (Powell, 2005). Companies often design dual-marketing strategies to reach children and youth with attractive product packaging and marketing communications that promote messages emphasizing taste, convenience, and fun whereas mothers are more often targeted with messages about the nutritional qualities such as the wholesomeness or health benefits of branded products (Schor, 2004).

The expenditures on food, beverage, and restaurant marketing are substantial. The advertising component alone amounted to industry expenditures of more than $11 billion in 2004, a sizable portion of which targets young people (Brown et al., 2005; Table 4-11). Of this, an estimated $5 to $6.5 billion was spent on televised food, beverage, and restaurant advertisements (Brown et al., 2005; Collier Shannon Scott and Georgetown Economic Services, 2004, 2005a), including about $1 billion to advertise directly to young consumers, primarily through television (McNeal, 1999). Additionally, more than $4.5 billion a year is spent on promotions such as premiums and coupons, $2 billion is spent on youth-targeted public relations including event marketing and school-based marketing, and $3 billion annually is spent on food product packaging designed for children and youth (McNeal, 1999). In all, an estimated more than $10 billion per year is now expended to market food, beverage, and restaurant products to children and youth (Brownell and Horgen, 2004).

Product Appeals

Fun, taste, and product performance are the predominant appeals used in children's food and beverage television advertising (Tseng, 2001). Television commercials use music and familiar songs and jingles to enhance the perceived quality of a brand and to serve as a vehicle for children to remember the name of a product (Scammon and Christopher, 1981; Schor, 2004). Child actors portrayed in food and beverage commercials have traditionally been depicted as having fun with their peers when they consume the advertised product (CSPI, 2003). Audiovisual production techniques accentuate and enhance positive feelings about products by using action, rapid pacing, loud music, animation mixed with live action, close-ups, and rapid cuts. Marketers also use food as entertainment where the product is linked to a desirable emotional state (CSPI, 2003; Samuels et al., 2003). Flavor, texture, and fun are the characteristics that foster brand appeal for products such as RTE sweetened breakfast cereals. Accompanying the close-ups of these food products are verbal references to product flavors or textures such as fruity or chocolaty, honey taste or marshmallow texture, crunchy or crispy. In many instances, the breakfast cereal product names reflect their contents (e.g., Frosted Flakes®, Frosted Mini Wheats®, Honey Comb®, Cocoa Pebbles®, Cookie Crisp®), underscoring and reinforcing sweet flavor qualities.

Branded Spokescharacters

Advertising approaches for breakfast cereals have generally revolved around characters that represented, promoted, or embodied specific brands. Many of the branded spokescharacters used today have been used for decades and often carry across several forms of communication including package designs, events, promotions, and advertising (Lawrence, 2003). The RTE breakfast cereal category represents a $6 billion annual business (Thompson, 2004). In 2004, the three major breakfast cereal companies—Kellogg Company, General Mills, and Kraft Foods—collectively invested $380 million in children's advertisements in the United States (Ellison, 2005). These companies have used spokescharacters to market and build brand awareness, appeal, and loyalty for their respective packaged products.

Spokescharacters symbolize brands, often with a particular demeanor intended to set a tone for the product (Enrico, 1999). These anthropomorphic figures are designed to be fun and friendly for children, and each is

TABLE 4-12 Spokescharacters for Selected Ready-to-Eat Breakfast Cereal Brands

The Kellogg's Company Cereals		Kraft Foods' Post Cereals
Cereal	Character	Cereal
Frosted Flakes®	Tony the Tiger™	Golden Crisp®
Froot Loops!®	Toucan Sam®	Honeycomb®
Kellogg's Smacks®	Dig 'Em™ Frog	Alpha-Bits®
Rice Krispies®	Snap! Crackle! Pop!®	Fruity Pebbles® and Cocoa Pebbles®

associated with the company's branded breakfast cereal. Table 4-12 shows spokescharacters for selected RTE cereal brands. Some of the characters have undergone physical transformations over the decades. For example, Tony the Tiger™ was created in 1951 to promote Kellogg's Sugar Frosted Flakes® that was later changed to Frosted Flakes®. More recently, he has been designed as slimmer and more muscular as Americans became more health conscious (Enrico, 1999). In 2005, the Tony the Tiger™ mascot was launched to reach 2- to 5-year-olds through a $20 million television and print campaign targeted to mothers as the household gatekeepers with a reformulated cereal as a "food to grow by" and to help active children "earn their stripes" (Thompson, 2004).

Real-life branded spokescharacters have also been used by companies to market their image and branded products. A clown named Ronald McDonald was created in 1963 and used as a spokescharacter to appeal to children, with the intent of associating him with a fun experience and the food offered at McDonald's (Enrico, 1999; Ritzer, 2004). Selected as the second most famous advertising image of the 20th century, after the Marlboro Man, Ronald McDonald's face is recognized by nearly 96 percent of American children, and is used to sell fast food for the QSR internationally in more than 25 languages (Enrico, 1999).

Employing the same type of advertising used for RTE breakfast cereals, manufacturers of bakery products such as snack cakes, cupcakes, and Twinkies used spokescharacters in enjoyable adventures. For example, Hostess uses Happy Hoho® and Captain Cupcake® (Hostess, 2005) and Nestlé uses the Nesquik Bunny™ to promote its chocolate-flavored beverage directly to children (Nestlé, 2004). Kool-Aid®, created in the 1920s, was promoted by two spokescharacters, the Smiling Face Kool-Aid® Pitcher, and in 1975, the Kool-Aid® Man (Hastings Museum of Natural and Cultural History, 2004; Kraft Foods, 2005b).

	General Mills' Cereals	
Character	Cereal	Character
Sugar Bear	Trix®	The Trix® Rabbit
Crazy Craver	Cocoa Puffs®	Sonny the Cuckoo Bird
Alpha-Bit Characters	Lucky Charms®	Lucky the Leprechaun
Fred Flintstone and Barney Rubble	Count Chocula®	Count Chocula®

Character Merchandising, Co-Branding, Cross-Promotions

Character merchandising, co-branding, and cross-promotions are techniques used to further the reach of brands by building brand awareness and brand loyalty. Character merchandising refers to the licensing of popular fictional characters, such as Harry Potter™, Spiderman®, Scooby-Doo®, SpongeBob Square Pants®, Winnie the Pooh®, Rugrats®, and Elmo® to promote the sale of many types of products (CSPI, 2003; Mintel International Group Ltd., 2003). Licensing is a contractual arrangement that allows copyright holders to loan their intellectual property to another company in exchange for payment (Allen, 2001). Co-branding is a technique where two companies partner to create one product. It is used to reach new customers and to extend a company's name and trademark to new areas of the consumer market (Pollack Associates, 2003). Cross-promotion is a technique in which a manufacturer sells a new product related to an existing product a consumer already uses or which the marketer has available. Cross-promotions have been mutually profitable and beneficial for companies that build business relationships across products and media.

In the children's media industries, companies may license the characters and images of their media products to other companies for a fee. The characters are taken from a variety of media sources including film cartoons, toy creations, live-action feature films, comic and fiction books, newspaper strip cartoons, video games, and advergames (Mintel International Group Ltd., 2003). The toy industry has benefited greatly from character licensing of children's movies and television. Other industries that have generated profits from character merchandising are snack food companies, QSRs, and clothing manufacturers that incorporate popular characters into their products to increase the likelihood that children or their parents will buy their products (Allen, 2001).

Certain licensed characters, such as Spiderman® and Scooby-Doo®, are designed to appeal to children and parents who remember them from their own childhoods (Mintel International Group Ltd., 2003). Many of the characters are found in multiple forms of media, such as Harry Potter™, a fictional character from a book, who also appears in live-action films and computer games (Mintel International Group Ltd., 2003). Different characters are used for various age groups depending on a child's cognitive abilities and the appeal of the character to children and to parents. For example, mothers tend to have a preference for gentle, one-dimensional, friendly, and safe characters such as Barney™, Mickey Mouse™, and Teletubbies™ (Hind, 2003; Lawrence, 2003). Marketers seek to establish positive relationships among a brand, the parent, and a very young child by developing programs with branded stories, in order to promote an ongoing relationship with the spokescharacter that endorses the brand and that also provides input to marketers for new product development targeted to young children (Hind, 2003).

By the time children reach the age of 6–7 years, they prefer humorous and sometimes more aggressive characters, such as Looney Tunes' Road Runner (Lawrence, 2003). As they get older, tweens ages 8–13 years prefer more complicated characters such as The Simpsons™. As their lifestyle interests broaden to include music and sports celebrities, cartoon characters become less important and certain brands are less appealing when compared to teen or adult brands (Lawrence, 2003). Based on these trends, it is apparent that different developmental stages carry the prospect of different responses to marketing by children and youth.

Character licensing has been a prominent means of cross-promoting and increasing product interest and brand awareness in foods and beverages either as versions of the product (e.g., SpongeBob SquarePants® Mac 'n Cheese), or as premiums (toys, prizes, or giveaways) associated with traditional products. Some companies develop business relationships with food and beverage companies and purchase registered trademarks, such as General Mills' Cheerios® and Kraft Foods' Oreos®, and use them under a license agreement to co-brand and market products such as books or toys to children under the age of 6 years. Children's books such as *Kellogg's Froot Loops!® Counting Fun Book* (Barbieri McGrath, 2000), *The Oreo™ Cookie Counting Book* (Lukas, 2000), *The M&M's® Brand Chocolate Candies Counting Board Book* (Barbieri McGrath, 1997), and the *Cheerios® Play Book* (Wade, 1998) are examples of licensing brands and co-branding aimed at young children. Products that have used cartoon characters on packaging to promote foods include Nabisco's Dora the Explorer® crackers and cookies, Edy's Fish 'N Chips® ice cream featuring Disney's *Finding Nemo* characters, Kellogg's Spiderman® Pop-Tarts®, and Kraft Macaroni and Cheese® with noodle shapes in SpongeBob SquarePants®, Rugrats®, and Scooby-Doo® varieties.

Licensed characters have only recently been used to market healthful food and beverage products that are designed for consumption by preschoolers. *Sesame Street* has licensed several of its characters to companies for products such as Apple & Eve *Sesame Street* Juices® (Apple & Eve, 2005), Earth's Best® line of organic breakfast foods and snacks (Earth's Best, 2005), and IN ZONE Brands' Tummy Tickler 100 percent fruit juices (IN ZONE Brands, 2004). IN ZONE Brands has also licensed the use of several other cartoon characters targeted at younger children including Bob the Builder™, Clifford the Big Red Dog™, Barney™, and Snoopy™ in programs such as *Baby Looney Tunes™*, *Dragon Tales™*, and *Land Before Time®* (IN ZONE Brands, 2004). The Fluid Milk Processor Promotion Board has used cartoon characters such as Garfield the cat, Superman™, Rugrats®, and Blue's Clues™ characters to promote the consumption of milk in children to promote bone health (Graetzer, 2005).

Cascadian Farm® promotes a high-fiber and reduced-sugar RTE breakfast cereal featuring Clifford the Big Red Dog™ (Cascadian Farm,

2003). Cascadian Farm built on its marketing of Clifford Crunch cereal to create "Clifford's Guide to the Guidelines." This online resource is an example of how some companies are reaching out to engage parents by providing tools for them to create healthful diets for their children. The guide was designed to help parents understand and follow the 2005 U.S. Department of Health and Human Services (DHHS)/USDA Dietary Guidelines for Americans when planning their children's meals (General Mills, 2005c; Chapters 2 and 3). Recently, Nickelodeon announced that it has begun licensing its popular cartoon spokescharacters, SpongeBob SquarePants® and Dora the Explorer®, to produce companies for promoting fruits and vegetables such as carrots and spinach, although it will still be used on less healthful branded processed food products (Smalls, 2005b). In addition, Sunkist® has recently collaborated with Sesame Workshop™ to encourage children and youth to choose citrus fruits as a healthful snack alternative, using *Sesame Street*'s Cookie Monster® (Sunkist, 2005). Long-term evaluations of the use of licensed characters are needed to assess the characters' appeal and influence on children's food preferences and consumption habits.

Food and beverage companies also use the highly profitable market of children's toys, books, and clothing to co-brand their products. In the toy market, Mattel's Barbie® doll has a variety of food-related dolls including McDonald's Fun Time™ Barbie (Mattel, 2001) and The Coca-Cola® Barbie® series (Mattel, 2005). Each of the dolls comes with the food company's logo and miniature examples of the company's products (CSPI, 2003; Samuels et al., 2003; Mattel, 2005). Hasbro offers several Play-Doh® play sets for children featuring familiar food brands such as Little Debbie®, Chuck E. Cheese®, and Lunchables®. Easy-Bake Oven® play sets from Hasbro provide children with real-life examples of branded foods. Examples feature Chips Ahoy®, Oreos®, Pizza Hut®, and M&M's® (Story and French, 2004).

Marketing tie-ins with children's movies and fast food are becoming more common (Lippman and McKay, 2001). For the first three Harry Potter™ movies, The Coca-Cola Company spent $287 million on a co-branding campaign (Walley, 2002), which guaranteed tie-ins with the movie and the character of Harry Potter™ in any promotional material through product packaging, games, the website, and in-store displays (Lippman and McKay, 2001). In partnership with DreamWorks entertainment company, Baskin-Robbins ran Sinbad-themed television spots endorsing its deep blue menace sundae and Sinbad's triple punch sherbet (PRIMEDIA Business Magazines & Media, 2004), and Masterfoods' M&M's® new color-changing candies, M&M's® Magic Minis, had Sinbad themes (PRIMEDIA Business Magazines & Media, 2004).

Two QSR chains, McDonald's Corporation and Burger King, maintain exclusive contracts with movie production companies. Burger King partners with DreamWorks and Nickelodeon for co-branding (Ordonez, 2001). In 1996, McDonald's Corporation signed a 10-year contract with Disney (McDonald's Corporation, 1996). It has also started a new multicategory licensing initiative called McKIDS™ that unifies its branded product line including toys, interactive videos, books, and DVDs to reflect active lifestyles (McDonald's Corporation, 2003). In 2005, the McKIDS™ line of products will offer branded bikes, scooters, skateboards, outdoor play equipment, and interactive DVDs.

Finding: The use of child-oriented licensed cartoon and other fictional or real-life spokescharacters has been a prevalent practice used to promote low-nutrient and high-calorie food and beverage products. Use of such characters to promote more healthful foods, particularly for preschoolers, is relatively recent.

Celebrity Endorsement

Manufacturers of CSDs have become highly competitive to capture the youth market, and youth appeal is being built into advertising targeted to broader audiences and specifically to adolescents. Celebrity endorsements of CSDs, such as the popular cola wars advertisement between Britney Spears, who advertised Pepsi®, and Christina Aguilera, who endorsed Coca-Cola®, links a brand to a fan base (TTT West Coast, 2002), and are designed to appeal to older children, tweens, and teens in the course of their exposure to advertising in adult and prime-time programming. Celebrity endorsement is also used for products from categories viewed as more healthful. Since 1994, the Fluid Milk Processor Promotion Board has sponsored the popular "Milk Mustache" celebrity advertising campaign that has featured entertainers and athletes promoting the benefits of milk and milk product consumption to promote bone health and to prevent osteoporosis, especially targeted to teens (Graetzer, 2005).

Premiums and Premium Advertising

Premium offers, such as toys or giveaways, are commonly used in children's food marketing. The Coca-Cola Company, which considered youth an important market for its drink by the early 1930s, was one of the first companies to use premiums to market to children and teens, which included special offers and premiums such as yo-yos, marbles, jump ropes, kites, whistles, wagons, and scooters provided by local bottlers (Petretti, 1992). Premiums are often used in RTE breakfast cereal marketing. The practice of providing product "news" on a cereal package was used as an added incentive to make the food product desirable with the premium centrally featured in an advertisement. The most successful RTE breakfast cereal premiums were "collectibles," such as action figures from a movie; children were encouraged to buy the same brand to acquire an entire collection. Premiums have included beauty kits (e.g., Brach's Rapunzel fruit snacks), trading cards (e.g., Nabisco Ritz crackers), dolls (e.g., Kellogg's Rice Krispies), and an E.T. Finger Flashlight (e.g., Kraft Food's Oreo O's cereal) (CSPI, 2003). At many QSR chains, meals are created and marketed as child-specific portion-sized meals that contain premiums and premium advertising inside the container to attract children and their parents to QSRs (Schlosser, 2001). In some cases, children are encouraged to purchase a product several times to obtain a toy or the other premium (CSPI, 2003). A variety of marketing opportunities promote collectible brands that increase in value over time (Neopets®, 2003). McDonald's Corporation celebrated its 25th anniversary of the Happy Meal by providing Ty Teenie Beanie Babies® as a collectible premium (McDonald's Corporation, 2004).

Media Use and Advertising Exposure

Information and data about the types and roles of the multiple media are changing rapidly, without common databases or categories. This means that there will inevitably be some uncertainty and some inconsistency in the ways available data may be interpreted. The descriptions that follow are intended to provide a general sense of the trends, in the face of the uncertainty.

Media Use Patterns

Television. Television advertising has been the largest media carrier of food and beverage marketing to children and adolescents. At the end of the 1950s, 87 percent of American households had televisions, which were the primary venues for advertising to children and parents (Alexander et al., 1998). Today, nearly all children ages 2–18 years live in households with a television—60 percent have three or more television sets (Roberts et al., 1999). Approximately 60 percent of all meals that the average family eats together are consumed while the television is on (Roberts et al., 2005). One-third (36 percent) of young children under age 6 years have a television in their own bedrooms (Rideout et al., 2003), as do two-thirds of those 8 years and older (Roberts et al., 1999; Roberts et al., 2005). Children and youth who have a television in their own bedrooms tend to watch more television than children who do not, and their parents have fewer rules about their children watching television (Roberts et al., 2005).

Television becomes a part of children's lives from infancy onward

(Rideout et al., 2003). Studies suggest that even 1- and 2-year-old children watch television regularly (Barr and Hayne, 1999; Meltzoff, 1988), and between the ages of 2 and 4, children view approximately 2 hours of television a day (Rideout et al., 2003). By elementary school, television viewing increases to more than 3 hours a day of "live" broadcasts, or more if videotaped watching is included (Comstock and Scharrer, 1999; Roberts and Foehr, 2005; Roberts et al., 2005). After age 14, "live" television viewing drops slightly to about 2.5 hours a day during late adolescence (ages 15–18) (Roberts and Foehr, 2005).

Although television viewing remains the vehicle through which children and youth spend a significant amount of their discretionary recreational time, they are also now using other types of electronic media, including video games, DVDs, computers, and wireless devices that provide access to the Internet (Rideout et al., 2003, 2005; Roberts et al., 1999, 2005; Rubin, 2004). In fact, it appears that, when given a choice, children and adolescents choose the Internet over television by a two-to-one margin (Gardner, 2000).

Computer use. Computer use begins early in life and increases rapidly. An estimated 21 percent of children under age 2, 58 percent of 3- to 4-year-olds, and 77 percent of 5- to 6-year-old children use a computer (Calvert et al., 2005; U.S. Department of Education, 2003). By the time they are 3 to 4 years old, many children can turn on a computer, point and click with a computer mouse, load a CD-ROM, and use or "surf" the Internet (Calvert et al., 2005).

From 2000 to 2005, the percentage of 8- to 18-year-olds who have computers in their homes increased from 73 percent to 86 percent, and three-quarters of them have Internet connections at home (Roberts et al., 2005). Between 1998 and 2001, the percentage of teens ages 14–18 years using the Internet increased from 51 percent to 75 percent, and the percentage of tweens ages 10–13 years using the Internet increased from 39 percent to 65 percent (U.S. Department of Commerce, 2002). One estimate suggests that more than 34 million children and youth ages 3 to 17 years in the United States use the Internet, representing 20 percent of the total Internet user population (Rubin, 2004). However, there is a difference in access and use of computers and the Internet, based on demographics and socioeconomic status. Among children ages 6 months to 6 years, Hispanics/ Latinos are less likely to have used a computer than African Americans or whites (Calvert et al., 2005). Use of both computers and the Internet is higher among whites and Asians than African American and Hispanic/ Latino children (U.S. Department of Education, 2003). Children and youth ages 5 to 17 years who live with more highly educated parents or in households with higher family incomes are more likely to use computers and the

Internet than those who live with less well-educated parents or in lower-income households (U.S. Department of Education, 2003). While Hispanic/Latino and African American children and youth ages 6–17 years have less Internet access at home than white children and youth of the same ages, they have increased access to the Internet at school (Rubin, 2004).

Other media use and multitasking. Total media exposure differs by age, ethnicity, and gender. When multitasking is considered, the combined screen time of 8- to 18-year-olds drops to an estimated 6.5 hours per day (Roberts et al., 2005). Older adolescents report watching television, videos/DVDs, and movies less than tweens or older children. Specifically, 8- to 10-year-olds report viewing 4.75 hours of screen time and 11- to 14-year-olds report viewing 4.5 hours of screen time. There is a significant drop to about 3.75 hours of viewing screen time for 15- to 18-year-olds (Roberts et al., 2005). There are social and ethnic differences in media use patterns. Among 8- to 18-year-olds, African American children and youth report the most screen time (e.g., representing television, videos, DVDs, and movies) at almost 6 hours per day; Hispanic/Latino children and youth follow at about 4.5 hours per day; and white children and youth report about 3.75 hours per day (Roberts et al., 2005). Time spent multitasking is a prominent characteristic of the media use patterns of youth ages 8–18—with multitasking an activity for 36 percent of African Americans, 27 percent of Hispanics/Latinos, and 21 percent of whites during media use time (Roberts et al., 2005).

There are also differences in how children and youth allocate their time to each individual medium. Table 4-13 highlights the percentage of time children and youth report use of budgeted screen time for different types of media by age. Older teens (ages 15–18 years) spent significantly less time

TABLE 4-13 Percentage of Time Children and Youth Report Using Budgeted Screen Time for Different Types of Media by Age

	Television (%)	Video/Movies (%)	Video Games (%)	Audio (%)	Computers (%)	Print (%)
Total sample	35	13	9	22	11	11
Age						
8–10	39	16	12	14	7	12
11–14	38	12	9	20	11	10
15–18	28	11	6	30	15	10

SOURCE: Roberts et al. (2005). Reprinted with permission. © 2005 by The Kaiser Family Foundation.

watching television or videos and significantly more time using computers or listening to audio media (e.g., radio, CD players, MP3 players, multimedia) than children and young teens. While older teens also spent more time on computers, they spent less time using video games than children ages 8–10 years (Roberts et al., 2005). Use of newer types of media, particularly computers, the Internet, and video games, appears to occur without a reduction in the time devoted to more traditional forms of media such as television, print, and music (Roberts et al., 2005). Video games are a primary activity of the 22.4 million 2- to 18-year-old children, tweens, and teens who use the Internet (Byrnes, 2000). The video game industry is now estimated to be between a $7–10 billion market (Entertainment Software Association, 2005; McCarthy, 2005). Console and personal computer-based video games surpassed movie-ticket box office sales worldwide in 2002 (Mack, 2004).

Youth are particularly adept at using wireless devices and incorporating them into their lifestyles. They provide social connectivity and entertainment, as a way to build relationships, convenience and multitasking capabilities, and fill in gaps of free time or boredom (Cheskin, 2001). Children ages 10 and older are projected to be one of the fastest growing markets for wireless voice and data services (Williamson, 2001). A 2001 survey of youth ages 12 and older reported that 63 percent owned at least one mobile device—58 percent owned a mobile phone, 13 percent owned a beeper or one-way pager, and 6 percent owned a hand-held personal digital assistant (PDA) (Upoc, 2002). African American and Hispanic/Latino youth markets have very high mobile device penetration rates—59 percent of 12- to 24-year-olds from these ethnic groups own a mobile phone and 11 percent own a two-way pager (Upoc, 2002). The fastest growing group of users of mobile data is children ages 10–14 years (Thomas, 2004). Cell phones may be increasingly attractive to marketers because they offer direct communication with young consumers, either through voice or touch-key interactive programs, and they bypass parental monitoring.

Television Advertising Exposure: Amount and Content

Estimates of the amount and trends in television advertising exposure, like all media use, vary substantially and use different data sources and analytic techniques. Some estimates show higher levels of exposure and trends that are flat or moderately increasing. Other assessments generally show lower levels of exposure, and trends that are decreasing. All analyses show substantial exposure to television advertising by children and youth.

Most of the available research about children's media use and advertising exposure is derived from studies of television viewing (Chapter 5). Although new media options are evolving at an unprecedented rate, the largest recent studies of children's media use concur that television remains the primary venue for reaching children and adolescents with marketing messages, especially younger children (Rideout et al., 2005; Roberts et al., 2005). Television receives the majority of advertising budgets as a measured media category because it reaches a larger proportion of a targeted audience compared to the newer interactive media (Stanley, 2004).

Since the Federal Trade Commission (FTC) first considered television advertising to children in 1978, researchers have tried to estimate accurately the extent of commercial content to which children are typically exposed. The methodology by which most estimates have been derived consists of integrating evidence about children's normative viewing patterns with evidence about the amount of commercial time contained in children's programming or overall television programming (including adult prime-time television viewing). There are varying estimates of the total number of commercials that are viewed by children. The data presented in this section provide a background to these estimates and support the view that children are heavily exposed to commercials. What is not reflected in the available data are children's long-term exposure to other forms of marketing techniques in television programming such as product placement in children's programs, product placement in adult television shows that children may co-view with their parents, and product placement in videos and DVDs viewed by children and adolescents.

Television advertising to children began in the 1950s when persuasive messages were placed on youth-oriented programs such as *Howdy Doody*, *The Mickey Mouse Club*, and *Roy Rogers* (Alexander et al., 1998). Saturday morning emerged as a time for children's programming on all three major networks—ABC, CBS, and NBC. The significance of Saturday morning programming was that it was the first time that mass media programming was specifically dedicated to the child audience. The emergence of a block of programs dedicated to children allowed marketers to target children with advertisements designed for and directed specifically at them. As early as the 1950s, the hosts of television programs were marketing products within these programs (Alexander et al., 1998). Television became a venue for 30-second commercials that had memorable jingles and lively spokescharacters that advertised food products such as RTE sweetened breakfast cereals (Kotz and Story, 1994). Other food products that were often marketed during youth television programming included candy, snacks, cookies, and sweetened CSDs. Few television commercials promoted food options such as fruits and vegetables or reduced-calorie and noncaloric beverages (Barcus, 1981; Kunkel and Gantz, 1992).

Children and adolescents have television viewing choices today that did not exist more than 35 years ago including syndicated and cable television. Nickelodeon (2005) is an example of the numerous children's programming networks that exist today. Other networks such as ABC Family, Discovery Kids, Cartoon Network, Fox Kids, and the Disney Channel target this age group by providing children and teens with a variety of programming options. Radio is another medium through which marketers reach to children and youth. Disney has made this medium a viable channel for advertising both to children and parents, who often listen to the radio together in the car. Radio Disney also offers promotions and contests that involve audiences in more active interactions with products advertised (Radio Disney, 2005).

The Federal Communications Commission's (FCC) regulation of commercial time through the Children's Television Act of 1990 limited commercial time on children's programs to 10.5 minutes per hour on weekends and 12 minutes per hour on weekdays. However, food is the most frequently marketed product in television advertisements during children's television programming, and accounts for 50 percent of the total advertisements viewed (Coon and Tucker, 2002; Gamble and Cotugna, 1999; Kotz and Story, 1994). Some estimates suggest that children view a food advertisement every 5 minutes of television viewing time (Kotz and Story, 1994).

Estimates of annual exposure to television advertising from nearly three decades ago indicated that an average viewer (child or adult) would be exposed to more than 20,000 television commercials per year (Adler et al., 1977). Subsequent data gathered between 1983 and 1987 indicated that the average child, watching roughly 4 hours of television per day, would see more than 30,000 commercials per year for all products, including food and beverages (Condry et al., 1988). Based on advertising content data gathered in 1990, and extrapolation using children's viewing patterns, some have estimated that children currently view as many as 40,000 commercials on television and cable per year (Kunkel and Gantz, 1992; Kunkel, 2001). The increasing estimates stem primarily from the growing trend of airing 15-second commercials, rather than longer 30- or 60-second commercials, as was common in the past (TV Bureau of Advertising, 2005). Taras and Gage (1995), for example, observed an increase of 11 percent in the number of commercials aired per hour of children's programming between 1987 and 1993, despite the fact that the total amount of advertising time remained relatively stable.

Given an apparent, albeit small, drop in children's time spent watching television in recent years (Zywicki et al., 2004), this estimate merits additional examination. Two preliminary unpublished analyses of primary data have been made public and suggest a possible reversal of the childhood advertising exposure trend. The first analysis is based on 4 weeks of Nielsen Monitor-Plus/Nielsen Media Research data for 1977 and 2004 examining children's programs and adult prime-time programs, advertisements, and audiences (e.g., children ages 2–11 and 12–17 years) (Ippolito, 2005). The first analysis reports that children ages 2–11 years viewed a total of 22,000 advertisements for all products in 1977 versus 23,530 in 2004 (Ippolito, 2005). These figures include paid advertisements, which decreased from 20,000 in 1977 to 17,507 in 2004, and promotional advertisements and public service announcements (PSAs), which increased from 2,000 in 1977 to 6,023 in 2004 (Ippolito, 2005).[10] The second analysis is also based on Nielsen Media Research data and measured total food, beverage, and restaurant commercials viewed per child from 1993 to 2004 (Collier Shannon Scott and Georgetown Economic Services, 2005b). This unpublished analysis reports that the number of food and beverage advertisements seen by children in programs where children are at least half the audience declined approximately 13 percent over this period.

Advertising on television overall has been about 11.5 minutes per hour since the mid-1980s (Cobb-Walgren, 1990). An industrywide survey conducted by MindShare, a widely recognized advertising firm, confirms that the level remained virtually unchanged in 2001, with an average of 11 minutes and 24 seconds per hour devoted to commercial messages (Downey, 2002). Thus, the data reviewed strongly support that U.S. children and youth are currently exposed to a large amount of commercial advertising on television.

For several reasons, it is difficult to identify with precision the total amount of time children are exposed to television advertising. There are both age-related and individual differences in the relative mix of programming types and times that children may view, as well as variability in the amount of commercial content presented across channel types, program genres, and times of day. There is also a lack of clarity about the precise amount of time currently devoted to advertising on children's programming. One study in the 1970s measured the time as approximately 12 minutes per hour (Barcus, 1981), but a study in the late 1980s measured only 8.3 minutes per hour (Condry and Scheibe, 1989). Although the FCC regulations of commercial programming through the Children's Television Act of 1990 provide maximum limits, there is some indication that the FCC's policies are not always followed. For example, in 2004, the FCC fined Nickelodeon $1 million for violating the per-hour time limit 591 times for

---

[10]The major broadcast networks (e.g., ABC, CBS, Fox, and NBC) donate an average of 17 seconds an hour to PSAs out of an average of 17 minutes and 38 seconds an hour of nonprogramming content. This represents a total of 48 minutes per week per network. In 2001, the Advertising Council estimated that it received nearly $400 million in donated online advertising space (Rideout and Hoff, 2002). Industry estimates of PSA expenditures are higher. In 2003, U.S. advertisers report spending more than $1.7 billion on PSAs—$1.6 billion for television and $100 million for cable networks (Brown et al., 2004).

advertising in children's programming (Broadcasting and Cable, 2004), and enforcement actions against other channels for excessive advertising time have occurred in the past.

Marketing of food products has been a common practice on children's programming since the early days of television. In a study examining 24 children's programs from the 1950s, 45 percent of all commercials observed were for sweetened breakfast cereals, confectionery, or snacks (Alexander et al., 1998). Starting in the 1970s, content analysis researchers began to produce a relatively clear picture of the overall profile of products typically presented in children's television advertising. Patterns in the distribution of product types promoted in commercials during children's shows demonstrate strong stability since regular measurement began approximately 30 years ago (Kunkel and McIlrath, 2003). In general, about half of all commercials during children's television programming have consisted of food and beverage products, primarily comprised of RTE sweetened breakfast cereals, candy, CSDs and sweetened drinks, and QSRs (Gamble and Cotugna, 1999). This pattern can be seen in Table 4-14, which compares findings from three of the largest studies of children's advertising, one each conducted in the 1970s, 1980s, and 1990s.

Although there has been a decline in the percentage of commercials for the food product categories from the 1970s to the 1990s (Ippolito, 2005), food product commercials predominate in the advertising directed to children. From a chronological perspective, Cotugna (1988) reports that 71 percent of all such commercials are food advertisements; Kotz and Story (1994) report 56.5 percent; Taras and Gage (1995) report 48 percent; Gamble and Cotugna (1999) report 63 percent; and Byrd-Bredbenner (2002) reports 78 percent. The samples for these smaller studies are typically in the range

TABLE 4-14 Common Types of Food Advertising as a Proportion of All Commercials in Children's Television Programming

Product Type	Barcus (1977)	Condry et al. (1988)[a]	Kunkel and Gantz (1992)[b]
Cereals	25%	25%	22%
Candies/snacks/beverages	29%	17%	18%
Fast food/restaurants	10%	10%	6%
Total of primary food categories	64%	52%	46%

[a]Percentages were derived by combining data reported for advertising sampled in 1983, 1985, and 1987.

[b]Kunkel and Gantz (1992) report data for broadcast networks that yielded a total of 72 percent for these three categories, but their overall totals included advertising on independent broadcast and cable channels, which were not surveyed by the previous studies.

of 10–20 hours each, which may account in part for the range of outcomes; nonetheless the pattern is clear that food commercials predominate in television advertising directed to children.

On the other hand, there continues to be some uncertainty about the trends for the actual numbers of television commercials seen by children. An analysis of Nielsen Media Research data conducted for the Association of National Advertisers (ANA) and GMA reports that the number of food, beverage, and restaurant commercial impressions viewed annually by children ages 2–11 years has declined from 5,909 in 1994 (or roughly 16 commercials a day) to 5,152 in 2004 (or roughly 14 commercials a day) (Collier Shannon Scott and Georgetown Economic Services, 2005b). This is the first study to indicate any reduction in the number of television commercials seen by children. Preliminary findings of an unpublished study similar to the ANA/GMA study were presented publicly at a joint workshop sponsored by the DHHS and the FTC. That comparison covers a longer period, from 1977 to 2004, and reports a larger decline with 34 percent fewer food and beverage advertisements in programs watched mainly by children (Ippolito, 2005). Others have found either stability or increases in the number of food and beverage commercials appearing in children's programming during this same period (Byrd-Bredbenner, 2002; Gamble and Cotugna, 1999; Story and French, 2004; Taras and Gage, 1995).

With respect to commercial content, the content analysis research indicates that the nutritional characteristics of the food advertised in children's programming are generally for high-calorie (e.g., high sugar or high fat) and low-nutrient foods and beverages. Applying nutritional categories, Kotz and Story (1994) found that 44 percent of all food advertising in a sample of children's television programming were in the "fats, oils, and sweets" food group, the category of foods recommended to be the smallest proportion of one's overall food consumption in the USDA food guidance system. Taras and Gage (1995) indicate that 85 percent of advertised RTE breakfast cereals were high in sugar, as were 100 percent of advertised candy and sweets. In a more recent analysis of food advertisements viewed by children, Harrison and Marske (2005) found that 83 percent were for convenience or fast foods and sweets. Another analysis showed that sugar and corn syrup are the most common ingredients in food products marketed to children (Gamble and Cotugna, 1999). Virtually all studies find limited commercial advertising of healthful food and beverage products to children and youth such as for fruits or vegetables.

Young viewers are also often exposed to general audience oriented shows and the advertising that accompanies them. For example, far greater numbers of children watch such programs as The Simpsons on Sunday evenings than view any Saturday morning children's show, despite the fact that the latter group has a much higher concentration of children in the audience although smaller numbers overall.

Similar findings for general audience programming that may be seen by children are reported by Kuribayashi et al. (2001), who compared commercials on Saturday morning children's shows to Saturday evening adult programs. These researchers categorized foods as "unhealthy" if they contained significant amounts of fat (30 percent or more), sodium (360 mg), cholesterol (35 mg), or sugar (33 percent of calories). Applying this definition, the researchers found that 78 percent of food advertising during evening programming was for less healthful food products, compared to 97 percent for the children's programs.

There are limited data for determining the types of food and beverage advertisements seen by children and youth of different racial and ethnic groups. Two content analysis studies found that food advertisements aired on prime-time television programs directed to African American households feature more high-calorie and low-nutrient food and beverage products than prime-time programs intended for white audiences (Henderson and Kelly, 2005; Tirodkar and Jain, 2003). There has been limited funding to support research to study the relationship between English-language and Spanish-language television viewing and Hispanic/Latino children and youth in the United States (Subervi-Velez and Colsant, 1993), despite a variety of Hispanic-oriented media (Endicott et al., 2005). There were no content analyses of food and beverage advertisements directed at Hispanic/Latino children and youth available to the committee. This is an important area for future research.

Finding: Children are exposed to extensive advertising for high-calorie and low-nutrient foods and beverages and very limited advertising of healthful foods and beverages during their daily television viewing.

Print Media

Children and teens read a variety of magazines, ranging from fashion, sports, and entertainment to automotive and electronic games (MPA, 2004a). Some of the more popular children's magazines are *Nickelodeon Magazine, Sports Illustrated for Kids,* and *Disney Adventures* (CSPI, 2003), and some popular teen magazines include *Teen People, Seventeen, CosmoGirl, Dirt Rider,* and *Boys' Life* (MPA, 2004a). Advertisers use the magazines as vehicles to market to teens according to life stage, interests, and gender (MPA, 2004a). Certain teen magazines focus on celebrities and the entertainment industry, and teen publications carry advertisements as well as product placement (KFF, 2004). A recent survey conducted by Neopets® (2003) showed that more than 30 percent of teens' purchases were directly influenced by magazine advertisements for music, games, makeup, and clothes. According to that survey, magazines have even more influence on entertainment choices, persuading 37 percent of teens to see a movie in the theater and 36 percent to purchase a video or DVD (Neopets®, 2003). Recently, teen magazines have started to use the Internet to recruit individuals to inform the magazine staff about emerging trends in youth culture (KFF, 2004). For example, *Teen People* accesses a network of 9,000 "trendspotters" across the United States who keep the editorial staff up to date on teen issues and concerns (KFF, 2004).

Other Marketing Strategies

Newer marketing approaches directed at children are beginning to appear in Internet applications and video games, including advergames. In an era of television advertisement-skipping technologies such as TiVo and audience fragmentation, the placement of products in venues (e.g., television, films, music, the Internet) that are not readily recognizable by consumers as marketing venues has become a growing practice, with products integrated seamlessly into programming content (Balasubramanian, 1994; Gardner, 2000; Mazur, 1996; PQMedia, 2005). There are also event and loyalty marketing such as kids' clubs, school-based marketing, and promotions and public relations. Interactive technologies, particularly the Internet, and the more recent wireless technologies such as cell phones, are emerging in new interactive marketing plans (Calvert, 2003).

Systematic and reliable estimates are not readily available for how much marketers are spending in the newer media channels, but the amounts are substantially less than for traditional television advertising. For example, Wild Planet Toys spent only $50,000 for a 4-month online promotion rather than a $2 million traditional television advertising campaign (Gardner, 2000). Similarly, Nabisco spent less than one percent of its advertising and marketing budget at its online site, and produced games that could later be exported (Gardner, 2000). Advertising in and around online games is still relatively rare but is expected to grow rapidly, expanding from a $77 million dollar budget in 2002 to an estimated $230 million dollars in 2007 (Mack, 2004).

Outdoor media include the use of billboards, buses, and projected images. This type of outdoor promotion goes well beyond the traditional roadside billboard. Companies and brands are finding new mechanisms for marketing such as hot air balloons, sides of buses, and "wrapping" buildings and cars with promotional material and signage to generate attention and interest among young people. In 1998, a study conducted by the J. Walter Thompson Media Research Group concluded that outdoor venues can have a significant impact on children, especially when familiar brands or familiar characters are used. In the study, a campaign by the Fox Kids Network found that awareness of the network among children rose by 27 percent as a result of using billboards (Freitas, 1998).

Event and Loyalty Marketing

Event sponsorships can occur in a variety of settings including schools, shopping malls, and county fairs. The practice enables children to have a fun experience with brands and often to sample new brands (CSPI, 2003). Kids' clubs organized by specific companies represent a vehicle for these companies to target the child and teen markets. Kids' clubs distribute coupons and catalogs after learning vital demographic and consumer profile information through "member" registration (Consumers Union, 1990). Baskin-Robbins offers a birthday club program for children, offering a free coupon for a kid-size scoop of ice cream on the child's birthday (Baskin-Robbins, 2005). Kids' clubs and birthday clubs target children through e-mail and direct mail to the home mailbox. Coupons and catalogs are forms of advertising and promotional efforts to encourage children to purchase items (CSPI, 2003; Consumers Union, 1990).

School-Based Marketing

Commercial activities in schools appear to be increasing, although published documentation is limited. In one survey of high school principals, half—51.1 percent—believed that corporate involvement in their school had increased within the previous 5 years (Di Bona et al., 2003), the largest involvement being in the form of incentive programs (41.4 percent). Such changes have been noted by the press. An analysis of media references to school commercialism has found significant increases over the past 6 years (Molnar, 2003). These trends have raised particular concerns due to the extent of the activities and the vulnerabilities of children (Palmer et al., 2004). Reasons for the increase of in-school marketing to children and adolescents include the desire to increase sales and generate product loyalty, the ability to reach large numbers of children and adolescents in a contained setting, and the financial vulnerability of schools due to chronic funding shortages (Story and French, 2004).

In-school commercial activities related to food and beverages include product sales, direct advertising, indirect advertising, and marketing research on students (GAO, 2000; Palmer et al., 2004; Story and French, 2004). Direct advertising seeks to gain students' discretionary money through a diversity of in-school venues, while indirect advertising and marketing conveys a favorable industry image to students which may influence their brand preferences, brand loyalty, and purchasing behaviors (GAO, 2000). Examples of marketing practices used in schools are shown in Table 4-15.

Multimillion-dollar contracts between manufacturers and school systems have become common. One of the most controversial contract practices is the "pouring contract" or "pouring rights" with school districts for the exclusive use of particular brands of beverages (Nestle, 2000). Many of these contracts are negotiated on a districtwide basis and offer a specified amount for signing a multiyear contract, with additional funds tied to success in meeting specified sales quotas (Nestle, 2000). In 1998, more than 100 schools or school districts had signed exclusive contracts to sell either Coke® or Pepsi®, and by 2000, there were an estimated 180 "pouring rights" contracts in 33 states (Nestle, 2000). In 2001, The Coca-Cola Enterprises had signed 20 exclusive multiyear contracts (McKay, 2001). Recent media attention about food and beverage marketing practices to children has led companies to change their school programs. The Coca-Cola Company and its bottlers have publicly stated that they have collaborated with leaders from major educational institutions to develop model guidelines for school beverage sales and partnerships (Short, 2005; The Coca-Cola Company, 2003). In 2005, the American Beverage Association (ABA) developed new school vending policy guidelines restricting the sale of beverages in elementary, middle, and high schools (ABA, 2005b), discussed later in the chapter.

Contract arrangements are also made with QSR chains to sell food on the school premises, a form of competitive foods to the National School Lunch Program (Chapters 3 and 6). Additional ways to raise funds for schools include cash and credit rebate programs in which stores or other businesses agree to donate a percentage of revenues generated by sales in the form of either cash or supplies and equipment. More traditional school fundraising activities include the sales of items such as candy by students or their parents (GAO, 2000).

Direct advertising seeks to gain the students' purchasing dollars through a diverse range of in-school marketing venues (e.g., billboards, posters, book covers, school buses, and kiosks). It also includes media-based advertising which goes directly into school classrooms, hallways, lunchrooms, and computer labs. Channel One has been the leading example of direct advertising in the classroom during school hours, providing schools free television equipment and satellite access in return for reaching approximately 8 million secondary students in 370,000 classrooms (Atkinson, 2005; GAO, 2000). Channel One was introduced in 1990 as a 10-minute originally produced news program that had content written specifically for teenage students and presented by young adult anchors and correspondents, accompanied by 2 minutes of commercials (Greenberg and Brand,

TABLE 4-15 Marketing Practices in U.S. Schools

Activities	Examples
Product Sales	
Food/beverage sales benefiting a district, school, or student activity	• Exclusive contracts or other arrangements between school districts, or schools and bottlers to sell soft drinks in schools or on school grounds
Branded fast food	• Contracts or other arrangements between districts or schools and fast food companies to sell food in schools or on school grounds
Cash or credit rebate programs	• Programs that award cash or equipment to schools in proportion to the value of store receipts or coupons collected by the schools (e.g., cereal box tops, food product labels)
Fundraising activities	• Short-term sales of candy, pizza, cookie dough, and other products by parents, students, or both to benefit a specific student population or club
Direct Advertising	
Advertising in schools, in school facilities, and on school buses	• Billboards and signs in school corridors, sports facilities, or buses
	• Product displays
	• Corporate logos or brand names on school equipment, such as marquees, message boards, scoreboards, and backboards
	• Advertisements, corporate logos, or brand names on posters, book covers, and student assignment books
Advertisements in school publications	• Advertisements in sports programs, yearbooks, school newspapers, and school calendars
Media-based advertising	• Televised advertisements aired by Channel One or commercial stations
	• Screen-saver advertisements, corporate logos, or brand names on computers
Samples	• Free snack foods or beverages
Indirect Advertising	
Industry-sponsored educational materials	• Teaching materials and nutrition education kits from food companies that incorporate the sponsor's products or promote the sponsor's brand
	• Nutrition information produced by trade associations (e.g., dairy, meat, egg, sugar association)
Industry-sponsored contests and incentives	• Pizza Hut's Book-It program, McDonald's McSpellIt Club
Industry grants or gifts	• Industry gifts to schools that generate commercial benefits to the donor
Marketing Research	
Surveys or polls	• Student questionnaires or taste tests
Internet panels	• Use of the Internet to poll students' responses to computer-delivered questions
Internet tracking	• Tracking students' Internet behavior and responses to questions at one or more websites

SOURCES: GAO (2000); Story and French (2004).

1993). A content analysis of commercials that aired on Channel One in the early 1990s revealed that in the commercials examined, 86 percent were for products (including candy, gum, and chips) and 14 percent were for PSAs (Wulfemeyer and Mueller, 1992). Its advertising revenue decreased from $50.2 million in 2002 to $39.1 million in 2004, in part due to decisions by companies such as Kraft Foods and the Kellogg Company to eliminate in-school marketing (Atkinson, 2005).

Indirect advertising in schools encompasses a range of activities. One of the most controversial forms of indirect advertising is industry-sponsored educational materials (SEMS), which are materials donated by corporations to supplement the curriculum. In its evaluation of 77 SEMS, Consumers Union found nearly 80 percent to be either biased or topically incomplete (Consumers Union, 1995). Other common forms of indirect advertising include the following: industry-sponsored contests or incentives (e.g., providing coupons for free pizza for reading a specified number of books); inclusion of brand-name products as examples in textbooks; provision of industry-sponsored teacher training; donation of hardware for computer labs; or branded scoreboards for gymnasiums or athletic fields.

The National Association of Secondary School Principals (NASSP) has developed guidelines for school beverage partnerships that apply to middle schools and high schools that address vending machine policies, use of logos and signage on school grounds, visibility of company logos, and product promotions and fundraising in schools (NASSP, 2005). Additionally, many state and local school districts have enacted legislation regarding the availability and nutritional quality of beverages sold in public schools (Chapter 6).

Finding: The competitive multifaceted marketing of high-calorie and low-nutrient food and beverage products in school settings is widely prevalent and appears to have increased steadily over the past decade.

New Venues and Vehicles

New and innovative marketing approaches that are used in the adult marketplace are now being adapted for children and youth (Kaikati and Kaikati, 2004), including marketing research. Emerging marketing practices often blur the line between product and content through practices such as product placement in movies, television programs, websites, or games; viral marketing; information collection from youth as they spend time on Internet websites; interactions with online dialogues; and video news releases (Gardner, 2000; Mazur, 1996). At home and in public, children and youth are surrounded by a mobile, fast-paced, high-tech world, which they find comfortable, easy to navigate, and populated with branded characters.

Many websites collect aggregate data from the children who visit them; however the Children's Online Privacy Protection Act (COPPA) requires parental permission before children ages 12 and younger can provide personal data that may be used in future advertisements directed to them (Montgomery, 2001; Chapter 5).

The Internet and Websites

The Internet is a form of measured media that provides many opportunities for marketers to reach children and adolescents about food choices. Online interactive technology provides the means for companies to attract and develop one-to-one relationships with youth through websites for games, contests, discounts, and prizes. Many websites require registration to visit; therefore, all personal information such as a child's or teen's e-mail address, home address, age, and phone number are stored. Children can be sent promotional items, such as newsletters and coupons, to their e-mail address for redemption. "Cookies" can also be placed on individual computers to trace the online activities of a child or adolescent. The tracking makes it relatively easy for marketers to connect advertising messages to youth at popular websites. Online advertising to older children and teens is becoming more common on sites where they purchase MP3 music files to download onto their digital music players. Websites with e-mail, chat rooms, and instant messaging capabilities are also very popular among adolescents and with marketers for targeting purposes. Nearly three-fourths of online teens use instant messaging (Lenhart et al., 2001).

With the advent of personal video recorders and TiVo that can limit exposure to, and the cost-effectiveness of, traditional commercials, creative alternatives are spawned. For example, many branded products marketed to youth maintain websites that are created to supplement traditional forms of mass media advertising, and they are much less expensive to create and sustain. These "branded environments" are popular with older children, tweens, and teens, and use a range of online activities to keep them on the website (Montgomery, 2001). Many popular youth television programs encourage children and youth to visit the website advertised during the end-of-show credits to provide an additional experience with the audience where they find tailored messages. These websites use attractive language, humor that appeals to teens, and interactive games that are likely to increase their appeal to underage youth (Williams et al., 1997). The video news release, in which companies circulate stories about its products, is another form of virtual advertising that is used on television by many news organizations (Mazur, 1996). This kind of technique is less expensive than traditional advertisements and not labeled as an advertisement for the public, which views it as a news program.

Product Placement Across Multiple Forms of Media

Product placement is a marketing strategy aimed at placing products in a visible setting outside a typical marketing context (PQMedia, 2005). Movie placement is a good example. Food product placement made its most prominent debut when Steven Spielberg's ET character ate Reese's Pieces® candy in the movie *ET*, and short-term national sales of the candy increased by 66 percent (Mazur, 1996).The role of product placement in television has become more popular over the past 5 years as an integral component of a larger marketing strategy (PQMedia, 2005). Product placements are increasingly being used across various media vehicles simultaneously including network and cable television programs; films; radio lyrics; pop, hip-hop, and rap music; videos and DVDs; comic strips; books; plays; video games; and advergames (Gupta and Gould, 1997; Holt, 2004; Mortimer, 2002). Marketers recognize the importance of product placement with children and youth who have grown up using technology and turn to other media outlets than television for entertainment and information.

Product placement is part of a broader segment of marketing services called branded entertainment (PQMedia, 2005). Although a product is visible in television shows or films, it is often not the focus, and fits seamlessly into the context of a story or program. Product integration is a special type of product placement where an advertised product is central to the program's content (PQMedia, 2005). Product placement is designed by media production agents to provide realism to movie and television scenes while attempting to influence viewers through increased brand awareness and product endorsement (Karrh, 1994).

Product placement in prime-time television programs and movies. Although product placement is prohibited by law in programs directed at children (Linn, 2004), it is common in prime-time television programming. There has been limited research investigating the frequency of placement of branded food and beverage products in television programming. One examination of their frequency on prime-time television programming found that nearly 3,000 brand appearances occurred in 154 prime-time programs over a week of programming aired in 1997 on the four major networks—ABC, NBC, CBS, and Fox (Avery and Ferraro, 2000). Some evidence shows that the amount of money spent on product placement for food and beverage products may be substantial. For example, The Coca-Cola Company paid $20 million for product placement on *American Idol*, a television program that is heavily viewed by tweens and teens (Linn, 2004).

Product placements are abundant in children's and teens' movies. In the 2002 film, *Spiderman®*, the action hero used his web-spinning capabilities to retrieve a can of Dr. Pepper® to quench his thirst. Heinz Ketchup® was featured in the movie, *Scooby Doo*. Another popular movie among children, *Spy Kids 2*, had a character opening a lunch box which included items such as a Big Mac®, french fries, and a CSD with the golden arches of the McDonald's Corporation prominently displayed. There has also been limited research on the effect of product placement in television or films on consumer behavior. In one study, children were shown amended versions of a brief film clip from a popular movie, half with a prominent branded CSD and half without the branded CSD. Those who had viewed the branded clip selected the branded beverage more frequently after the viewing (Auty and Lewis, 2004).

Product placement in music. The inclusion of branded beverage products into popular songs is emerging as a new type of product placement. Certain media and entertainment companies actively seek brand-spot placements on their CDs and DVDs while a growing number of industry sponsors seek product placements in hip-hop lyrics and music videos (Holt, 2004; Kaikati and Kaikati, 2004).

Product placement in video games and advergames. Product placement is also a growing phenomenon on the Internet. Companies typically retain a product placement agency for an annual fee, then pay additional fees for actual placements, with the cost dependent on whether the product just appears or if the product is actually used and labeled (Mazur, 1996). Video game manufacturers previously paid companies for use of their logos and brands in video games. Now the practice is reversing as video game revenues rival those for movies. It is estimated that industry sponsors will spend $750 million to embed products in electronic games including advergames and video games. Online advergaming revenue (including both traditional advertising and advertising within games) is estimated to increase from $134 million in 2002 to $774 million by 2006 (Fattah and Paul, 2002).

Although it is difficult to assess the impact that advergames (see below) may have on consumers' brand loyalty, a distinct advantage of embedding products within video games is brand repetition. The average online gamer spends 5 to 7 minutes on an advergaming site, which is an estimated 14 times the amount of time spent watching a television commercial (Fattah and Paul, 2002). Additionally, the nature of the interaction with product brands online compared with a television commercial is very different. An online user is an active receiver of marketing messages, whereas a television viewer may look away or leave a room during a television commercial (Fattah and Paul, 2002; CSPI, 2003). Companies survey consumers to determine positive brand impressions and branded product recall. Product recall demonstrates the effectiveness of this embedding. When players were interviewed, they generally did not find the product embedding intrusive or offensive (Fattah and Paul, 2002; Kaikati and Kaikati, 2004).

Food marketers are increasingly building brand awareness and loyalty through product placement through video games on CD-ROMs, consoles, or the Internet (Freeman, 1998). A successful game, regardless of the platform, is equivalent to a successful product because the consumer is engaged, interested, and focused on the product (Mack, 2004). Games offer the capacity to foster and enhance chat room "buzz" and "word of mouth," thereby compounding its promise as a marketing technique. Brands are placed in realistic situations within the video game to simulate their real-world use, to enhance branding, and to increase interest in specific products (Mack, 2004).

Traditional console or hand-held games are a more expensive venue for product placement than are online venues. In a console game, planning must be done in advance, and once it appears on the market, the product placement cannot be changed. Although slower than console games, simple flash animation games, available only on the Internet, can be created and updated rather quickly as one online version can simply replace an earlier version (Mack, 2004).

Advergames are Internet-based video games with a subtle or overt commercial message (Eisenberg et al., 2002). A recent unpublished analysis of Nielsen Media Research and Nielsen//NetRatings data examined the exposure of children ages 2–11 years to Internet entertainment sponsored by 23 food and restaurant companies. Findings suggested that entertainment content on food and restaurant websites accounted for a very small amount (0.025 percent) of the combined total Internet and television impressions for these companies (Collier Shannon Scott and Georgetown Economic Services, 2005b).

However, advergames are a way to build brand awareness and brand loyalty, ensuring that immersive branding occurs through extended periods of time of exposure versus an "impression," so that children and teens may develop favorable views and memories of specific branded products (Calvert, 2003). Food marketers are building brand awareness and loyalty with advergames such as "Big G All-Stars vs. Major League Baseball," a CD-ROM game in which cereal characters from General Mills play against major league baseball teams (Freeman, 1998). The Hostess Company has a website featuring interactive advergames with the Twinkie® brand intended for children ages 7 to 11 years. Although the website does not sell products or provide information about the products, it serves to imprint the brand name and build brand loyalty among children (Hunter, 2002). Advergaming has also reached toddlers and infants with familiar rhymes within carefully designed Internet-based games (Friedman, 2001).

While gaming has generally been favored by boys more than girls (Subramanyam et al., 2001), most companies now attempt to attract both genders through a branded advergame that revolves around action or role play (Mack, 2004). Websites that are popular with tween girls, such as Neopets.com®, use marketing techniques such as product placement and immersive advertising, which integrates sponsors' products or services into activities available on a website (Fonda and Roston, 2004; Neopets®, 2005). In the land of Neopia®, children create pets with cuddly names and the play with them (Snider, 2002). In the Neopia® food shop, young children can "spend" their Neopoints to purchase Uh Oh Oreo® cookies, Nestlé Swee-Tarts®, and Laffy Taffy® candy. They can gain Neopoints by viewing cereal advertisements and Disney movie trailers and participate in marketing surveys. Tie-ins to new CDs and other products are also featured. Neopets® advertisers include Discovery Kids Channel, Disney, Frito-Lay, General Mills, Hasbro, Kellogg Company, Kraft Foods, Mars, McDonald's Corporation, Nabisco, Nestlé, Universal Studios, and Warner Brothers (Neopets®, 2005). Although Neopets® was initiated in 2000, the company describes itself as "the world's largest and fastest growing youth entertainment network on the Internet" (Neopets®, 2005). Neopets® describes itself as having pioneered the technique called "immersive advertising," which seamlessly integrates sponsors' products or services into activities available on the Neopets.com® website (Neopets®, 2005). Neopets® reports that it has 30 million members, 39 percent under 13 years of age, and 40 percent between 13–17 years of age (Neopets®, 2005). Postopia.com® is another website. Hosted by Viacom International, the parent company of Nickelodeon, it features Kraft Foods' food and beverage brands (Viacom International, 2005). Another website, Candystand.com®, is hosted by various companies that make confectionery such as Life Savers® and provides arcade games, card games, and downloads (Skyworks Technologies, 2004).

Digital Television

A new marketing technique called "interactive product placement" merges television and the Internet through channels such as digital television and Web television. With these technologies becoming more available, products are expected to become featured as part of program stories and will be available for purchase by clicking a mouse that is connected to a television screen (Montgomery, 2001). This type of interactive media that allows the purchase of merchandise through television using a remote control is also called "t-commerce" or "embedded commerce," and is currently available on websites of television programs. A new form of technology will provide a one-click ordering opportunity from the television screen for all products including food and beverage products (Children Now, 2005;

Tarpley, 2001). This type of technology may also allow marketers to track and store users' personal data for marketing purposes (Children Now, 2005).

Viral Marketing

Viral marketing is a form of "under the radar" marketing (sometimes called "stealth marketing" in popular vernacular), which represents the "buzz" or "word of mouth," which occurs when people talk about a product to one another, either with real words or through virtual communication through an electronic platform (Henry, 2003; Kaikati and Kaikati, 2004). Viral marketing may be effective with teens, particularly if discounts, desirable products, and free premiums are provided (Schor, 2004). Buzz or viral marketing functions in the electronic marketplace through trendsetters who "seed" messages, brand preferences, and incentives (e.g., gift coupons for websites, product samples) (Gladwell, 2000). In some instances, the trendsetters may receive training and be aware of their role. In other instances, it is entirely web-based communication, creating a "blogging network." The buzz tools are Internet chat rooms, news groups, and "blogs" (e.g., personal online journals; the term is short for "web logs") (Kaikati and Kaikati, 2004).

With viral marketing, a company may hire young actors who sign a confidentiality agreement and then interact with unsuspecting consumers in a popular or public gathering spot. Music industry marketers have used the approach by sending pairs of young, trend-conscious consumers into stores to talk about a new CD or DVD to each other, knowing that they are overheard by unsuspecting customers (Kaikati and Kaikati, 2004). Although the strategies vary in venues and demographics, they share the same basic approach and goals, which are to arouse curiosity and encourage consumers to develop a focused interest in a specific product they may otherwise not have considered purchasing (Kaikati and Kaikati, 2004). Buzz marketing is often a component of an integrated media and marketing mix (Henry, 2003). The potential utility of viral marketing for food and beverage promotion is just emerging, in particular for CSDs, but its effectiveness is not yet known (Holt, 2004).

Mobile Marketing

Cellular telephones are now ubiquitous in the United States. Most cell phones are now able to process data services such as text messaging, information, Internet access, and entertainment. The Mobile Marketing Association has established a voluntary code of conduct for wireless marketing campaigns. One of the code's requirements is that consumers must select all marketing programs or be able to easily decline certain programs; however, not all marketers have followed the standards (Joyce, 2004). Although marketing through a cell phone can be legally achieved only with a recipient's consent, technological developments with cell phones and marketing efforts to older children and youth may significantly change this premise in the future. For example, The Coca-Cola Company launched a marketing campaign in Germany that allows consumers to send text message codes found under bottle caps in return for receiving a branded cellphone game (Red Herring, 2005). Young consumers are also enthusiastic adopters of text messaging and other mobile features such as transmitting electronic games on the Internet between friends (Calvert, 2003). Many marketers believe that the relative ease with which teens and tweens use mobile technology offers a large, untapped potential market (Preschel, 2005; Thomas, 2004).

In 2005, Nickelodeon and Verizon Wireless launched the Nick Mobile, which brings Nickelodeon video content to users of Verizon Wireless's V CAST wireless phones (Verizon Wireless, 2005). A selection of 1- to 3-minute Nickelodeon videos that have recognizable characters from *Dora the Explorer*, *Blue's Clues*, and *LazyTown* are available to view on cell phones (Verizon Wireless, 2005), and these videos may contain embedded food and beverage products.

Cell phones are also equipped with global positioning satellite tracking capabilities and will be able to provide businesses and companies with the ability to "find" consumers anywhere and tailor advertising messages to them. For example, it is possible that an individual walking the streets of a major city may someday receive advertisements by cell phone instantly when passing by a store. Cell phones may also be used to allow young consumers to purchase products without using cash (Calvert, 2003), already occurring outside the United States. For example, consumers in Japan are able to use their mobile phones to purchase products from Coca-Cola™'s "Cmode" vending machines (Red Herring, 2005).

Adult cell phone users are able to download store merchandise coupons, instant-win games, and sweeps, and these features could potentially be used when marketing to children. Current mobile phone owners ages 12 and older were surveyed about their willingness to accept and use wireless coupons or special offers. Of those polled, 79 percent of African Americans ages 12–34 years and 61 percent of Hispanics/Latinos ages 12–34 years were somewhat or very likely to use wireless coupons or special offers (Upoc, 2002).

Finding: Food and beverage marketing is increasingly delivered through integrated vehicles other than the traditional television advertising (e.g., Internet, event sponsorships, outdoor media, kid's clubs, video games, advergames, product placement, music, and schools) that are especially appealing to children and youth.

COMPANY AND INDUSTRY GUIDELINES AND POLICIES

Self-Regulation: Children's Advertising Review Unit

Mindful of the need for responsible practices in marketing food and beverage products to children and youth, the industry has developed its own program of self-regulation that has two basic elements: (1) a code of practice, representing a set of ethical guidelines that provide oversight for the content of advertising activities, and (2) a process for implementing, reviewing, and enforcing the code of practice. The purpose of industry self-regulation is to ensure that advertising messages directed to young children are truthful, accurate, and sensitive to this audience, thereby "preserving their freedom to direct their messages to young children" (CARU, 2003b). To administer the industry program of self-regulation, the Children's Advertising Review Unit (CARU) was formed in 1974 to promote "responsible children's advertising." CARU is part of an alliance with the major advertising trade associations through the National Advertising Review Council (NARC), which is the body that establishes the policies and procedures for CARU. NARC members include the Association of National Advertisers (ANA), the American Association of Advertising Agencies (AAAA), the American Advertising Federation (AAF), and the Council of Better Business Bureaus (CBBB) (CARU, 2003a).

CARU's board consists of academic and business members. It is financed entirely by the business community, and receives support from the various sectors that advertise to children, including advertising agencies, toy and video game manufacturers, food and beverage companies, QSRs, and Internet providers (CARU, 2003b). CARU is the investigative arm of the advertising industry's voluntary self-regulation program for children and youth. Cases are brought to the attention of these two entities from competitive challenges from other advertisers, and also from self-monitoring traditional and newer media, including the Internet (CARU, 2003b).

CARU's *Self-Regulatory Guidelines for Children's Advertising* include seven basic principles for responsible advertising directed to children under the age of 12 years that relate to specific advertising techniques, such as advertising that involves endorsement and promotion by program or spokescharacters (Box 4-1). The CARU guidelines are adopted voluntarily and emphasize nondeceptive communication for children; however, CARU does not have oversight of product content or services being advertised (CARU, 2003a).

BOX 4-1
CARU's Principles in Advertising to Children

1. Advertisers should always take into account the level of knowledge, sophistication and maturity of the audience to which their message is primarily directed. Younger children have a limited capacity for evaluating the credibility of information they receive. They also may lack the ability to understand the nature of the personal information they disclose on the Internet. Advertisers, therefore, have a special responsibility to protect children from their own susceptibilities.

2. Realizing that children are imaginative and that make-believe play constitutes an important part of the growing up process, advertisers should exercise care not to exploit unfairly the imaginative quality of children. Unreasonable expectations of product quality or performance should not be stimulated either directly or indirectly by advertising.

3. Products and content which are inappropriate for children should not be advertised or promoted directly to children.

4. Recognizing that advertising may play an important part in educating the child, advertisers should communicate information in a truthful and accurate manner and in language understandable to young children with full recognition that the child may learn practices from advertising which can affect his or her health and well-being.

5. Advertisers are urged to capitalize on the potential of advertising to influence behavior by developing advertising that, wherever possible, addresses itself to positive and beneficial social behavior, such as friendship, kindness, honesty, justice, generosity and respect for others.

6. Care should be taken to incorporate minority and other groups in advertisements in order to present positive and pro-social roles and role models wherever possible. Social stereotyping and appeals to prejudice should be avoided.

7. Although many influences affect a child's personal and social development, it remains the prime responsibility of the parents to provide guidance for children. Advertisers should contribute to this parent–child relationship in a constructive manner.

SOURCE: CARU (2003a).

CARU's guidelines are formally supported by many food, beverage, and QSR member companies, including General Mills, Kellogg Company, Kraft Foods, McDonald's Corporation, Nestlé, and PepsiCo (CARU, 2003b). Many companies and trade associations representing the food and beverage industry have adopted some of these principles in their own sets of standards, such as accurate and age-appropriate advertising, acknowledgment of children's imaginations, and attention to the fact that children are often unable to distinguish a commercial from information. For example, in January 2005, Kraft Foods publicly clarified existing policies and announced changes in the company's product portfolio and advertising policies to children under 12 years of age. The company stated that it does not advertise to children ages 6 years and younger on television, radio, and print media; it discontinued advertising and promotion in schools, including Channel One; and it had developed nutrition standards for all products sold through vending machines in schools (Friedmann, 2005).

An independent assessment of company compliance with the CARU guidelines across a sample of 10,000 advertisements directed to children in the early 1990s found a high overall rate of adherence (Kunkel and Gantz, 1993). An assessment conducted by NARC (2004) suggested that within its designated technical purview, the CARU guidelines have been generally effective in enforcing voluntary industrywide standards for traditional advertising, and that the number of advertisements that contain words and images that directly encourage excessive food consumption in children has been reduced. Implicit in these findings, however, is their limited scope. The guidelines do not address issues related to the volume of food advertising targeted to children, the broader marketing environment, or the many alternative integrated marketing approaches that are rapidly increasing as primary strategies for reaching children and youth.

There has been growing concern among consumer advocacy groups about CARU's ability to monitor children's food and beverage advertising and newer forms of marketing across several types of media. In response to this concern, the Grocery Manufacturers Association (GMA, 2005a) recently proposed several changes to enhance CARU's resources, transparency, and enforcement capacity to strengthen the CARU self-regulatory system (GMA, 2005d). GMA's proposal includes provisions that would (1) expand CARU's advisory board to support the monitoring and review process; (2) allow CARU to work with advertisers to develop approaches that would encourage constructive and consistent healthy lifestyle messages; (3) strengthen voluntary pre-dissemination review of advertisements; (4) expand CARU's guidelines to address advertising contained in commercial computer games, video games, and interactive websites where children and teens are exposed to advergames; (5) prohibit paid product placement on children's programming; and (6) use third-party licensed characters appropriately in children's advertising. GMA also proposed two recommendations for the government. The first calls on the private sector to build a closer relationship with the FTC and DHHS to strengthen the voluntary self-regulatory system. The second is for the government to support the private-sector initiatives. GMA suggested that the DHHS develop an awards program that would recognize companies for promoting healthy lifestyles in such areas as consumer communications, employee health and wellness, community activities, product development, and public–private partnerships (GMA, 2005d).

Finding: Efforts by the Children's Advertising Review Unit have influenced certain elements of traditional advertising within its designated purview, but these standards do not address the impact of the volume of advertising, the appeal of its association with other elements of the popular culture for children and youth, or the influences of rapidly increasing marketing approaches. Furthermore, there is a need for a more formal evaluation of the effectiveness of its impact and enforcement capacity.

Food and Beverage Companies

Individual companies, and industry collectively, are motivated to make changes in their product portfolios toward more healthful choices in the marketplace for a variety of reasons, including expanding their market share, displaying social responsibility, avoiding regulation, and avoiding litigation. In terms of expanding market share, some companies are taking advantage of consumer interest in nutrition and health by developing and promoting new food and beverage products, and reformulating existing products, to meet specific nutritional guidelines. Several are also creating new packaging to reduce portion sizes of certain products, supporting community health and wellness initiatives, promoting nutrition education and physical activity in schools, initiating consumer research to develop more effective ways to convey nutrition information, and delivering information about more healthful company products to consumers. By manifesting social responsibility through the marketing of healthier products, companies anticipate strengthening both their market position and their credibility with consumers. Although hardly a mainstream practice, some early positive signs suggest the possibility for leading companies to serve as role models for the entire industry sectors (e.g., food and beverage companies, restaurants, entertainment sector).

Recent statements made by theAmerican Council for Fitness and Nutrition and GMA have acknowledged that the food and beverage industry can play a positive role in assisting children, youth, their families, and communities to lead more healthful lives (ACFN, 2004; GMA, 2005b). GMA's public statements also underscore a commitment to reverse the obesity trend in the United States, and acknowledges that the solution will involve a long-term investment as well as multiple and integrated strategies across many sectors (GMA, 2005b).

There is some indication that several of the leading food and beverage companies are reformulating some popular brands to eliminate or reduce *trans* fats and saturated fats as well as to develop reduced sugar, low-fat, or fat-free choices, and higher nutrient products, and to shift overall product portfolios toward healthier options on a small scale (Collier Shannon Scott and Georgetown Economic Services, 2005c; Friedmann, 2005; GMA, 2004; PepsiCo, 2004a; Powell, 2005; Taaffe, 2005). The shift in product portfolios has been stimulated in part by competition. Some companies have set internal goals to ensure that increasing portions of their revenues come from either new or reformulated products in response to consumers' growing interest in healthful options and concern about less healthful products. Several large companies have targeted their product research and development for all age groups. Consumer demand will assist in the development and reformulation of existing company products to more nutritious foods and beverages. A major challenge for these companies is to develop marketing plans and communication strategies that complement efforts undertaken by government and nonprofit groups to educate consumers about the distinguishing nutrition and health-related features of their particular brands within the context of general nutrition education, and how these messages fit into a healthful diet balanced with physical activity.

One strategy employed by several companies seeking to market more specifically on health grounds, has been the development of proprietary logos or icons that communicate the nutritional qualities of their branded products. PepsiCo uses the *SmartSpot*™ logo, Kraft Foods uses the *Sensible Solution*™ logo, General Mills promotes 14 different *Goodness Corner* icons, and the Kellogg Company promotes its *Healthy Beginnings Program* and its *Breakfast Nook* logo on packages to identify their products and convey nutritional content information to consumers (Collier Shannon Scott and Georgetown Economic Services, 2005c; Friedmann, 2005; Powell, 2005; Taaffe, 2005). Typically, such products are given "healthier" icons by the companies if they provide key nutrients at targeted levels, meet FDA specifications for "reduced," "low" or "free" in calories, fat, saturated fat, sugar, or sodium, or contribute to some functional benefit such as promoting heart health or hydration. While representing important steps toward drawing attention to more nutritious products, the array of categories, icons, and other graphics, as well as the different standards employed may introduce some confusion, particularly for young consumers, raising the need for standard and consistent approaches.

An example of work to embed an icon initiative in a larger effort is Kraft Foods' announcement of marketing changes to enhance the visibility of the healthier choices in its product line. Emphasizing the *Sensible Solution*™ labeling icon that provides a "flag" on food and beverage products that meet specific "better-for-you" criteria, Kraft announced a shift in the mix of products it advertises in television, radio, and print media viewed primarily by children ages 6–11 years during children's programming. The company has committed to advertising, over the course of 2005, only those products that meet its *Sensible Solution*™ criteria. In this plan, products not meeting these criteria (e.g., Kool-Aid® beverages, Oreos®, and Chips Ahoy!® cookies, and many types of Post breakfast cereals and Lunchables®) would no longer be advertised and would be progressively phased out in marketing communications in 2006 (Kraft Foods, 2005c). The company also announced that only the products that meet the *Sensible Solution*™ criteria will appear on company websites that primarily reach children ages 6–11 years, and it released a new line of Nabisco 100 percent whole grain cookies and crackers (Kraft Foods, 2005d). Still to be addressed are issues such as advertising to youth, ages 12–17 years, and application of the marketing guidelines to the use of fictional or cartoon spokescharacters on product packages, contests, premiums, and advergames on the Internet (CSPI, 2005).

In a narrower example, PepsiCo has announced an initiative focused on schools, in which it will provide 100 percent *SmartSpot*™ products and less-than-150-calorie single-serve packages in elementary school vending machines (Taaffe, 2005). For middle and high schools, it will provide 50 percent *SmartSpot*™ products that meet company-designated nutrition criteria of "good for you" or "better for you", and 50 percent "fun-for-you" products (that do not have any nutritional qualities) (Taaffe, 2005).

In addition to branded products, there are potential opportunities for packaging innovations for usually unbranded products to meet the de-mands of consumer convenience while meeting the goals laid out in the Dietary Guidelines for Americans. Fresh and dried fruits, vegetables, and whole grains have not been marketed extensively, perhaps because most are not branded products (Gallo, 1999). Due to the increasing concern about childhood obesity, new product and packaging innovations are expanding the availability of fruits, vegetables, and whole grain products to children and adolescents. The introduction of time-saving products such as bagged, prewashed lettuce and salad ingredients and "snack pack" shaved baby carrots have provided adult consumers and their children with convenient preparations and take-out options (Guthrie et al., 2005).

Finding: The consistency, accuracy, and effectiveness of the proprietary logos or icons introduced by several food companies as positive steps to communicate the nutritional qualities of some of their branded products to consumers have not been evaluated. Without an empirically validated industrywide rating system and approach, efforts to use such graphic por-trayals on food labels may fall short of their potential as guides to better food and beverage choices by children, youth, and their parents.

Full Serve and Quick Serve Restaurants

Some QSRs are also exploring ways they might market healthier products. For example, the largest QSR, McDonald's, announced both that it would seek to transform Ronald McDonald into a spokesperson advocating physical activity, and to introduce and promote some healthier food and beverage options that are lower in total calories and fat at its QSR franchises. Happy Meals now offer the choice of apple dippers (fresh, peeled apple slices) served with a low-fat caramel dipping sauce as an alternative to french fries, and beverages include apple juice and low-fat white and chocolate milk served in child-friendly containers (McDonald's Corporation, 2004). The company has also begun offering a range of premium salads that are lower in calories than burgers, french fries, and CSDs (McDonald's Corporation, 2005a; Warner, 2005). Additionally, McDonald's has announced that it will add nutritional information on its food packaging starting in 2006 (Barrionuevo, 2005). On the other hand, McDonald's also points out that their initiative is contingent upon consumer demand. An additional challenge is the special handling and packaging that the new offerings require due to a shorter shelf life (Plunkett Research Ltd., 2005).

The SUBWAY® chain restaurants developed the F.R.E.S.H. Steps initiative that was inspired by children and adults requesting healthier meals. The initiative was advertised as helping children and their parents to pledge to living more healthfully by being physically active and eating a variety of nutritious choices. The restaurant also offers voluntary nutrition information about their menu options, and lower-calorie options through the SUBWAY® Kids' Pak® meal that has less fat, saturated fat, and cholesterol than the burger and french fries. The sandwiches can be custom made to children's needs (Subway, 2005).

While the healthier menu options are gaining media attention, most QSRs continue to offer choices that are predominantly high in total calories, saturated fat, sugar, and salt. For example, Ruby Tuesday's operates a fast-growing chain of family-style restaurants known for their salad bar, sandwiches, soups, burgers, and platters. In 2003, the restaurant chain developed a program to provide consumers with nutrition information to make healthier choices at point-of-purchase. However, like other QSR and casual dining restaurant chains, they are gradually reintroducing high-calorie, high-fat choices on their menus because customers are not ordering the healthier low-calorie selections (Pressler, 2005). Many QSRs point out that since consumer demand is the true test of a healthier food and beverage initiative, their success is dependent upon a broader-based sustained societal effort focused on healthier choices.

Finding: Certain food and beverage companies and quick serve restaurants with products prominently consumed by children are actively exploring more balanced and health-promoting product development and marketing strategies. Prevailing industry practices, guidelines, and efforts remain limited.

Food and Beverage Retailers

Supermarkets and other venues such as convenience stores, drug stores, superstores, and warehouse clubs all influence consumers' choices through their display of healthful foods, beverages, and meals. Activities and changes implemented by some food retailers include offering products that are healthier, less costly, and packaged in smaller portions; promoting healthier products for children through special displays, shelf markers, cross-merchandising, incentives and premiums, in-store product samples, and related activities and events; and sponsoring school nutrition tours, Web and nutrition information on health and weight management, menu planning for children, and in-store health checkups including determinations of children's Body Mass Index levels (Childs, 2005). Nonetheless, a typical retailer is more likely to flag such items as CSDs, ice cream, and cookies in their promotions (Information Resources, 2005).

It has been suggested that retailers have both profit and public relations incentives to help consumers purchase and consume a healthful diet and to demonstrate that industry can be responsive to public concerns (IOM, 2005). Public-sector initiatives at the federal, state, and local levels might also facilitate activities undertaken by food retailers that support healthful diets, including public recognition, company awards for excellence, competitions, and performance-based tax breaks.

Finding: The food retail sector has taken some steps to promote healthful products to young consumers and their families, but there are abundant opportunities to do more to promote child-oriented foods and beverages that are healthful, visually accessible, and economically affordable.

Trade Associations

Trade associations represent the interests of food and beverage companies, restaurants, the entertainment industry, and the advertising and marketing sector. The GMA has taken steps to survey its member companies with regard to product development, product packaging innovations, providing consumer information resources, public–private partnerships, and the promotion of healthful lifestyles, employee wellness, and public health initiatives (GMA, 2004). GMA has also developed guidelines for competitive foods and beverage provisions in schools and advertising to children, emphasizing products in schools that meet the Dietary Guidelines for Americans; adhere to an age-appropriate product mix as determined by school systems; and ensure school administrators' control over vending machines, including choices of food offerings, locations, and times of operation (GMA, 2005b,c; Chapter 6). Although the GMA also has an active Food and Health Strategy Group and it endorses stronger CARU guidelines, as noted earlier in this chapter, it has not yet developed or institutionalized formal company guidelines, best practices, competitions, incentives, or recognition programs that encourage and reward its members to develop and promote healthier food and beverage products. Government agencies could provide technical assistance to help ensure the consistency of these efforts with sound nutrition principles, as well as to help in monitoring compliance and publicizing results.

The largest food and beverage trade association, the Food Products Association (FPA, formerly the National Food Processors Association), uses its scientific and laboratory capacity to provide technical support to member companies in their efforts to improve the safety and nutritional quality of their products, as well as to help them in the application of relevant policies—such as the Dietary Guidelines, *MyPyramid*, and food labeling requirements—to their product lines. FPA has also implemented various food and nutrition labeling education initiatives to help families and educators assist in making wise food choices, and FoodFit.com, a website devoted to promoting and enhancing the health of consumers through healthful eating and active living. It places an emphasis on advocacy for nutrition and health claims on food products to benefit consumer food choices, and has, in this respect, the potential to facilitate public–private collaboration on industrywide standards and graphic representation for products that support healthful diets (FPA, 2005).

The American Marketing Association (AMA) has developed its own guidelines regarding how its members conduct promotional activities. The AMA has stated that it is committed to clear communication and full disclosure of product risks, and its ethical guidelines for members emphasize that marketers must do no harm; marketers must foster trust in the marketing system; and marketers must embrace, communicate, and practice the fundamental ethical values that will improve consumer confidence in the integrity of the marketing exchange system (AMA, 2005b). Unlike CARU, the AMA guidelines are designed to govern the marketing practices of professionals rather than to encourage self-regulation by the food and beverage industry.

The American Beverage Association, representing distributors, bottlers, and vending machine companies, developed school vending policy guidelines in 2005 to limit the availability of CSDs in schools, and increase the availability of lower calorie and higher nutrient beverages.

Under the new voluntary industry-supported policy: (1) elementary schools would only make available water and 100 percent juice; (2) middle schools would only provide low-calorie or noncaloric beverages such as water, noncaloric CSDs, low-calorie juice drinks, 100 percent juice, and sports drinks during school hours and no full-calorie CSDs or full-calorie juice drinks with 5 percent or less juice until after school hours; and (3) high schools would provide a variety of beverage choices including bottled water, 100 percent juice, sports drinks, and juice drinks, with no more than 50 percent of the vending selections dedicated to CSDs (ABA, 2005b). The guidelines are supported by 20 companies comprising 85 percent of the U.S. school vending beverage sales by bottlers. Because the implementation of the policy is voluntary, determination of its effectiveness will depend on monitoring.

Media and Entertainment Industries

The media and entertainment industries have a powerful impact and important potential to change the social norms around food choices and physical activity behaviors. The news and entertainment media can potentially reach children, teens, and their parents through print, broadcast (television and radio), cable, music, and Internet-based programming that incorporates healthy dietary messages, images, and placements. Through news reporting, the media also has potential to strengthen their capacity to serve as interpretive and monitoring authorities with respect to the meaning of emerging findings in nutrition, the truthfulness of various nutrition claims, and the implications of developments for the nutrition and physical activity status of children and youth. Although various consumer groups have suggested certain criteria for media and entertainment practices related to food and nutrition, including the use of cartoon spokescharacter licensing and celebrity endorsements, the entertainment industry has not yet developed specific guidelines for their licensing companies. Similarly, the interactive video game industry as yet lacks standards that might guide food and beverage encouragement in the games used by children and teens (Walsh et al., 2004).

Several steps are under consideration by certain companies reaching large numbers of children. Nickelodeon, for example, supports balanced programming, which means that advertisements for food products should depict food and beverages within a healthful lifestyle. In 2005, Nickelodeon has reportedly implemented a companywide policy to discontinue advertisements that do not meet these standards (Smalls, 2005a). Nickelodeon is also changing the way their characters and brands can be used, limiting promotions that contradict messages that do not promote healthful life-styles, and eliminating the use of food in promotional activities including prizes in game shows and sweepstakes (Smalls, 2005a).

Health and Wellness Advisory Groups

A number of food and beverage companies, including Kraft Foods, PepsiCo, and McDonald's Corporation, have established advisory groups as a step to respond to a variety of marketing concerns. These advisory groups are intended to help the companies to develop strategies to promote more healthful food and beverage product options to consumers that are also economically viable. Examples include PepsiCo's Blue Ribbon Advisory Board (PepsiCo, 2004b), McDonald's Corporation's Global Advisory Council on Balanced Lifestyles (McDonald's Corporation, 2005b), and Kraft Foods' Worldwide Health & Wellness Advisory Council (Kraft Foods, 2005e). Members are intended to offer expertise in health and wellness disciplines that include nutrition, obesity, physical activity, public health, human behavior, and the impact of media on child development, and they are to assist the companies in developing policies, standards, and measures for implementing specific health-related initiatives. The long-term impact of these advisory groups is undetermined.

Public–Private Partnerships

Developing and sustaining partnerships that foster community-based health and wellness programs is an important component of promoting marketing of more healthful products to children and youth. A number of food, beverage, and restaurant companies have developed partnerships with sports, educational institutions, or scientific institutions to promote and encourage children and youth to lead more active lifestyles (Collier Shannon Scott and Georgetown Economic Services, 2005c). There are multiple examples. PepsiCo has developed a partnership with the University of North Carolina to promote a $4 million campaign called *Get Kids in Action* to reduce and prevent childhood obesity; a partnership with America on the Move called *Balance First* to disseminate lesson plans that teach the concept of energy balance in elementary and middle schools, with the goal of reaching 2.5 million U.S. students; and a partnership with the School Nutrition Association to develop wellness solutions in schools. General Mills has developed a partnership with the President's Council on Physical Fitness and the American Dietetic Association to promote *The Champions Program*. Kraft Foods has a partnership with the Latino Children's Institute to promote *Salsa Sabor y Salud*. The Coca-Cola Company has developed

Live It!, a health and fitness school partnership initiative advertised as helping sixth graders build healthier lifestyles (The Coca-Cola Company, 2005b). The impact and reach of these programs is undetermined.

Industry Coalitions

Many in the food and beverage industry are actively involved in various coalitions to promote healthier choices and lifestyles for U.S. children, youth, and their parents, and they have widely differing perspectives and strategies. The American Council for Fitness and Nutrition (ACFN) is a nonprofit coalition formed by more than 90 food and beverage companies, trade associations, and professional health and nutrition societies, including the American Dietetic Association and the American Association of Diabetes Educators, with the goal of promoting comprehensive and achievable solutions to the growing obesity rates in the United States (ACFN, 2004). ACFN members work in support of the CARU guidelines and initiatives that emphasize motivation rather than economic and regulatory incentives in child nutrition (ACFN, 2004).

The Advertising Council, a nonprofit member of the ANA, formed the Coalition for Healthy Children in 2005, also including the food, beverage, restaurant, and advertising industries. This coalition works to engage members to address childhood obesity by harnessing key messages into their internal communications programs as well as their advertising, packaging, websites, community-based programs, and marketing events with consistent key messages (Ad Council, 2005).

The Alliance for American Advertising (AAA) consists of a variety of food and beverage companies, and advertising and media associations, that works to discourage government regulation of advertising, and supports its members' ability to advertise to all people, including children (ANA, 2004). Members of the coalition include the American Advertising Federation, American Association of Advertising Agencies, ANA, General Mills, Kellogg Company, Kraft Foods, PepsiCo, GMA, and the Snack Food Association (Office of the Clerk, U.S. House of Representatives, 2004). The ANA describes the coalition members as supporting CARU's self-regulatory approach to advertising, public education approaches for addressing the causes of obesity, and supporting effective ways to reverse the obesity trend (ANA, 2004).

SUMMARY

Food and beverage products are among the products most heavily marketed to children and youth in the United States. The increased purchasing power, and influence of young people has drawn more and more industry attention, creativity, and resources to the production and marketing of food and beverages for children and youth. Product branding has become a normalized part of the lives and culture of American children and youth, and the majority of food and beverage marketing practices promote branded products instead of unbranded food groups. Marketers use a range of strategies to build brand awareness and brand loyalty early in life that is intended to be sustained into adulthood.

The growth rate in recent years in new product introductions for both food and beverage products targeted to children and adolescents, is greater than the growth rate for food and beverage products targeted to the general market. The majority of these new food and beverage products were branded products that are high in total calories, sugar, salt, fat, and low in nutrients.

Television remains the primary promotional medium for measured media marketing of food and beverage marketing to children and youth, but a shift is occurring toward other sales promotion such as product placement, character licensing, the Internet, advergames, in-school marketing, and special events marketing. Viral marketing and product placement that traverse many types of media are newer marketing strategies being used more commonly to reach consumers. Commercial and noncommercial content are becoming more indistinguishable, sophisticated, and blended, presenting a special challenge, given the limited capacity of younger children to process these messages cognitively. Guidelines developed by the National Advertising Review Council and administered by the Children's Advertising Review Unit have contributed to the enforcement of industrywide standards for traditional advertising. However, these standards have not kept pace with the expanded forms of marketing communication.

The heightened public interest in health and wellness and increased concern about obesity presents certain marketing risks—such as increased costs associated with developing, reformulating, packaging, test marketing, and promoting food and beverage products, as well as uncertainty related to creating and sustaining consumer demand for these new products—as well as potentially profitable yet unexplored marketing opportunities. Food and beverage manufacturers can compete for and expand their market share for healthier food and beverage product categories, be role models for the industry by substantially shifting overall product portfolios toward healthier products, and serve as socially responsible corporate stakeholders in the response to childhood obesity. In making positive changes that expand consumers' selection of healthier foods and beverages, despite the challenges of market forces and the marketplace, companies may avoid the risk of either government regulation or litigation.

Leading food, beverage, and restaurant companies have taken certain, limited constructive steps to develop more balanced and health promoting-strategies, such as reformulating or developing new products, changing product packaging to reduce portion sizes, establishing health and wellness councils, developing public–private partnerships to promote energy balance education in schools, and supporting community-based health and wellness initiatives. Still, the food and beverage industry, restaurants, entertainment and media companies, the food retail sector, and trade associations remain far short of their full potential to do much more to develop and consistently promote healthful food, beverage, and meal options to children and youth.

REFERENCES

ABA (American Beverage Association). 2004. *It's a "Bevolution": National Soft Drink Association Changes Name to American Beverage Association to Reflect Wide Range of Beverages Industry Produces.* [Online]. Available: http://www.ameribev.org/pressroom/111104namechange.asp [accessed June 12, 2005].

ABA. 2005a. *What is ABA?* [Online]. Available: http://www.ameribev.org/about/ [accessed June 12, 2005].

ABA. 2005b. Beverage industry announces new school vending policy: Plan calls for lower-calorie and/or nutritious beverages in schools and new limits on soft drinks. *News Release.* August 16. [Online]. Available: http://www.ameribev.org/pressroom/2005_vending.asp [accessed September 20, 2005].

ACFN (American Council for Fitness and Nutrition). 2004. *Tipping the Scales on Obesity: Meeting the Challenges of Today for a Healthier Tomorrow.* [Online]. Available: http://www.acfn.org/resources/TTS.pdf [accessed July 12, 2005].

ACNielsen. 2004. *Consumer Insight. Eighth Annual ACNielsen Consumer and Market Trends Report.* Schaumburg, IL: ACNielsen.

Ad Council. 2005. Ad Council announces collaboration to combat childhood obesity "coalition for healthy children." *News Release.* July 13. [Online]. Available: http://www.adcouncil.org/about/news_071305/ [accessed September 20, 2005].

Adler R, Friedlander B, Lesser G, Meringoff L, Robertson T, Rossiter J, Ward S. 1977. *Research on the Effects of Television Advertising to Children: A Review of the Literature and Recommendations for Future Research.* Washington, DC: U.S. Government Printing Office.

Alexander A, Benjamin L, Hoerrner K, Roe D. 1998. We'll be back in a moment: A content analysis of advertisements in children's television in the 1950s. *Journal of Advertising* 27(3):1–9.

Allen JC. 2001. The economic structure of the commercial electronic children's media industries. In: Singer D, Singer J, eds. *Handbook of Children and the Media.* Thousand Oaks, CA: Sage Publications.

AMA (American Marketing Association). 2005a. *Marketing Definitions.* [Online]. Available: http://www.marketingpower.com/content4620.php [accessed May 23, 2005].

AMA. 2005b. *Ethical Norms and Values for Marketers.* [Online]. Available: http://www.marketingpower.com/content435.php [accessed July 10, 2005].

ANA (Association of National Advertisers). 2004. *ANA Compendium of Legislative, Regulatory and Legal Issues.* [Online]. Available: http://www.ana.net/govt/2004_compendium.pdf [accessed June 29, 2005].

Apple & Eve. 2005. *Just for Kids.* [Online]. Available: http://www.appleandeve.com.kids.asp [accessed June 20, 2005].

Atkinson C. 2005. Channel One hits bump, losing ads and top exec. *Advertising Age* 76(11): 3–38.

Austin SB, Rich M. 2001. Consumerism: its impact on the health of adolescents. *Adolesc Med* 12(3):389–409.

Auty S, Lewis C. 2004. Exploring children's choice: The reminder effect of product placement. *Psychol Marketing* 21(9):697–714.

Avery R, Ferraro R. 2000. Verisimilitude or advertising? Brand appearances on prime-time television. *J Consum Affairs* 34(2):217–244.

Babin LA, Carder ST. 1996. Viewers' recognition of brands placed within a film. *Int J Ad* 15(2):140–151.

Balasubramanian SK. 1994. Beyond advertising and publicity: Hybrid messages and public policy issues. *J Advertising* 23(4):29–46.

Barbieri McGrath B. 1997. *The M&M's Brand Chocolate Candies Counting Board Book.* Watertown, MA: Charlesbridge Publishing.

Barbieri McGrath B. 2000. *Kellogg's Froot Loops! Counting Fun Book.* New York: Harperfestival.

Barcus FE. 1977. *Children's Television: An Analysis of Programming and Advertising.* New York: Praeger.

Barcus F. 1981. The nature of television advertising to children. In: Palmer E, Dorr D, eds. *Children and the Faces of Television.* New York: Academic Press. Pp. 273–285.

Barr R, Hayne H. 1999. Developmental changes in imitation from television during infancy. *Child Dev* 70(5):1067–1081.

Barrionuevo A. 2005. McDonald's to add facts on nutrition to packaging. *NY Times.* October 25.

Baskin-Robbins. 2005. *Baskin-31-Robbins® Birthday Club.* [Online]. Available: http://www.baskinrobbins.com/BDayClub/ [accessed June 7, 2005].

Beverage Digest. 2004. *Special Issue: Top-10 U.S. Carbonated Soft Drink Companies and Brands for 2003.* [Online]. Available: http://www.beverage-digest.com/pdf/top-10_2004.pdf [accessed June 10, 2005].

Boone LE, Kurtz DL. 1998. *Contemporary Marketing Wired.* 9th ed. Orlando, FL: The Dryden Press.

BrandWeek. 2005. *A Special Report: Superbrands. Plus: America's Top 2000 Brands.* [Online]. Available: http://www.brandweek.com [accessed August 8, 2005].

Broadcasting and Cable. 2004. Breaking . . . ABC family, Nick fined by FCC. *Broadcasting & Cable* October 25. P. 394.

Brown K, Endicott RC, Macdonald S, Schumann M, Macarthur G, Sierra J, Matheny L, Green A, Ryan M. 2004. 100 leading national advertisers. *Advertising Age* June 28. Pp. 1–83.

Brown K, Endicott RC, Macdonald S, Schumann M, Macarthur G, Sierra J, Matheny L, Green A, Ryan M. 2005. 50th annual 100 leading national advertisers. *Advertising Age* June 27. Pp. 1–84. [Online]. Available: http://www.adage.com/images/random/lna2005.pdf [accessed September 16, 2005].

Brownell KD, Horgen KB. 2004. *Food Fight: The Inside Story of the Food Industry, America's Obesity Crisis, and What We Can Do About It.* New York: The McGraw-Hill Companies.

Business Insights. 2005a. *The Top 10 Global Leaders in Food.* Brochure. [Online]. Available: http://www.globalbusinessinsights.com/etwodir/mailings/rc412/rc412pdfs/rc412j-brochure.pdf [accessed June 3, 2005].

Business Insights. 2005b. *New Profit Opportunities in Health and Nutrition to 2009.* [Online]. Available: http://www.globalbusinessinsights.com/etwodir/mailings/rc445/rc445pdfs/rc445e-brochure.PDF [accessed August 29, 2005].

Business Wire. 2005. *Mars, Incorporated Announces New Nutrition-Focused Business.* June 30.

Buzz Marketing Group. 2004. *Blue Fusion Releases National Youth Survey on the Brand Loyalty of Teens.* Press Release. [Online]. Available: http://buzzmg.com/pressrelease/040217.pdf [accessed July 12, 2005].

Byrd-Bredbenner C. 2002. Saturday morning children's television advertising: A longitudinal content analysis. *Fam Consum Sci Res J* 30(3):382–403.

Byrnes N. 2000. Babes in virtual toyland. *Business Week* 3672:62–64.

Calvert SL. 2003. Future faces of selling to children. In: Palmer EL, Young BM, eds. *The Faces of Televisual Media.* Mahwah, NJ: Lawrence Erlbaum Associates. Pp. 347–357.

Calvert SL, Rideout VJ, Woolard JL, Barr RF, Strouse GA. 2005. Age, ethnicity, and socio-economic patterns in early computer use. A national survey. *Am Behav Scientist* 48(5):590–607.

Cannondale Associates. 2005. *Cannondale Study Identifies Trade Promotion Best Practices.* Press Release. November 25. [Online]. Available: http://www.cannondaleassoc.com/upload/61525-39.doc [accessed July 28, 2005].

CARU (Children's Advertising Review Unit). 2003a. *Self-Regulatory Guidelines for Children's Advertising.* 7th ed. New York: Council of the Better Business Bureaus.

CARU (Children's Advertising Review Unit). 2003b. *About the Children's Advertising Review Unit (CARU).* [Online]. Available: http://www.caru.org/ [accessed November 10, 2005].

Cascadian Farm. 2003. *Cascadian Farm® Products.* [Online]. Available: http://www.cascadianfarm.com/cfarm/products/product_detail.asp?category=8 [accessed June 20, 2005].

Chaplin H. 1999. Food fight. *Am Demographics* 21(6):64–65.

Cheskin. 2001. *The Wireless Future: A Look at Youth Unplugged.* [Online]. Available: http://www.cheskin.com/docs/Sites/1/wirelessexecsumm.pdf [accessed September 11, 2005].

Children Now. 2005. *Interactive Advertising and Children: Issues and Implications.* [Online]. Available: http://www.childrennow.org/assets/pdf/issues_media_dtv_brief1.pdf [accessed October 11, 2005].

Childs N. 2005. *Selected opportunities for food retailers to address childhood obesity.* Presentation at the DHHS-FTC Workshop about Perspectives on Marketing, Self-Regulation, and Childhood Obesity. July 14–15. [Online]. Available: http://www.ftc.gov/bcp/workshops/foodmarketingtokids/index.htm [accessed September 23, 2005].

Cobb-Walgren CJ. 1990. The changing commercial climate. *Current Issues and Research in Advertising* 13(1-2):343–368.

Collier Shannon Scott, PLLC, Georgetown Economic Services, LLC. 2004. *Television Advertising for Food and Restaurants: Total Expenditures and Number of Commercials Seen by Children. A Report to The Grocery Manufacturers of America and The Association of National Advertisers.* October 1.

Collier Shannon Scott, PLLC, Georgetown Economic Services, LLC. 2005a. *Report Methodology Presented to the IOM Committee on Food Marketing and the Diets of Children and Youth for Television Advertising for Food and Restaurants: Total Expenditures and Number of Commercials Seen by Children.* April 11.

Collier Shannon Scott, PLLC, Georgetown Economic Services, LLC. 2005b. *Television Advertising and Internet Viewing of Food and Restaurant Messages: Total TV Ad Expenditures, Total Screen Time, TV Commercials and Web Pages Seen by Children.* May 13.

Collier Shannon Scott, PLLC, Georgetown Economic Services, LLC. 2005c. *Issues in Advertising and Promotion of Food and Health—IOM Panelists' Response to IOM Questions.* May 12.

Comstock G, Scharrer E. 1999. *Television: What's On, Who's Watching, and What It Means.* San Diego, CA: Academic Press.

ConAgra Foods. 2004. *Kid Cuisine Product Fact Sheet.* [Online]. Available: http://www.conagrafoods.com/brands/kid_cuisine.jsp [accessed May 8, 2005].

Condry J, Bence P, Scheibe C. 1988. Nonprogram content of children's television. *J Broadcasting Electronic Media* 32(3):255–270.

Condry J, Scheibe C. 1989. Nonprogram content of television: Mechanisms of persuasion. In: Condry J, ed. *The Psychology of Television.* Hillsdale, NJ: Lawrence Erlbaum Associates. Pp. 173–231.

Consumers Union. 1990. *Selling America's Kids: Commercial Pressures on Kids of the 90s.* [Online]. Available: http://www.consumersunion.org/other/sellingkids/ [accessed September 19, 2005].

Consumers Union. 1995. *Captive Kids: Commercial Pressures on Kids at School.* Yonkers, NY: Consumers Union Education Series. P. 29.

Coon K, Tucker K. 2002. Television and children's consumption patterns: A review of the literature. *Minerva Pediatrician* 54(5):423–436.

Cotugna N. 1988. TV ads on Saturday morning children's programming—What's new? *J Nutr Ed* 20(3):125–127.

CSPI (Center for Science in the Public Interest). 2003. *Pestering Parents: How Food Companies Market Obesity to Children.* Washington, DC: CSPI. [Online]. Available: http://www.cspinet.org/new/200311101.html [accessed September 19, 2005].

CSPI. 2005. Kraft advertising-to-kids policy applauded. *News Release.* January 12. [Online]. Available: http://cspinet.com/new/200501125.html [accessed September 22, 2005].

Dannon. 2005. *Our Products.* [Online]. Available: http://www.dannon.com/dn/dnstore/cgi-bin/ProdSubEV_Cat_240859_NavRoot_200.htm [accessed June 5, 2005].

DataMonitor. 2004. *Company Overviews.* [Online]. Available: http://www.DataMonitor.com [accessed July 19, 2005].

DataMonitor. 2005. *Company Overviews.* [Online]. Available: http://www.DataMonitor.com [accessed October 27, 2005].

Deutche Bank Securities. 2004. *Why TV Advertising Doesn't Work for Mature Brands.* May 18. Pp. 1–18.

Di Bona J, Chaudhuri R, Jean-Baptiste J, Menachem P, Wurzburg M. 2003. Commercialism in North Carolina high schools: A survey of principals' perceptions. *Peabody Journal of Education* 78(2):41–62.

Doss VS, Marlowe J, Godwin DD. 1995. Middle-school children's sources and uses of money. *J Consum Affairs* 29(1):219–241.

Downey K. 2002. *Clutter Rises Even in Weak Ad Economy.* April 5. [Online]. Available: http://www.medialifemagazine.com/news2002/apr02/apr01/5_fri/news2friday.html [accessed July 11, 2005].

Earth's Best. 2005. *Let's Make a Great Start to a Lifetime of Good Health.* [Online]. Available: http://www.earthsbest.com/sesame_street/ [accessed June 20, 2005].

Eisenberg D, McDowell J, Berestein L, Tsiantar D, Finan E. 2002. It's an ad, ad, ad, ad world. *Time* 160(10):38–41.

Ellison S. 2005. Divided, companies fight for right to plug kids' food. *The Wall Street Journal* January 26. P. B-1.

Endicott RC, Brown K, MacDonald S, Schumann M, Ryan M, Sierra J, Wentz L. 2005. Hispanic Pact Pack. *Advertising Age* (Supplement) July 18. Pp. 1–51. [Online]. Available: http://www.adage.com/images/random/hispfactpack05.pdf [accessed September 16, 2005].

Enrico D. 1999. Top 10 advertising icons. The Advertising Century: Special Issue. *Advertising Age* vol 43. [Online]. Available: http://www.adage.com/century/century.html [accessed April 11, 2005].

Entertainment Software Association. 2005. *Computer and Video Game Software Sales Reach Record $7.3 Billion in 2004.* [Online]. Available: http://www.theesa.com/archives/2005/02/computer_and_vi.php [accessed March 10, 2005].

ERS/USDA (Economic Research Service/United States Department of Agriculture). 2004. *Food CPI, Prices, and Expenditures. Food and Alcoholic Beverages: Total Expenditures.* [Online]. Available: http://www.ers.usda.gov/Briefing/CPIFoodAndExpenditures/Data/table1.htm [accessed June 17, 2005].

ERS/USDA. 2005a. *Food CPI, Prices, and Expenditures.* [Online]. Available: http://www.ers.usda.gov/Briefing/CPIFoodAndExpenditures/ [accessed October 27, 2005].

ERS/USDA. 2005b. Food expenditures. In: *Agricultural Outlook: Statistical Indicators.* [Online]. Available: http://www.ers.usda.gov/Publications/Agoutlook/AOTables/ [accessed July 7, 2005].

Fattah H, Paul P. 2002. Gaming gets serious. *Am Demographics.* 24(5):38–44.

FitchRatings. 2004. *Can Coca-Cola Products Be Replaced? The Future of the Beverage Industry and the Effect of Consumer Dietary Trends.* November 16.

FMI (Food Marketing Institute). 2003. *Shopping for Health: Whole Health for the Whole Family.* Washington, DC: FMI and Prevention Magazine.

FMI. 2004. *Supermarket Facts: Industry Overview 2004.* [Online]. Available: http://www.fmi.org/facts_figs/superfact.htm [accessed May 3, 2005].

Fonda D, Roston E. 2004. Pitching it to kids. *Time* 163(26):52–54.

Food Engineering. 2004. *The World's Top 100 Food and Beverage Companies.* [Online]. Available: http://www.foodengineeringmag.com/FILES/HTML/PDF/Top100chart.pdf [accessed July 12, 2005].

FPA (Food Products Association). 2005. [Online]. Available: http://www.fpa-food.org/ [accessed November 19, 2005].

Freeman L. 1998. Selling kids (building brand loyalty among children). *Food and Beverage Marketing* 17(6).

Freitas S. 1998. Reflecting America's Changing Face. *Advertising Age* 69(29):A6.

Friedman W. 2001. Nestle goes gaming. *Advertising Age* 72(43):50.

Friedmann L. 2005. *Marketing Strategies That Foster Healthy Food and Beverage Choices in Children and Youth.* Presentation at a Workshop for the Committee on Food Marketing and the Diets of Children and Youth. Washington, DC, January 27.

Friend B, Stapylton-Smith M. 1999, April. *Through the Eyes of Children.* Presentation at the ESOMAR Marketing in Latin America Conference. Santiago, Chile.

Gallo AE. 1999. Food advertising in the United States. In: Frazao E, ed. *America's Eating Habits: Changes & Consequences.* Washington, DC: U.S. Department of Agriculture.

Gamble M, Cotugna N. 1999. A quarter century of TV food advertising targeted at children. *Am J Health Behav* 23:261–267.

GAO (U.S. General Accounting Office). 2000. *Commercial Activities in Schools.* GAO/HEHS-00-156. Washington, DC: GAO. [Online]. Available: http://www.gao.gov/archive/2000/he00156.pdf [accessed May 3, 2005].

Gardner E. 2000. Understanding the net's toughest customer. *Internet World* 6(3):66–72.

Gatorade. 2004. *The Gatorade Story.* [Online]. Available: www.gatorade.com [accessed November 10, 2005].

General Mills. 2005a. *Brands: Yoplait and Columbo.* [Online]. Available: http://www.generalmills.com/corporate/brands/product.aspx?catID=55# [accessed June 5, 2005].

General Mills. 2005b. *New Go-GURT Smoothie Introduced By Yoplait.* [Online]. Available: http://www.generalmills.com/corporate/health_wellness/in_the_news_detail.aspx?itemID=8156&catID=7586&section=news [accessed June 12, 2005].

General Mills. 2005c. *Cascadian Farm Unveils Guide to the Guidelines to Educate Parents About Kid Nutrition. Clifford the Big Red Dog Goes to Washington D.C. to Bring Fun to the Breakfast Table.* [Online]. Available: http://www.generalmills.com/corporate/health_wellness/in_the_news_detail.aspx?itemID=9695&catID=7586&section=news [accessed June 20, 2005].

Gladwell M. 2000. *The Tipping Point: How Little Things Can Make a Big Difference.* Boston, MA: Back Bay Books.

GMA (Grocery Manufacturers of America). 2002. New survey shows national brand loyalty high among american consumers. *News Release.* [Online]. Available: http://www.gmabrands.com/news/docs/NewsRelease.cfm?DocID=971& [accessed July 12, 2005].

GMA. 2004. *GMA Members: Part of the Solution.* October 2004.

GMA. 2005a. *Grocery Manufacturers Association.* [Online]. Available: http://www.gmabrands.com/ [accessed July 22, 2005].

GMA. 2005b. *GMA Board Statement and Guiding Principles for the Food and Beverage Industry on Diet, Physical Activity and Health.* Washington, DC: GMA.

GMA. 2005c. *Industry Position Statement on School Wellness Policy.* Washington, DC: GMA.

GMA. 2005d. GMA statement regarding proposals to strengthen advertising self-regulation. *News Release.* July 15. [Online]. Available: http://www.gmabrands.com/news/docs/NewsRelease.cfm?DocID=1542& [accessed July 22, 2005].

GMA Forum. 2005. *Cannondale Trade Promotion Study 2005. Saying No to the Status Quo.* Second Quarter. Pp. 72–84.

Graetzer K. 2005. *Comments of the MilkPEP Board Concerning Advertising and Marketing Strategies Effective in Fostering Healthy Food Choices in Children and Youth.* IOM Committee on Food Marketing and the Diets of Children and Youth. June 2.

Greenberg BS, Brand JE. 1993. Television news and advertising in schools: The "Channel One" controversy. *J Commun* 43(1):143–151.

Grier SA. 2005. *The Past, Present, and Future of Marketing of Foods to Children.* Presentation at the DHHS-FTC Workshop about Perspectives on Marketing, Self-Regulation, and Childhood Obesity. July 14–15. [Online]. Available: http://www.ftc.gov/bcp/workshops/foodmarketingtokids/index.htm [accessed July 27, 2005].

Grier SA, Brumbaugh AM. 2004. Consumer distinctiveness and advertising persuasion. In: Williams JD, Lee W-N, Haugtvedt CP, eds. *Diversity in Advertising.* Hillsdale, NJ: Lawrence Erlbaum Associates, Inc.

Guest LP. 1955. Brand loyalty—twelve years later. *J Appl Psychol* 39:405–408.

Gupta P, Gould S. 1997. Consumers' perceptions of the ethics and acceptability of product placement in movies: Product category and individual differences. *J Current Issues and Res Ad* 19(1):37–50.

Guthrie JF, Lin BH, Reed J, Stewart H. 2005. Understanding economic and behavioral influences on fruit and vegetable choices. *Amber Waves* 3(2):36–41. [Online]. Available: http://www.ers.usda.gov/AmberWaves/April05/pdf/april05_feature_fruitsandvegetables.pdf [accessed April 14, 2005].

Harris JM. 2002. Food manufacturing. In: Harris J, Kaufman P, Martinez S, Price C. 2002. *The U.S. Food Marketing System, 2002.* Agricultural Economic Report No. (AER811). Washington, DC: Economic Research Service, U.S. Department of Agriculture. Pp. 3–11. [Online]. Available: http://www.ers.usda.gov/publications/aer811/aer811.pdf [accessed May 2, 2005].

Harris JM. 2005. Companies continue to offer new foods targeted to children. *Amber Waves* 3(3):4. [Online]. Available: http://www.ers.usda.gov/AmberWaves/June05/pdf/FindingsDHJune05.pdf [accessed June 6, 2005].

Harrison K, Marske AL. 2005. Nutritional content of foods advertised during the television programs children watch most. *Am J Public Health* 95(9):1568–1574.

Hastings Museum of Natural and Cultural History. 2004. *Hey Kool-Aid®!* [Online]. Available: http://www.hastingsmuseum.org/koolaid/history.htm [accessed June 11, 2005].

Henderson VR, Kelly B. 2005. Food advertising in the age of obesity: Content analysis of food advertising on general market and African American television. *J Nutr Educ Behav* 37:191–196.

Henry A. 2003. How buzz marketing works for teens. *Advertising & Marketing to Children*. World Advertising Research Center. Pp. 3–10.

Hind A. 2003. Brands for the under-3s: Teletubbies, a case study. *Advertising & Marketing to Children*. World Advertising Research Center. Pp. 25–33.

Holt DB. 2004. *How Brands Become Icons: The Principles of Cultural Branding*. Boston, MA: Harvard Business School Press.

Hostess. 2005. *Planet Twinkie*. [Online]. Available: http://www.twinkies.com/index.asp [accessed May 8, 2005].

Hunter BT. 2002. Marketing foods to kids: Using new avenues. *Consumers' Research* Pp. 23–25.

Information Resources. 2005. *Time and Trends: A Snapshot of Trends Shaping the CPG Industry*. [Online]. Available: http://www.gmabrands.com/publications/gmairi/2005/may/may.pdf [accessed June 20, 2005].

IN ZONE Brands. 2004. *Tummy Tickler Products*. [Online]. Available: http://www.tummytickler.com/products.htm [accessed June 20, 2005].

IOM (Institute of Medicine). 2005. *Preventing Childhood Obesity: Health in the Balance*. Washington, DC: The National Academies Press.

Ippolito PM. 2005. *TV Advertising to Children 1977 v. 2004*. Presentation at the DHHS-FTC Workshop about Perspectives on Marketing, Self-Regulation, and Childhood Obesity. July 14–15. [Online]. Available: http://www.ftc.gov/bcp/workshops/foodmarketingtokids/index.htm [accessed July 27, 2005].

Jekanowski MD. 1999. Causes and consequences of fast food sales growth. *Food Review.* 22(1):11–16.

Joyce K. 2004. MMA in the News. *PROMO Magazine*. [Online]. Available: http://mmaglobal.com/modules/news/print.php?storyid=26 [accessed July 26, 2005].

JP Morgan. 2003. *Food Manufacturing. Obesity: The Big Issue. European Equity Research.* April 16.

Kaikati AM, Kaikati JG. 2004. Stealth marketing: How to reach consumers surreptitiously. University of California, Berkeley: *California Management Review* 46(4):6–22.

Karrh JA. 1994. Effects of brand placements in motion pictures. In: King AW, ed. *Proceedings of the 1994 American Academy of Advertising*. Athens, GA: American Academy of Advertising.

Kaufman PR. 2002. Food retailing. In: Harris J, Kaufman P, Martinez S, Price C. *The U.S. Food Marketing System.* Agricultural Economic Report No. (AER811). Washington, DC: Economic Research Service, U.S. Department of Agriculture. [Online]. Available: http://www.ers.usda.gov/publications/aer811/aer811.pdf [accessed May 2, 2005].

Kelley B, Graham L, Quinn T, Sears B. 2004. *Changes in the Confectionery Industry*. 2004 All Candy Expo®. [Online]. Available: http://www.allcandyexpo.com/industry_forum.cfm [accessed June 16, 2005].

KFF (Kaiser Family Foundation). 2004. *Tweens, Teens and Magazines Fact Sheet*. [Online]. Available: http://www.kff.org/entmedia/loader.cfm?url=/commonspot/security/getfile.cfm&PageID=47098 [accessed May 3, 2005].

Kotler P, Armstrong G. 2004. *Principles of Marketing*. 10th Edition. Upper Saddle River, NJ: Pearson Education/Prentice Hall.

Kotz K, Story M. 1994. Food advertisements during children's Saturday morning television programming: Are they consistent with dietary recommendations? *J Am Diet Assoc* 94(11):1296–1300.

Kraft Foods. 2004. *Form 10-K Annual Report for the Fiscal Year Ended December 31, 2004.* [Online]. Available: http://kraft.com/pdfs/KraftAR04_10K.pdf [accessed June 6, 2005].

Kraft Foods. 2005a. *Our Products: Lunchables®.* [Online]. Available: http://www.kraftfoods.com/om/bn/c_Products/Lunchables.htm [accessed June 3, 2005].

Kraft Foods. 2005b. *Kool-Aid Man.* [Online]. Available: http://www.kraft.com/100/innovations/koolaidman.html [accessed June 11, 2005].

Kraft Foods. 2005c. Kraft Foods announces marketing changes to emphasize more nutritious products. [Online]. *News Release.* January 12. Available: http://www.kraft.com/newsroom/01122005.html [accessed September 21, 2005].

Kraft Foods. 2005d. Kraft Foods announces healthy lifestyle initiatives at California summit on health, nutrition and obesity. *News Release.* January 12. [Online]. Available: http://www.kraft.com/newsroom/09152005.html [accessed September 22, 2005].

Kraft Foods. 2005e. *Obesity Initiatives.* [Online]. Available: http://www.kraft.com/obesity/advisory.html [accessed November 15, 2005].

Kunkel D. 2001. Children and television advertising. In: Singer D, Singer J, eds. *Handbook of Children and the Media.* Thousand Oaks, CA: Sage.

Kunkel D, Gantz W. 1992. Children's television advertising in the multi-channel environment. *J Commun* 42(3):134–152.

Kunkel D, Gantz W. 1993. Assessing compliance with industry self-regulation of television advertising to children. *J Applied Communication* 21(2):148–162.

Kunkel D, McIlrath M. 2003. Message content in advertising to children. In: Palmer E, Young B, eds. *Faces of Televisual Media: Teaching, Violence, Selling to Children.* Mahwah, NJ: Erlbaum Associates. Pp. 287–300.

Kuribayashi A, Roberts MC, Johnson RJ. 2001. Actual nutritional information of products advertised to children and adults on Saturday. *Children's Health Care* 30(4):309–322.

Lauro PW. 2002. Swanson focuses on its new, fashionable TV dinner. *The New York Times* October 30. [Online]. Available: http://inventors.about.com/od/inventionsalphabet/a/tv_dinner.htm [accessed May 8, 2005].

Lawrence D. 2003. The role of characters in kids marketing. *Advertising & Marketing to Children.* World Advertising Research Center. 4(3):43–48.

Lenhart A, Rainie L, Lewis O. 2001. *Teenage Life Online: The Rise of the Instant-Messaging Generation and the Internet's Impact on Friendships and Family Relationships.* Pew Internet & American Life Project. [Online]. Available: http://www.pewinternet.org/pdfs/PIP_Teens_Report.pdf [accessed July 9, 2005].

Lewis LB, Sloane DC, Nascimento LM, Diamant AL, Guinyard JJ, Yancey AK, Flynn G. 2005. African Americans' access to healthy food options in South Los Angeles restaurants. *Am J Public Health* 95(4):668–673.

Linn S. 2004. Food marketing to children in the context of a marketing maelstrom. *J Public Health Policy* 25(3/4):24–35.

Lippman J, McKay B. 2001. Warner Bros. choose Coke to bestow marketing magic on Harry Potter film. *Wall Street Journal.* P. A3.

Lukas C. 2000. *The Oreo Cookie Counting Book.* New York: Little Simon.

Mack A. 2004. Gaming scores with advertisers. *Media Week* 14(26):18–20.

Marketing Intelligence Service. 2005. *ProductScan® Online Database of New Products.* [Online]. Available: http://www.productscan.com [accessed April 30, 2005].

Mattel. 2001. *Barbie® Doll Puts on Another Famous Uniform to Serve Up Smiles.* [Online]. Available: http://www.shareholder.com/mattel/news/20010501-43068.cfm [accessed June 5, 2005].

Mattel. 2005. *Barbie® Collector.* [Online]. Available: http://www.barbiecollector.com [accessed June 5, 2005].

Mazur L. 1996. Marketing madness. *Environ Magazine* 7(3):36–41.

McCarthy M. 2005. Disney plans to mix ads, videogames to target kids, teens. *USA Today*. [Online]. Available: http://usatoday.com/money/media/2005-01-17-disney-advergaming_x.htm [accessed March 15, 2005].

McDonald's Corporation. 1996. The power of our global brand. In: *1996 Summary Annual Report*. [Online]. Available at: http://www.mcdonalds.com/corp/invest/pub/annual_rpt_archives/1996_annual.html [accessed April 11, 2005].

McDonald's Corporation. 2003. McDonald's™ introduces new McKIDS™ multi-category, worldwide licensing program. *News Release*. [Online]. Available: http://www.media.mcdonalds.com/secured/news/pressreleases/2003/Press_Release11132003.html [accessed July 10, 2005].

McDonald's Corporation. 2004. *McDonald's® Celebrates 25 Years of Happy Meals with the Return of Ty Teenie Beanie Babies®*. [Online]. Available: http://www.mcdonalds.com/usa/news/2004/conpr_07222004.html [accessed July 5, 2005].

McDonald's Corporation. 2005a. *McDonald's Press Release*. [Online]. Available: http://www.mcdonalds.com/usa/news/current/conpr_05042005.html [accessed July 8, 2005].

McDonald's Corporation. 2005b. *Global Advisory Council on Balanced Lifestyles*. [Online]. Available: http://www.mcdonalds.com/corp/values/socialrespons/resrecog/expert_advisors0/advisory_council_on.html [accessed July 8, 2005].

McGinn D. 2003. Pitching to kids. *Boston Globe*. [Online]. Available: www.boston.com/globe/magazine/2003/0416/kids.html [accessed February 20, 2005].

McKay B. 2001. Coke finds its exclusive contracts aren't so easily given up. *Wall Street Journal (Eastern Edition)* June 26. Pp. B1, B4.

McNeal JU. 1964. *Children as Consumers*. Austin: Bureau of Business Research, University of Texas at Austin.

McNeal JU. 1998. Tapping the three kids' markets. *Am Demographics* 20(4):37–41.

McNeal JU. 1999. *The Kids Market: Myth and Realities*. Ithaca, NY: Strategist.

Meltzoff A. 1988. Imitation of televised models by infants. *Child Development* 59(5): 1221–1229.

Mintel International Group Ltd. 2003. *Character Merchandising in Food and Drink–UK*. [Online]. Brief summary of full report. Available: http://www.the-infoshop.com/study/mt17377_food_drink.html [accessed June 6, 2005].

Molnar, A. 2003. *No Student Left Unsold: The Sixth Annual Report on Trends in School-house Commercialism 2002–2003*. [Online]. Available: http://www.asu.edu/educ/epsl/CERU/CERU_Annual_Report.htm [accessed November 19, 2005].

Montgomery K. 2001. Digital kids: The new online children's consumer culture. In: Singer DG, Singer JL, eds. *Handbook of Children and the Media*. Thousand Oaks, CA: Sage Publications. Pp. 625–650.

Montgomery K, Pasnik S. 1996. *Web of Deception*. Washington, DC: Center for Media Education.

Moore ES, Wilkie WL, Lutz RJ. 2002. Passing the torch: Intergenerational influences as a source of brand equity. *J Marketing* 66(2):17–37.

Mortimer, R. 2002. Box office brand bonanzas. *Brand Strategy* 166:25.

MPA (Magazine Publishers of America). 1999. *Highlights of Sales Scans*. [Online]. Available: http://www.magazine.org/content/Files/Sales%5FScan%5FHighlights.pdf [accessed June 20, 2005].

MPA. 2004a. *Teen Market Profile*. [Online]. Available: http://www.magazine.org/content/files/teenprofile04.pdf [accessed April 24, 2005].

MPA. 2004b. *African American Market Profile*. [Online]. Available: http://www.magazine.org/content/files/market_profile_black.pdf [accessed June 18, 2005].

MPA. 2004c. *Hispanic/Latino Market Profile*. [Online]. Available: http://www.magazine.org/content/Files/MPAHispMktPro.pdf [accessed June 17, 2005].

NARC (National Advertising Review Council). 2004. *Guidance for Food Advertising Self-Regulation.* New York: NARC. [Online]. Available: http://www.narcpartners.org/NARC_White_Paper_6-1-04.pdf [accessed April 10, 2005].

NASSP. 2005. *NASSP Guidelines for Beverage-Provider Business Agreements.* [Online]. Available: http://www.principals.org [accessed October 27, 2005].

Neal WD. 2005. *Principles of Market Segmentation.* [Online]. Available: http://www.marketingpower.com/content1006.php# [accessed June 14, 2005].

Nebenzahl ID, Secunda E. 1993. Consumers' attitudes toward product placement in movies. *Int J Ad* 12(1):1–11.

Neopets®. 2003. *Youth Study 2003.* [Online]. Available: http://demo.neopets.com/presskit/articles/research/ym2003.html [accessed July 7, 2005].

Neopets®. 2005. *Corporate Fact Sheet.* [Online]. Available: http://demo.neopets.com/presskit/compinfo.html [accessed July 3, 2005].

Nestlé. 2004. *Nesquik.* [Online]. Available: http://www.nestle.com/Our_Brands/Beverages/Nesquik/ [accessed June 6, 2005].

Nestle M. 2000. Soft drink "pouring rights": Marketing empty calories. *Public Health Reports* 115(4):308–319.

Nestle M. 2002. *Food Politics: How the Food Industry Influences Nutrition and Health.* Berkeley, CA: University of California Press.

Nestle M, Wing R, Birch L, DiSogra L, Drewnowski A, Middleton S, Sigman-Grant M, Sobal J, Winston M, Economos C. 1998. Behavioral and social influences on food choice. *Nutr Rev* 56(5):S50–S74.

Nickelodeon. 2005. *All Nick TV Shows.* [Online]. Available: http://www.nick.com/all_nick/ [accessed May 28, 2005].

Nielsen Monitor-Plus. 2005. *National Cable Television Advertising Spending (NAN, NICK, TOON, TDSN), Full Day.* January 1, 2003–December 31, 2004.

NRA (National Restaurant Association). 2005. *Restaurant Industry Fact Sheet 2005.* [Online]. Available: http://www.restaurant.org/pdfs/research/2005factsheet.pdf [accessed June 15, 2005].

Office of the Clerk, U.S. House of Representatives. 2004. *Alliance for American Advertising House ID Numbers.* [Online]. Available: http://clerk.house.gov/pd/houseID.html?reg_id=37455 [accessed July 27, 2005].

Ordonez J. 2001. Burger King pairs with DreamWorks and Nickelodeon. *Wall Street Journal.* P. B2.

Palmer E, Cantor J, Kunkel D, Dowrick P, Linn S, Wilcox B. 2004. *Psychological Implications of Commercialism in Schools.* Washington, DC: American Psychological Association Task Force on Advertising and Children.

PBS (Public Broadcasting System) Frontline. 2001. *Merchants of Cool.* [Online]. Available: http://www.pbs.org/wgbh/pages/frontline/shows/cool/etc/script.html [accessed June 5, 2005].

Peleo-Lazar M. 2005. *McDonald's Presentation at the IOM Workshop on Strategies That Foster Healthy Food and Beverage Choices in Children and Youth.* Committee on Food Marketing and the Diets of Children and Youth. Washington, DC, January 27.

PepsiCo. 2004a. *Sustainable Advantage.* Annual Report 2004. [Online]. Available: http://www.pepsico.com/investors/annual-reports/2004/247528PepsicoLR.pdf [accessed July 3, 2005].

PepsiCo. 2004b. *Blue Ribbon Advisory Board.* [Online]. Available: http://www.smartspot.com/commitment_to_health/420.php [accessed July 8, 2005].

Petretti A. 1992. *Coca-Cola Collectibles Price Guide.* 8th Edition. Hackensack, NJ: Nostalgia Publications.

Pinnacle Foods Corporation. 2003. *Swanson 50th Anniversary Celebration.* [Online]. Available: http://www.swansonmeals.com/50th/ [accessed May 6, 2005].

Plunkett Research Ltd. 2005. *Food Industry Almanac 2005.* Brief Summary. [Online]. Available: http://www.mindbranch.com/products/R207-0054.html [accessed September 21, 2005].

Pollack Associates. 2003. *Special Report: 2003. Supermarkets: Brands & Private Label.* New York, NY. [Online]. Available: http://www.supermarketalert.com/pdf%20docs/3BrandsPriLabel.pdf [accessed September 16, 2005].

Pollack Associates. 2004. *Special Report: 2004. Private Label & Branding.* New York. [Online]. Available: http://www.supermarketalert.com/pdf%20docs/04specrptsfr03/4prilabel-web.pdf [accessed September 16, 2005].

Powell K. 2005. *Fostering Healthy Choices.* Presentation at the IOM Workshop on Strategies that Foster Healthy Food and Beverage Choices in Children and Youth. Committee on Food Marketing and the Diets of Children and Youth. Washington, DC, January 27.

PQMedia. 2005. *Product Placement Spending in Media 2005: Executive Summary.* [Online]. Available: http://www.pqmedia.com/product-placement-spending-in-media.html [accessed June 10, 2005].

Preschel S. 2005. *Backpacks, Lunch Boxes and Cells? . . . Nearly Half of U.S. Teens and Tweens Have Cell Phones, According to NOP World mKids Study.* New York. [Online]. Available: http://www.nopworld.com/new.asp?go=news_item&key=151 [accessed July 26, 2005].

Pressler MW. 2005. Hold the health, serve that burger: Restaurant chains find low-fat means lean sales. *Washington Post.* August 18.

Prichard J. 2003. Kellogg's popular, pioneering Pop-Tarts turn 40 this year. *The Detroit News.* [Online]. Available: http://www.detnews.com/2003/business/0304/06/business-128483.htm [accessed June 5, 2005].

PRIMEDIA Business Magazines & Media. 2004. *DreamWorks Brings Back Partners for Sinbad DVD.* [Online]. Available: http://promomagazine.com/deals/marketing_dreamworks_brings_back/ [accessed July 7, 2005].

QuickMBA. 2004. *Market Segmentation.* [Online]. Available: http://www.quickmba.com/marketing/market-segmentation/ [accessed June 14, 2005].

Radio Disney. 2005. *Radio Disney.* [Online]. Available: http://radio.disney.go.com/music/projectfamily/ [accessed July 7, 2005].

Red Herring. 2005. *Brand-name companies have caught on to the interactive power of mobile phone marketing. Is it a new advertising medium, or just glorified spam?* [Online]. Available: http://www.redherring.com/PrintArticle.aspx?a=12506&sector=Industries [accessed July 26, 2005].

Rideout V, Hoff T. 2002. *Shouting to Be Heard: Public Service Advertising in a New Media Age.* Menlo Park, CA: Henry J. Kaiser Family Foundation.

Rideout VJ, Vandewater EA, Wartella EA. 2003. *Zero to Six: Electronic Media in the Lives of Infants, Toddlers and Preschoolers.* Menlo Park, CA: Henry J. Kaiser Family Foundation.

Rideout V, Roberts DF, Foehr UG. 2005. *Executive Summary: Generation M: Media in the Lives of 8–18 Year Olds.* Menlo Park, CA: Henry J. Kaiser Family Foundation.

Ritzer G. 2004. *The McDonaldization of Society.* Thousand Oaks, CA: Sage Publications, Inc.

Roberts D, Foehr U. 2005. *Kids and Media in America.* Cambridge, UK: Cambridge University Press.

Roberts D, Foehr U, Rideout V, Brodie M. 1999. *Kids and Media @ the New Millennium: A Comprehensive National Analysis of Children's Media Use.* Menlo Park, CA: Kaiser Family Foundation.

Roberts DF, Foehr UG, Rideout V. 2005. *Generation M: Media in the Lives of 8–18 Year Olds.* Menlo Park, CA: Henry J. Kaiser Family Foundation.

Roberts K. 2004. *Lovemarks: The Future Beyond Brands.* New York: PowerHouse Books.

Roper Youth Report. 2003. *American Youth Wielding More Household Buying Power.* New York. [Online]. Available: http://www.nopworld.com/news.asp?go=news_item& key=59 [accessed April 11, 2005].

Rubin R. 2004. *Kids vs. Teens: Money and Maturity Guide Online Behavior.* eMarketer. [Online]. Available: http://www.emarketer.com/Report.aspx?kids_may04 [accessed November 21, 2005].

Samuels SE, Craypo L, Dorfman L, Purciel M, Standish MB. 2003. *Food and Beverage Industry Marketing Practices Aimed at Children: Developing Strategies for Preventing Obesity and Diabetes.* A report on the proceedings from a meeting sponsored by The California Endowment held in San Francisco in June 2003.

Scammon DL, Christopher CL. 1981. Nutrition education with children via television: A review. *J Advertising* 19(2):26–36.

Schlosser E. 2001. *Fast Food Nation.* New York: Houghton Mifflin Company.

Schor JB. 2004. *Born to Buy: The Commercialized Child and the New Consumer Culture.* New York: Scribner.

Short D. 2005. When science met the consumer: The role of industry. *Am J Clin Nutr* 82(suppl):256S–258S.

Siegel DL, Coffey TJ, Livingston G. 2001. *The Great Tween Buying Machine.* Ithaca, NY: Paramount Market Publishing, Inc.

Skyworks Technologies. 2004. *Life Savers Candystand.* [Online]. Available: http://candystand. com [accessed July 10, 2005].

Smalls M. 2005a. *Moving the Needle.* Presentation at the IOM Workshop on Strategies that Foster Healthy Food and Beverage Choices in Children and Youth. Committee on Food Marketing and the Diets of Children and Youth. Washington, DC, January 27.

Smalls M. 2005b. *Current Media Efforts to Foster Healthier Choices for Children.* Presentation at the DHHS-FTC Workshop about Perspectives on Marketing, Self-Regulation, and Childhood Obesity. July 14–15. [Online]. Available: http://www.ftc.gov/bcp/work-shops/foodmarketingtokids/index.htm [accessed July 27, 2005].

Smith JW, Clurman A, Wood C. 2005. *Coming to Concurrence: Addressable Attitudes and the New Model for Marketing Productivity.* Evanston, IL: Racom Communications.

Snider M. 2002. Hey kids! Let's play adver-games! *Maclean's* 115(51):36–37.

Stanley T. 2004. Marketers aim for parents via TV. *Advertising Age* 75(40):75.

Stewart H, Blisard N, Bhuyan S, Nayga RM Jr. 2004. *The Demand for Food Away from Home. Full Service or Fast Food?* Agricultural Economic Report No. 829. Washington, DC: Economic Research Service, U.S. Department of Agriculture. [Online]. Available: http://www.ers.usda.gov/publications/aer829/aer829.pdf [accessed September 17, 2005].

Stipp H. 1993. New ways to reach children. *Am Demographics* 15(8):50–56.

Story M, French S. 2004. Food advertising and marketing directed at children and adolescents in the US. *Int J Behav Nutr Phys Act* 1(1):3–20. [Online]. Available: http://www.ijbnpa. org/content/1/1/3 [accessed April 11, 2005].

Strasburger VC. 2001. Children and TV advertising: Nowhere to run, nowhere to hide. *J Dev Behav Pediatr* 22(3):185–187.

Subervi-Velez FA, Colsant S. 1993. The television world of Latino children. In: Berry GL, Asamen JK. *Children & Television: Images in a Changing Sociocultural World.* Newbury Park, CA: Sage Publications.

Subramanyam K, Greenfield P, Kraut R, Gross E. 2001. The impact of computer use on children's and adolescents' development. *J Appl Dev Psychol* 22(1):7–30.

Subway. 2005. *F.R.E.S.H. Steps Initiative.* [Online]. Available: http://www.subway.com/ subwayroot/MenuNutrition/index.aspx [accessed October 27, 2005].

Sunkist. 2005. *"C" is for Citrus as Sunkist and Sesame Workshop Announce Healthy Habits for Life Partnership.* [Online]. Available: http://www.sunkist.com/press/release.asp?id=72 [accessed November 18, 2005].

Survey Value. 2005. *Brand Loyalty.* [Online]. Available: http://www.surveyvalue.com [accessed July 12, 2005].

Swinburn BA, Caterson I, Seidell JC, James WPT. 2004. Diet, nutrition and the prevention of excess weight gain and obesity. *Pub Health Nutr* 7(1A):123–146.

Taaffe E. 2005. *PepsiCo Health & Wellness: Capturing Growth at the Intersection.* Presentation at the IOM Workshop on Strategies that Foster Healthy Food and Beverage Choices in Children and Youth. Committee on Food Marketing and the Diets of Children and Youth. Washington, DC, January 27.

Taras HL, Gage M. 1995. Advertised foods on children's television. *Arch Pediatr Adolesc Med* 149(6):649–652.

Tarpley T. 2001. Children, the Internet, and other new technologies. In: Singer D, Singer J, eds. *Handbook of Children and the Media.* Thousand Oaks, CA: Sage.

Teenage Research Unlimited. 2004. *The TRU Study.* [Online]. Available: http://www. teenresearch.com/PRview.cfm?edit_id=168 [accessed May 3, 2005].

Teenage Research Unlimited. 2005. Weekly spending. *TRU Study Update.* [Online]. Available: http://www.teenresearch.com/view.cfm?page_id=87&txt=txt1.cfm&pic=tru1.cfm [accessed September 24, 2005].

Teinowitz I, MacArthur K. 2005. McDonald's ads target children as young as 4. Government food marketing hearing told of elementary school programs. *Advertising Age.com.* January 28.

The Coca-Cola Company. 2003. *Model Guidelines for School Beverage Partnerships.* Atlanta, GA: Coca-Cola Company. [Online]. Available: http://www2.coca-cola.com/ourcompany/hal_school_beverage_guidelines.pdf [accessed July 7, 2005].

The Coca-Cola Company. 2005a. *Brand Fact Sheets.* [Online]. Available: http://www. virtualvender.coca-cola.com [accessed November 10, 2005].

The Coca-Cola Company. 2005b. *Live It!* Press Release. [Online]. Available: http://www2. coca-cola.com/presscenter/nr_20050526_americas_liveit.html [accessed October 19, 2005].

The Hershey Company. 2005. *Company Profile.* Available: http://www.thehersheycompany. com/about/profile.asp [accessed October 31, 2005].

The Intelligence Group/Youth Intelligence. 2005. *Nickelodeon/Youth Intelligence Tween Report 2004.* [Online]. Available: http://www.youthintelligence.com/cassandra/cassarticle. asp?cassArticleId=3 [accessed September 16, 2005].

Thomas D. 2004. *Teens Driving Mobile Data Market. Operators Should Target Kids, Not Business Users, Says Research.* Vnunet.com. [Online]. Available: http://www.vnunet.com/articles/print/2125293 [accessed July 26, 2005].

Thompson S. 2004. Kellogg pounces on toddlers. *Advertising Age.* December 6. P. 1.

Tillotson JE. 2004. America's obesity: Conflicting public policies, industrial economic development, and unintended human consequences. *Annu Rev Nutr* 24:617–643.

Tirodkar MA, Jain A. 2003. Food messages on African American television shows. *Am J Public Health* 93(3):439–441.

Tseng ES. 2001. Content analysis of children's television advertising today. Austin, TX: The University of Texas at Austin. Unpublished manuscript. [Online]. Available: http://www.ciadvertising.org/student_account/fall_01/adv392/estseng/ContentAnalysis/ContentAnalysis.html-72k [accessed February 22, 2005].

TTT West Coast. 2002. Cola wars: Britney vs. Christina. *News Release.* March 29. [Online]. Available: http://extratv.warnerbros.com/reframe.html?http://extratv.warnerbros.com/dailynews/pop/03_01/03_29a.html [accessed July 9, 2005].

TV Bureau of Advertising. 2005. [Online]. Available: http://www.tvb.org/nav/build_frameset. asp?url=/rcentral/index.asp [accessed October 27, 2005].

UBS Warburg. 2002. *Absolute Risk of Obesity. Global Equity Research.* November 27.

Upoc. 2002. *Snapshot of the U.S. Wireless Market.* [Online]. Available: http://www. genwireless.com/downloads/mobilestatssummary020802.ppt [accessed June 29, 2005].

U.S. Census Bureau. 2000. *Sex by Single Years of Age (PCT12).* [Online]. Available: http:// www.census.gov/census2000/states/us.html [accessed August 26, 2005].

U.S. Census Bureau. 2001. *National Intercensal Estimates (1990–2000).* [Online]. Available: http://www.census.gov/popest/archives/EST90INTERCENSAL/US-EST90INT-04.html [accessed March 7, 2005].

U.S. Census Bureau. 2004. *Annual Estimates of the Population by Sex and Selected Age Groups for the United States: April 1, 2000 to July 1, 2003.* [Online]. Available at: http://www.census.gov/popest/national/asrh/NC-EST2003/NC-EST2003-02.pdf [accessed March 7, 2005].

U.S. Department of Commerce. 2002. *A Nation Online: How Americans Are Expanding Their Use of the Internet.* [Online]. Available: http://www.ntia.doc.gov/ntiahome/dn/html/anationonline2.htm [accessed April 9, 2005].

U.S. Department of Education. 2003. *Computer and Internet Use by Children and Adolescents in 2001.* NCES 2004-014. Washington, DC: National Center for Education Statistics.

U.S. Department of Labor. 2004. *Consumer Expenditures in 2002.* Report 974. Washington, DC: U.S. Department of Labor. [Online]. Available: http://www.bls.gov/cex/csxann02. pdf [accessed October 26, 2005].

U.S. Market for Kids' Foods and Beverages. 2003. 5th edition. Report summary. [Online]. Available: http://www.marketresearch.com/researchindex/849192.html#pagetop [accessed May 3, 2005].

Valdés MI. 2000. *Marketing to American Latinos: A Guide to the In-Culture Approach.* Part 1. Ithaca, NY: Paramount Market Publishing, Inc.

Variyam JN. 2005a. The price is right. *Amber Waves.* February. Pp. 20–27.

Variyam JN. 2005b. *Nutrition Labeling in the Food-Away-From-Home Sector.* Economic Research Report No. 4. Washington, DC: Economic Research Service, U.S. Department of Agriculture. [Online]. Available: http://www.ers.usda.gov/publications/err4/err4.pdf [accessed April 30, 2005].

Verizon Wireless. 2005. Nickelodeon and Verizon Wireless launch Nick Mobile on V CAST, bringing kid TV favorites to Verizon Wireless V CAST phones. *News Release.* [Online]. Available: http://news.vzw.com/news/2005/05/pr2005-05-05.html [accessed July 11, 2005].

Viacom International. 2005. *Welcome to Postopia!* [Online]. Available: http://www.postopia. com [accessed July 9, 2005].

Wade L. 1998. *The Cheerios® Play Book.* New York: Little Simon.

Walley W. 2002. Taubin has Warner executives raving, "I'm Just Wild about Harry." *Advertising Age* 73(12):S10.

Walsh D, Gentile D, Gieske J, Walsh M, Chasco E. 2004. *Mediawise Video Game Report Card.* [Online]. Available: http://www.mediafamily.org/research/2004_VGRC.pdf [accessed July 7, 2005].

Warner M. 2005. You want any fruit with that Big Mac? *The New York Times.* February 20.

Williams J. 2005a. *Advertising of Food and Beverage Products to Children, Teen, and Adult Multicultural Markets.* University of Texas at Austin Working Paper.

Williams J. 2005b. *Product Proliferation Analysis for New Food and Beverage Products Targeted to Children 1994–2004.* University of Texas at Austin Working Paper.

Williams JD, Tharp MC. 2001. African Americans: Ethnic roots, cultural diversity. In: Tharp MC, ed. *Marketing and Consumer Identity in Multicultural America*. Thousand Oaks, CA: Sage Publications. Pp. 165–211.

Williams W, Montgomery K, Pasnik S. 1997. *Alcohol and Tobacco on the Web: New Threats to Youth*. Washington, DC: The Center for Media Education.

Williamson. 2001. Creating a Better Brighter Smarter Internet. *Interactive Week* 8(39):26–29.

Wulfemeyer KT, Mueller B. 1992. Channel One and commercials in classrooms: Advertising content aimed at students. *Journalism Quarterly* 69(3):724–742.

Yankelovich. 2003. *Youth Monitor™. Youth Today: Shaping Tomorrow*. Chapel Hill, NC: Yankelovich Partners, Inc.

Yankelovich. 2005. *Youth Monitor™*. [Online]. Available: http://www.yankelovich.com/products/youth2005_ps.pdf [accessed May 3, 2005].

Zywicki TJ, Holt D, Ohlhausen M. 2004. *Obesity and Advertising Policy*. George Mason Law and Economics Research Paper No. 04-45. [Online]. Available: http://papers.ssrn.com/sol3/papers.cfm?abstract_id=604781 [accessed June 7, 2005].

5

Influence of Marketing on the
Diets and Diet-Related Health
of Children and Youth

INTRODUCTION

This chapter identifies and assesses the research on the influence of food and beverage marketing on the diets and the diet-related health of U.S. children and youth. The work of this chapter should be understood within the context of what is known about these two areas. Chapter 1 describes the breadth and complexity of these factors as well as their multidirectional quality. Chapter 2 discusses the strong evidence that the food and beverage consumption patterns of U.S. children and youth do not meet recommendations for a health-promoting diet and that an estimated 16 percent are obese. Increasing numbers of children and youth also have a variety of physical and psychosocial problems associated with diet and weight.

Chapter 3 discusses the various factors that influence young people's food and beverage consumption habits. Chapter 4 reviews the ways in which young people are targeted for food and beverage marketing of both product categories and new product lines. A substantial proportion of such marketing is for high-calorie and low-nutrient foods and beverages. The corporate investment in advertising and other marketing practices is aimed at promoting consumer purchases—which are presumably related to consumption of the product advertised and the dietary practices and diet-related health profiles of today's children and youth.

This chapter reviews and assesses the evidence that explores various aspects of marketing's influence on the diets and diet-related health of our young people. The three core sections in the middle of the chapter present the results of a systematic evidence review of peer-reviewed literature in the area. They include enough of the technical and analytic detail to support the committee's findings about the contributions of marketing. Prior to these three sections are several that explain how the systematic evidence review was conducted, and following them are sections that address related elements such as comparison with other recent reviews and needed research. Throughout the chapter, care is taken to consider the role of marketing as one of multiple factors influencing diet and diet-related health.

The chapter begins with a description of the systematic evidence review undertaken to assess the influence of marketing on the diet and diet-related health of children and youth, including how it was organized, the criteria used for including evidence, the dimensions addressed, the coding process, the nature of the evidence examined, and the process used to review this evidence. This is followed by three sections that present the results of the systematic evidence review relevant to three relationships: (1) the relationship between marketing and precursors of diet, (2) the relationship between marketing and diet, and (3) the relationship between marketing and diet-related health. The role of factors with the potential to moderate these three relationships is then discussed. Finally, the systematic evidence review and its findings are considered in relationship to the results of other recent reports, and areas for future research are identified. A summary of the key findings concludes the chapter.

SYSTEMATIC EVIDENCE REVIEW

The committee conducted a systematic evidence review in order to investigate and summarize the empirical evidence that is directly relevant to the core question: What is the influence of food and beverage marketing on the diets and diet-related health of children and youth? The committee's review included 123 published empirical studies identified from a set of nearly 200 in the published literature. Systematic evidence reviews are qualitatively different from meta-analyses or traditional narrative reviews (Petticrew, 2001). Systematic evidence reviews do not involve the statistical synthesis of a set of studies, the technique of meta-analyses, but rather attempt to reduce the inevitable bias from narrative reviews by developing explicit and systematic criteria for study inclusion and for assessing the level of evidentiary support provided by each study. As a result, systematic evidence reviews sometimes include far fewer studies than traditional narrative reviews, but they also typically include more than just randomized controlled trials. For example, this review includes not only many controlled experimental studies, but also many observational studies—both cross-sectional and longitudinal—on the influence of food and beverage marketing on the diets and diet-related health of children and youth.

In addition to supporting a rigorous assessment of a comparatively large body of research, a systematic evidence review is well suited for finding and describing any major gaps in the existing evidence base. The influence of television advertising intended for children, for example, has been studied fairly extensively by academic researchers. However, the influence of Internet marketing techniques, such as advergaming—developed specifically for older children and growing rapidly, unlike television advertising—has not been the subject of a single peer-reviewed, published academic study. A section at the end of the chapter presents recommended research directions derived largely from the committee's systematic evidence review process.

The Analytic Framework

A five-element causal framework (Figure 5-1) was used in assessing the research evidence that related marketing to the diets and diet-related health of children and youth. These elements relate to the marketing-associated elements of the overall ecological schematic presented in Chapter 1.

The arrows in this framework are meant to represent potential causal mechanisms by which marketing might affect diet and diet-related health.[1] At the outset, the framework was created from the committee's identification of likely variables, relationships, and processes if food and beverage marketing were to have an effect on young people's diet and diet-related health. For each of the major elements in the framework, multiple variables were identified to support the widest possible search for relevant research. As research was identified and reviewed, the framework was revised to better reflect what has been studied.

In the resulting framework, the initiating or exogenous factors are *marketing* variables. Marketing variables involve the product, such as differences in product formulation, packaging, or portion size; place, such as placement of items at eye level on supermarket shelves or availability in vending machines, convenience stores, or quick serve restaurants; price, such as the price of healthful food in a school vending machine versus the price for less healthful options; and promotion, such as television or billboard advertising. The systematic evidence review focused on marketing intended for young people ages 18 years and younger rather than on the parents of these young people. At the same time, research was included when it addressed marketing techniques that could engage either or both

---

[1]The problems of causal inference are discussed in the section on Causal Inference Validity below.

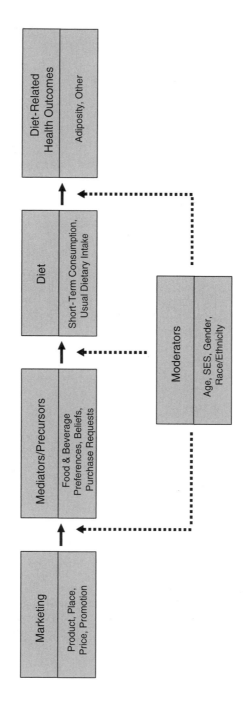

FIGURE 5-1 The five-element causal framework used to organize the systematic evidence review.

young people and their parents (e.g., product placement in a popular movie that both young people and parents would watch) if the research reported results for young people.

Marketing might affect diet through a variety of *mediators* or *precursors* of diet. In general, a mediator/precursor is a factor through which causal influence passes. For example, if watching television increases obesity, this influence might be mediated by decreasing physical activity, or it might be mediated by increasing calorie intake, or by both. In the causal framework in Figure 5-1, mediators/precursors of diet are intended to capture the factors that could be directly affected by marketing and that in turn might have a direct effect on diet, but which themselves do not involve directly obtaining or consuming food. For example, television advertisements for sweetened cereals aimed at young children are effective when they cause the child to make a request to the person who purchases food for the family. Thus a common mediator to consuming food or beverage products at home is food purchase requests. Other marketing approaches aim to change purchasing behavior through influencing beliefs about what is "cool" to drink, what provides energy, or what constitutes a balanced breakfast. Still other marketing efforts seek to influence a child's preferences for a product through its association with a well-known character, such as Darth Vader or Tony the Tiger®. Of the studies the committee reviewed on the relationship between a specific marketing factor and a precursor to diet, the great bulk involved food or beverage preferences, beliefs, or purchase requests. Thus the second element in the causal framework consists of a family of factors identified as precursors of diet. Those factors primarily include food and beverage preferences, beliefs, or purchase requests.

The third element in the causal framework is *diet*. For the committee's task, diet refers to the distribution and amount of food consumed on a regular basis. Unfortunately, not all studies measured diet comprehensively in this way. Many measured some short-term dietary behavior, such as the number of pieces of fruit or candy consumed in a child-care setting during an afternoon following an exposure to television advertising for fruit or candy that morning. Short-term effects on consumption may or may not translate into longer term effects on a young person's dietary patterns. Thus, it is important to distinguish studies that considered short-term dietary effects from those that attempted to relate marketing to a more comprehensive measure of diet. Experimental studies tended to focus on short-term consumption following some controlled exposure; cross-sectional and longitudinal studies employed broader measures of usual dietary intake, though they rarely assessed diet comprehensively.

The fourth element in the framework is diet-related health such as obesity, the metabolic syndrome, or type 2 diabetes. Nearly all the empirical research relating some marketing factor to diet-related health considered some version of the relationship between direct or indirect measures of body fat (adiposity) and television viewing. For simplicity, the term adiposity is used in this chapter to encompass the range of measures in the research reviewed.

The fifth element in the framework is *moderators*, variables that might alter the cause and effect relationships described in the path from marketing to diet-related health. In this domain, the committee identified age, gender, race/ethnicity, socioeconomic status, as well as whether a young person has the opportunity to make independent food purchases, can understand the persuasive intent of advertising, and has accurate nutritional knowledge as a potential moderator.

In general, a moderator is a factor that changes the nature of the causal relationship between two other factors. In the most extreme and simple case, the state of a flashlight's batteries moderates the influence of the switch on the state of the light. When the batteries are charged, the state of the switch fully determines the state of the light. When the batteries are dead, the switch has no effect whatsoever on the light. In another example, genetic or congenital factors moderate the influence of certain drugs on their intended outcome. For example, the effect of penicillin is quite different among those not allergic. Similarly, certain factors might moderate the effect of marketing on precursors, diet, or diet-related health. For example, the influence of television advertisements on food and beverage preferences might be moderated by cognitive development, as indexed by age. Children under about age 8 generally do not understand the persuasive intent of advertising or the implications of persuasive intent for the nature of the advertising they encounter (Blosser and Roberts, 1985; Donohue et al., 1978; Robertson and Rossiter, 1974; Ward et al., 1977). Presumably, they are more readily influenced by advertising and other forms of marketing than are children older than about 8 years. Income or socioeconomic status might also moderate the effects of marketing on diet. For those in a low-income family, for example, the effect of price might be much stronger than it is for those in a high-income family. Because foods such as fruits and vegetables cost more per calorie than do French fries or cheeseburgers, socioeconomic status may be an important moderator of the influence of fruit and vegetable marketing strategies. In another example, gender may moderate teens' reactions to marketing for sweet or high-fat foods and beverages. By early adolescence, many girls are concerned about their weight (Story et al., 1995) and, assuming that teens know that consuming sweets and high-fat foods leads to weight gain, they might be more resistant to the marketing of those foods than adolescent boys.

The arrows in the framework are not meant to reflect quantitative strength, only the possibility of a causal element, and are primarily meant to provide a guide with which to review the relevant research. Nor is the framework meant to be exhaustive. The causal relationships flow only in one direction: from marketing through precursors and so on to diet and diet-related health. Clearly, however, the variables included in the framework might also relate bidirectionally. For example, consumer preferences for sweets or high-fat foods can clearly influence marketing strategies, among other things, influencing product formulation or the product qualities emphasized in advertising. Or, as another example, public concern about diet-related health outcomes such as nutritional inadequacies or obesity can impact product formulation and advertising claims, such as emphasizing fortified, low-fat, or whole-grain products. Such bidirectional relationships require more academic research, and their existence underlines the dynamic complexities noted in ecological perspective presented in Chapter 1.

The framework, then, provides both a causal perspective for the committee's examination of evidence on the influence of marketing on young people's diet and diet-related health, and a structure for organizing the empirical research on this topic. Many studies have examined the relationship between a marketing factor and a mediator/precursor. Many others ignored mediators/precursors and examined the relationship between a marketing factor and a measure of diet, and still others ignored precursors and diet, but examined the relationship between a marketing factor and some aspect of diet-related health. The analysis of the evidence presented later in this chapter is organized along these lines: evidence for a causal connection between marketing and mediator/precursor factors first, then evidence for a causal connection between marketing and diet, and finally, evidence for a causal connection between marketing and diet-related health.

Identification of Research for the Review

Unlike narrative reviews, a systematic evidence review includes explicit criteria for which studies to include and which to exclude. In establishing these criteria, the committee sought to create a body of evidence that would be both extensive and directly relevant to its charge of assessing the effects of food and beverage marketing on the diets and diet-related health of children and youth. The committee identified four distinct foci of existing research: industry and marketing sources and peer-reviewed literature; marketing and television advertising; television advertising and media use; and marketing of products other than foods and beverages. These had implications for the criteria used to determine what research was included in the systematic evidence review.

Industry and Marketing Sources and Peer-Reviewed Literature

Marketing research is carried out by many different people and organizations for many different purposes. For ease of discussion, the committee characterized them broadly into two categories: industry and marketing information and peer-reviewed literature. There are some notable differences between them. A large amount of industry and marketing information related to foods and beverages promotion to children and youth is not publicly available, but peer-reviewed literature is in the public domain. Additionally, industry and marketing sources usually focus on specific products or brands, often in comparison to other product categories or brands, whereas peer-reviewed literature is usually directed at understanding the marketing process and related effects across a wide range of product categories.

Marketing and Television Advertising

A large amount of the research about the effect of marketing on young people's diet and diet-related health examines food and beverage advertising on television. This might be explained by three realities:

1.   Advertising is the most visible and measurable component of promotion, one of the classic four marketing practices, the others being product, place, and price;
2.   Advertising consumes a substantial and specific portion of a firm's marketing budget; and
3.   Of all food and beverage advertising encountered by children and adolescents, the majority occurs when they are viewing broadcast television and cable television programs.

Understanding the effects of televised advertising in today's food and beverage marketing on young people's diets and diet-related health contributes substantially to understanding the effects of broader marketing. Fuller understanding would come with research on other types of promotion in addition to advertising, other venues for advertising in addition to television and cable television, and other types of marketing in addition to promotion (i.e., product, place, and price). The marketing arena is complex and ever changing (see Chapter 4). Considerable work is still needed to develop a full understanding of marketing's current role, its likely future role, and important options for enhancing its positive role in influencing young people's diet and diet-related health. For the systematic evidence review, the committee established criteria that included all forms of marketing in all venues and vigorously searched for research about marketing other than television advertising.

Television Advertising and Media Use

A number of research studies deliberately use overall amount of television viewing time (primarily at home) as a measure of overall exposure to television advertising, on the assumption that advertising is a part of virtually all television viewing. Measuring home viewing assesses naturally occurring behavior and aggregates it over the many hours a day every day that most young people are watching television. Along with these benefits of measuring overall viewing come various measurement and inference challenges. In assessing the evidence on marketing's effects, attention was given to the extent to which the measurement and inference problems were addressed when overall television viewing was used intentionally to assess overall exposure to television advertising.

A number of other studies consider overall amount of television viewing per se as an independent variable, particularly in relationship to adiposity. Many are not explicit about the exact mechanisms by which television viewing relates to adiposity or they discuss several different possibilities, often but not always including exposure to advertising for foods and beverages. For example, some of the studies specify that a measure of television viewing is meant to reflect absence of physical activity. The committee established criteria by which all such studies could be included in the evidence base. In these studies, if a relationship was found between television viewing and the outcome of interest, such as adiposity, the reason for the relationship had several plausible explanations for it. Exposure to advertising is one. The committee's task was to determine for each study of this type whether there was good support for arguing that the relationship of television viewing to the outcome was, indeed, attributable in some degree to exposure to advertising during viewing.

Marketing of Products Other Than Foods and Beverages

There is a substantial body of research on the effect of marketing products other than foods and beverages to children and youth. In general, this research indicates that marketing can influence young people's beliefs, actions, and preferences. Much of the research has focused on television advertising for toys, but it has also included work on advertising for cigarettes and alcohol, as well as other products and services. A discussion of some of this body of research is included elsewhere in the report, but it was not formally evaluated by the committee for the systematic evidence review because it does not directly assess the effects of food and beverage marketing.

Final Criteria for Research Included in the Systematic Evidence Review

Based on considerations such as these, the committee's review was limited to publicly available, scientific studies involving quantitative data on the relationship between (1) a variable involving marketing relevant to young people ages 18 years and younger, and (2) either a variable involving a mediator/precursor, or a variable involving diet, or a variable involving diet-related health.[2] Studies that only considered the effect of a moderator variable and had no data pertinent to the relationship between a marketing variable and a precursor, diet, or diet-related health variable were not included. For example, if a study examined the effect of income on attitudes toward fruit and vegetables and had no measure of a marketing variable such as price or placement, then it was not included. Any study that met the inclusion criteria and employed measures that could be interpreted as assessing a marketing variable was included, whether or not the researchers intended the measure to represent that variable. For example, studies were included that used amount of television exposure as the independent variable, or that used attending a high school with Channel One programs (a specially produced high school news program that includes food and beverage advertisements) and examined precursors, diet, or diet-related health.

The criteria for a study to be included in the committee's systematic evidence review were therefore as follows:

1. Only peer-reviewed, published research that included a full description of methods and results or that directed the reader to another publicly available report that provided the full description of methods. This research could have appeared in print books and journals or e-books and e-journals.
2. Only research reports written entirely in English.
3. Any country as the location for the research.
4. Any publication date.
5. Only original research, no review articles.
6. Only research that reported a quantitative relationship between a variable involving marketing relevant to young people (as opposed to parents only) and a variable involving a mediator/precursor, or diet, or diet-related physical health outcome for young people (as opposed to parents).

---

[2]Diet-related health was defined as physical health not psychosocial health.

7.   Any research that used an independent variable that could be interpreted as a measure for some aspect of marketing.

Only published, peer-reviewed research literature was used in this review. There are certain constraints in this respect that apply to any literature review of this sort. It is possible, for example, that investigators have not submitted for publication the results of studies in which the relationship between food and beverage marketing and a pertinent outcome was not statistically significant. In addition, peer reviewers and journal editors may have had a bias to favorably review only those studies in which the results are statistically significant. If so, then the published studies represent only a sample of all studies that have been done, and this sample is biased in the direction of statistically significant relationships between food and beverage marketing and the outcome of interest. However, if such a bias does exist, the direction of that bias should not be assumed as either an increase or decrease in the influence of marketing on the measured precursors, diet, or diet-related health.

Although a publication bias is possible in the research reviewed below, the committee considered the bias, if it exists, to be small. As will be displayed, nonsignificant results have been published in numerous and diverse sources. Moreover, an early examination of unpublished theses, dissertations, and conference papers revealed relatively few nonsignificant findings. Given the importance of the issues, the committee considered it unlikely that well-conceived and well-executed studies were not submitted or were rejected on the grounds that the results were not statistically significant.

Finding the Research

Using the guidelines described above and the many possible variables identified with the initial proposed causal framework, extensive and iterative searches for relevant literature were conducted. Briefly, the quest included an online bibliographic search of several databases, outreach to experts in relevant fields, examining published literature reviews, recourse to committee members' personal and university libraries, and pursuing references cited in articles that were being coded for the systematic evidence review.

A two-stage process determined whether each item was included in the final systematic evidence review. One or more committee members read the titles and abstracts of more than 200 items and removed any that clearly did not meet one or more of the inclusion criteria. Many review articles, opinion pieces, studies involving adults only, and studies that did not include a marketing "causal" variable and an "effect" variable that represented a precursor to diet, diet, or diet-related health were removed. The remaining studies were assigned to two people (drawn from committee members and university students commissioned to assist in this process) for complete coding. If the two coders subsequently agreed the item did not meet the inclusion criteria, it was discarded. In the end, the systematic evidence review included 155 research results from 123 studies.

To place this collection of evidence in context, it is helpful to compare this systematic evidence review of the effects of food and beverage marketing on children and youth with the previous most extensive effort. That work, commissioned by the U.K. Food Standards Agency, reflected similar goals and identified 55 articles or entries describing 51 relevant studies for systematic review (Hastings et al., 2003). Building on the base of that work, and applying even more stringent criteria for the publication quality of the studies reviewed, we have been able to identify and assess an even larger body of evidence. Hence, this committee's review of the evidence represents the most comprehensive and rigorous assessment to date of food and beverage marketing's influence on children and youth.

Dimensions of the Review

Each research study that met the committee's inclusion criteria was reviewed and then "coded" on several dimensions that were used in the systematic evidence review for the relationships between the following factors:

1. *Marketing* and a *precursor to diet*
2. *Marketing* and *diet*
3. *Marketing* and a *diet-related health outcome*

If more than one relationship was examined in a published study, a separate entry in the evidence table was created for each such relationship. In some cases this resulted in multiple results for one study. For example, one study examined four matched schools, two of which had Channel One and two of which did not (Greenberg and Brand, 1993). Outcomes measured included the students' news knowledge, their attitudes toward foods and beverages advertised by Channel One, and their purchases of foods and beverages advertised by Channel One. For the committee's purposes, student news knowledge was dropped from further consideration, and two entries for the evidence table were created: one representing results for a precursor study of the relationship between Channel One television advertising and food and beverage preferences, and one representing results for a diet study of the relationship between Channel One television advertisements and usual dietary intake as measured by recent food and beverage purchases.

There were also three other circumstances under which a single publication could contribute more than one result to the evidence table. If a publication reported more than one complete study, each study was represented by at least one result in the evidence table even if each study addressed the same relationship. If a publication employed two or more entirely different samples to test the same question (not to test whether the samples were different), each sample was entered separately into the evidence table. Finally, if a publication utilized different research methods (e.g., both cross-sectional and longitudinal in a panel design) to test the same question, results from each method were entered separately into the evidence table.

Other variations that could have been treated as separate entries in the evidence table were instead incorporated into a single entry. If multiple measures were used in a study to examine a putative result of marketing, then the different measures were described, but only one result—precursor to diet, diet, or health (diet-related health outcome)—was entered into the evidence table. For example, if both skinfold thickness and body mass index (BMI) were used as measures assessing an influence of television advertising, then the entry into the evidence table was "health." If the research participants came from different age groups from among infants and toddlers, younger children, older children, and teens, the groups were described within one result. If outcomes varied for different subgroups or different measures, they were also described within one result. In assessing the research evidence, it was at times appropriate to consider differences such as these; for example, the relationship of advertising to diet should be examined separately for children and teens. In these cases, the number of items considered in the data tables will be larger than the total number of results in the systematic evidence review table.

Each result in the evidence table was identified by author(s) and publication date of the item in which the result appeared. Its basic characteristics were then coded, three ratings were judged, a mini-abstract was written, and any coder comments were added. Coding the basic characteristics and rating the relevance of the research to the committee's purposes are described in the next two sections.

Coding the Basic Characteristics

The marketing factor studied was recorded as the "cause" variable, and the precursor, diet, or diet-related health factor studied was recorded as the "effect" variable. For example, in Bao and Shao's (2002) study of the effect of radio advertisements for the Cheerwine beverage, "radio advertisements" was recorded as the cause variable, and in the Storey et al. (2003) study of the effect of television viewing on obesity, "obesity" was recorded as the effect variable. If the putative cause variable was television advertising and it was measured by overall television viewing, a special note was made in the coding.

The methods by which the cause and effect variables were measured were also recorded. For example, in Yavas and Abdul-Gader (1993), the cause variable was television advertisements, and its measure was "self-reported average number of advertisement breaks seen each evening." Its effect variable was food purchase requests, and its measure was "self-reported frequency of advertised product requested (Likert-scale)." In the Storey et al. (2003) study of the effect of television viewing on obesity, obesity was measured by BMI calculated from self-reported height and weight, whereas in the Stettler et al. (2004) study, obesity was measured by BMI calculated from physical measures of height and weight taken by a trained technician and by skinfold thickness measured by the technician in various parts of the body. During assessment of the evidence from the body of research in the systematic evidence review, the cause and effect variables were placed into a small number of conceptual categories, and these were added into the final evidence table.

The kind of research study design was coded. For example, some studies were experiments, a few were natural experiments, many were cross-sectional (observational) studies, and some were longitudinal studies. Also coded were the sample size of the study, the age group(s) of the young people studied, and whether the relationship between the marketing variable and the effect variables was statistically significant at the 0.05 level or better. For all statistically significant results, the relationship was in the expected direction and so not explicitly coded.

Rating the Relevance of the Evidence

Relevance of the evidence for the committee's tasks was assessed as high, medium, or low on three key dimensions: (1) the strength of the evidence for a causal relationship between a marketing variable and an outcome precursor, diet, or diet-related health variable (causal inference validity), (2) the quality of the measures used in the study, and (3) the degree to which the results in the study generalize to everyday life (ecological validity).

These criteria are *not* meant to assess the scholarly quality of the research reviewed. It was assumed that the peer-review process screened for this in order for the work to be published. A large, longitudinal study of television viewing and obesity might be designed and executed with impeccable care, but because the researchers were interested in establishing an association rather than a cause–effect relationship, its relevance to the committee's purpose—which prioritizes the ability to make causal inferences—would result in a low rating on causal inference validity. Similarly, a carefully designed and conducted experiment on advertising and children's product evaluation for two competing brands might be rated high on causal inference validity but, because the experiment was conducted in laboratory conditions quite different from everyday life, it might be rated low on ecological validity. Clearly, such low ratings do not reflect the quality of the research conducted; they reflect the relevance of the research to the committee's charge to assess the effects of food and beverage marketing on young people's diet and diet-related health. The two relevance ratings, which will be explained next, both required consideration of the nature and quality of the measures. Measure quality was, therefore, also rated, using the same high, medium, low system used for the two relevance ratings, and it also will be explained below.

Causal Inference Validity Rating. Philosophers, statisticians, economists, epidemiologists, and other social scientists have not yet achieved consensus on the definition of causation, and this debate is likely to go on for some time.[3] Agreement is much more substantial, however, on the issue of causal inference, that is inferring from statistical studies the existence or absence of a causal relationship between two particular quantities, such as hours of television watched and calories expended from vigorous physical activity.[4]

---

[3]There are two major schools of thought on causation in the statistical literature, a counterfactual account mostly due to Rubin (1974), and an intervention/manipulability account due to Spirtes et al. (2000) and Pearl (2000). In the counterfactual account, one makes explicit the difference between the observed value of a response variable and the value that *would have been* observed had an alternative value for treatment been assigned to a given individual. The assumptions required to make the inference from the data actually observed to the data one would have seen had every individual been assigned every possible treatment condition is, in this perspective, the problem of causal inference. See Sobel (1996) for an excellent introduction to the topic from this perspective. In the intervention account, one variable X is a direct cause of another Y relative to a system of variables including Z just in case there is some set of values one could hold Z fixed at such that the probability of Y conditional on *setting* (intervening or manipulating) $X = x1$ is different from the probability of Y conditional on *setting* X $= x2$, $x1 \neq x2$. In this paradigm, one models a causal system with a directed graph in which each edge $X \rightarrow Y$ represents that X is a direct cause of Y relative to the other variables Z in the system under study, and many of the problems of causal reasoning can be characterized qualitatively using such nonparametric graphical formulations. See Spirtes et al. (2004) for an account of causal inference from this perspective.

[4]See, for example, Glymour and Cooper (1999), Holland (1986), Pearl (2000), Robins (1988), Rosenbaum (2002), Rubin (1974), Sobel (1996), Spirtes et al. (2000, 2004), Wasserman (2004).

Put another way, accounts of causal inference tend to stress the same points regardless of the precise definition of causation utilized.

The evidence for interpreting an association as causal is entirely distinct from the evidence used to judge whether an association is statistically significant. For example, the evidence required for concluding that a statistical association exists between exposure to television advertising and calories consumed is distinct from the evidence required for concluding that an increase of exposure to television advertising causes an increase in calories consumed. To underscore this distinction, the committee explicitly created two dimensions for each study in the evidence review: one to record whether the statistical evidence for an association was significant, and another to record the evidence for concluding the existence of a causal relation.

The evidence for the existence of a causal relation is a function of the study design, the measures used, and the background knowledge that is credible. The classic design for inferring causation is the randomized experimental trial. Treatment is assigned randomly, and the outcome is measured by some device or person blind to the treatment assigned. If dropout was low, or was independent of treatment, and the outcome was measured validly, then the study provides strong evidence for causality. Experimental studies on the influence of food and beverage marketing were rated high on causal inference validity if treatment was assigned randomly, dropout was not a factor, and the measures used were valid.

In an observational study, that is, a study in which the treatment, or cause variable, was not assigned but rather just passively observed, an association between a putative cause X and a putative effect Y might be explained in three ways: (1) X is a cause of Y, (2) some third factor (confounder) is a common cause of both, or (3) Y is a cause of X. The overall assessment of causal inference validity for such studies rides on how convincingly the study eliminates possibilities 2 and 3.

Time order between the putative cause and effect is the most common reason for eliminating the third possibility, and statistically adjusting, or controlling, for potential confounders is the most common methodology for eliminating the second possibility. To have confidence that statistical controls are adequate, it is important to know both that all important confounders were included in the study and, just as importantly, that all important confounders were measured with high validity, reliability, and precision (see below for explanation). Thus, observational studies were rated high on causal inference validity if the measures of the cause and effect were valid, if all plausible confounders were included and measured validly, reliably, and precisely; and if some reason could be given to eliminate the possibility that the observed association was not due to causation opposite to that predicted, that is, the putative effect causing the putative cause.

To summarize, causal inference validity of each result in the evidence table was scored as high, medium, or low on the basis of the study design, the quality of the measures employed, the drop out rate, the statistical controls used, and the background knowledge available. Because some studies did not aim to make a case for causality, and others faced extremely difficult measurement challenges, judgments about causal inference validity do not and should not coincide with judgments about the scholarly quality of a study. More detail on the criteria used for rating causal inference validity is provided in the codebook (see Appendix F-1).

Measure Quality Rating. Clearly, measurement figures heavily in these judgments. So heavily, in fact, that the quality of measures was explicitly rated as high, medium, or low for each result entered into the evidence table. The measures used in each study were rated taking into consideration three dimensions: validity, reliability, and precision. Validity refers to the extent to which a measure directly and accurately measured what it intended to measure. For example, examining grocery store receipts is a valid measure of food purchased over a week, whereas asking someone to list the food he or she intends to buy over the next week is not. Reliability assesses the extent to which the same measurement technique, applied repeatedly, is likely to yield the same results when circumstances remain unchanged. For example, measuring a 6-year-old's cumulative exposure to lead by taking a single blood sample is highly unreliable; such measurements fluctuate markedly from day to day. Chemically determining the concentration of lead in discarded baby teeth is much more reliable (ATSDR, 2002). Precision refers to the fineness or coarseness of a measure. For example, measuring family income in number of dollars is precise, but measuring it as low, medium, or high is not.

Ecological Validity Rating. Ecological validity refers to the extent to which a study's results are likely to generalize to the naturally occurring world of marketing and young people's diets and diet-related health. An investigation's research setting might be quite dissimilar to the natural system being studied. For example, a study in which 6-year-olds are removed from class and taken to a trailer near their school, shown 7 minutes of commercials, and then asked to make a series of binary choices from photographs of item-pairs is low in ecological validity. A study in which mother–child pairs are surreptitiously observed in the supermarket and each food purchase request is recorded is more ecologically valid. Also high in ecological validity are studies in which daily television viewing is measured from the use of viewing diaries or program check-off lists. The measure quality may not be high but the ecological validity is high because everyday behavior over a period of time is being measured.

Research on marketing and behavior involves a tension between causal inference validity and ecological validity. Studies that carefully isolate a small number of causal factors in a laboratory setting tend to be high on causal inference validity, but low on ecological validity. Studies that observe young people in their natural environment tend to be high on ecological validity but low on causal inference validity. Rarely do studies score high on both measures.

The Coding Process

Using these dimensions for recording characteristics and for rating measure quality and relevance, the committee constructed an initial codebook and an evidence table. Several iterations of trial coding removed ambiguities from the codebook, calibrated and refined the evaluative criteria employed, and guided final choices about the set of coding dimensions. The final codebook is available in Appendix F-1.

Two coders were assigned to each article identified as relevant to the committee's purposes. They worked independently and resolved disagreements by discussion. If consensus was not readily obtained, other committee members were consulted. After agreement, both coders' comments on the article along with an abstract for the piece were included, and the final coding results were compiled into an evidence table that could be sorted on any categorical coding dimension (a condensed version of the evidence table is available in Appendix F-2). Coders were drawn from committee members and selected university students commissioned to assist in this process. All received training to ensure consistency in perspectives and process. In general, coders agreed with each other. Later reviews of the evidence table suggested that both the recording and rating functions were executed consistently by all coders.

Characteristics and Relevance of Research in the Systematic Evidence Review

The systematic evidence review is based on results from published original research about the relationship of commercial food and beverage marketing to diet indirectly through mediators (or precursors), to diet directly, and to diet-related health directly. The descriptive and evaluative characteristics for all the results included in the systematic evidence review are presented in Tables 5-1 and 5-2, respectively, according to whether the result pertained to the relationship of marketing to precursor, marketing to diet, or marketing to diet-related health.

Overall, the results are drawn from many different studies rather than from a few. In total, 123 different published reports of original research

TABLE 5-1 Descriptive Characteristics of Research in the Systematic Evidence Review for the Relationship of Marketing to Precursors of Diet, Marketing to Diet, and Marketing to Diet-Related Health

Characteristic	Marketing and Precursors of Diet	Marketing and Diet	Marketing and Diet-Related Health
Total Results*	45	36	74
Decade Published			
1970	6	0	0
1980	21	10	4
1990	10	13	25
2000	8	13	45
Research Design			
Experimental	25	10	1
Natural experiment	1	3	0
Longitudinal	2	2	17
Cross-sectional	17	21	56
Age Group			
Infants and toddlers (under 2)	0	0	1
Younger children (2–5)	23	12	17
Older children (6–11)	28	22	58
Teens (12–18)	6	10	33
Sample Size			
0–49	8	4	1
50–99	10	6	6
100–499	24	16	21
500–999	1	2	11
1,000 or more	2	8	35
Type of Marketing			
TV ads: experimental treatment	24	9	0
TV ads: observed in natural setting	0	0	2
TV ads: TV viewing only	15	22	56
TV ads: TV campaign	2	1	0
TV ads: TV viewing and other media use	0	2	16
All other marketing	4	2	0
Type of Outcome			
Preferences	27	0	0
Purchase requests	14	0	0
Beliefs	13	0	0
Short-term consumption	0	9	0
Usual dietary intake	0	27	0
Adiposity	0	0	73
Other	1	0	2

NOTE: Other types of marketing for precursors of diet were print ads, radio ads, multimedia campaign, and price and promotion. Other types of marketing for diet were product placement in film, and price and promotion. Other outcomes for precursors of diet were perceived intent and credibility of ads. Other outcomes for diet-related health were cholesterol levels and cardiovascular fitness.

*One result in the evidence table could be about more than one age group or type of marketing.

TABLE 5-2 Evaluative Characteristics of Research in the Systematic Evidence Review for the Relationship of Marketing to Precursors of Diet, Marketing to Diet, and Marketing to Diet-Related Health

Characteristic	Marketing and Precursors of Diet	Marketing and Diet	Marketing and Diet-Related Health
Total Results	45	36	74
Quality of Measures			
High	5	10	0
Medium	27	14	32
Low	13	12	42
Causal Inference Validity			
High	11	11	1
Medium	20	9	18
Low	14	16	55
Ecological Validity			
High	13	24	63
Medium	19	10	9
Low	13	2	2

contributed 155 different results to the systematic evidence review. On average, then, each publication accounted for 1.26 results in the evidence table. Across all three relationships, no single publication accounted for more than two results in the evidence table. When analyses delved into possible differences by age or by type of outcome, one publication could contribute more than two data points if it involved more than one age group or type of outcome. As will be discussed later, there is a clear need for more research in several areas. However, any finding that can be drawn from the research that has been done to date is based on a diverse set of studies conducted by different researchers. This fact enhances the credibility of the results.

The research spans four decades. During that time, issues addressed early on have also been addressed recently. The first few publications appeared in the 1970s, many appeared in the 1980s and 1990s, and many more have appeared halfway through the 2000s. For any of the three relationships for which findings can be drawn based on early research, there is also recent research that supports the finding and thereby reduces concern that earlier results on any of the three relationships might be different now due to societal changes (e.g., in the nature of food products or of beverage advertising).

All three main types of research designs have been used to study the direct relationship of marketing to precursors, diet, and diet-related health. For any one relationship, at least two experimental, cross-sectional, and longitudinal research designs have been employed in sufficient numbers so that the usual limitations of one design are generally counterbalanced by the usual strengths of another design. This is true particularly in terms of the ability to determine cause and effect relationships (causal inference validity) and to relate research results to phenomena in everyday life (ecological validity).

Overall, quality and relevance are reasonably good for the research included in the systematic evidence review. Earlier in this chapter the use of high, medium, and low ratings of measure quality, ability to infer causality, and similarity to everyday life was described. These three ratings were made for every result for each of the three relationships examined. Considering the three rating scales and three relationships together, with one exception, the number of medium and high ratings is greater than or about the same as the number of low ratings. The one exception is the causal inference validity rating for research on the relationship of marketing to diet-related health. About three-quarters of the results had low causal inference validity. Thus, it was much harder to arrive at findings about the relationship of marketing to diet-related health than it was to arrive at findings for the relationship of marketing to precursors of diet or to diet itself.

In social science research in general, it is difficult—but not impossible—to achieve in the same study high ability both to determine cause and effect relationships and to relate results to everyday life. It is true as well in the specific area of the relationship of marketing to the precursors of diet, the diets of young people, and their diet-related health. In fact, just 5 (3 percent) of the 155 results had high ratings for both causal inference validity and ecological validity. Three different high relevance studies (French et al., 2001a; Gorn and Goldberg, 1982; Greenberg and Brand, 1993) each contributed one result about the relationship between marketing and diet, and one (Robinson, 1999) contributed one result about the relationship between marketing and diet and one result about the relationship between marketing and diet-related health. Because of this pattern of rather inverse relevance ratings for causal inference validity and ecological validity, which is characteristic of research addressing many different social issues, findings must be carefully drawn from all available research, weighing the contribution of each result and the characteristics and relevance of the research in which it was reported.

Research samples ranged in size from a low in the 30s to a high of more than 15,000, with the majority either in the low 100s or more that 1,000. Overall, older children were the most frequently studied, but different age groups were studied for the three relationships. For the relationship of marketing to precursors of diet, most of the research involved younger (ages 2–5 years) and older children (ages 6–11 years), with some work with teens (ages 12–18 years). For the relationship of marketing to diet, most of the work involved older children, with quite a bit of work equally with younger children and teens. For the relationship of marketing to diet-related health, most of the work involved older children, then teens, and then younger children. The one study with infants and toddlers (under 2 years) was in this last area, diet-related health. Because of these variations in the ages of research participants and the possibility that age might moderate the relationships between marketing and precursors, diet, or diet-related health, findings were limited to those age groups for which enough research had been conducted.

Nearly all the research was about television advertising, which is the most prominent and frequent type of marketing young people encounter. Just 6 results (Auty and Lewis, 2004; Bao and Shao, 2002 [2 results]; French et al., 2001a; Macklin, 1990; Norton et al., 2000) of the 155 total were about any other type of marketing. The main types of outcomes were food and beverage preferences, purchase requests, and beliefs for the precursors of diet; short-term consumption and usual dietary intake for diet; and adiposity for diet-related health.

Overall the research included in the systematic evidence review was of sufficient size, diversity, and quality to support the derivation of several findings about the influence of marketing, specifically television advertising, on the precursors of children's and teens' diet, on their current diet, and on their diet-related health. Following a discussion of how the results in the evidence table were interpreted, the evidence and findings from it will be presented in three sections, first for the precursors of diet, then for diet, and finally for diet-related health.

Interpretation of the Results

Many factors were brought into play in deriving findings from the systematic evidence review. The quantity, variety, and statistical significance of results and the research from which they came influenced whether any finding was drawn and how definitive it was held to be. Pertinent results needed to be available from several different studies conducted by different researchers using different research populations and measures. A preponderance of pertinent results had to support the finding. In addition, any consistent differences between results supporting and not supporting the finding had to be taken into account. If a cogent explanation could be provided for results supporting and not supporting the finding, then the finding would need to be qualified accordingly.

Because of the committee's charge, particular attention was given to assessing cause and effect relationships and to establishing the degree to which such relationships are likely also to occur in everyday life in the United States. Useful findings might describe relationships between marketing and precursors, diet, or diet-related health, without being certain that one causes the other. Useful findings also might describe cause and effect relationships, without being certain that they would occur in everyday life. The most useful findings will describe the ways in which various aspects of marketing influence various aspects of precursors of diet, diet, or diet-related health, and do so with some confidence that these effects occur in the everyday lives of our young people.

In deriving findings from the systematic evidence review, the committee used a three-step process. First, it determined whether there were enough research results from which to derive a finding about a particular topic. For example, regarding the influence of televised food and beverage advertising on children's and teens' short-term consumption, the committee concluded there was enough evidence for both younger and older children, but "an absence of evidence" for teens. Second, for those topics for which there was sufficient evidence, the committee drew on all aspects of the evidence to decide whether there was a relationship between the marketing variable and the outcome variable. For example, there was sufficient evidence to reach findings about the relationship of televised food and beverage advertising on children's and teens' usual dietary intake. For younger and older children, on balance, the evidence supported the finding that advertising influenced intake, whereas for teens, on balance, the evidence supported the finding that advertising did not influence intake. Third, the committee provided a sense of the strength of the research support for the finding, using the terms "strong," "moderate," and "weak." For example, for the findings regarding advertising's influence on usual dietary intake, there was moderate evidence for such influence for younger children (ages 2–5 years), weak evidence for such influence for older children (ages 6–11 years), and weak evidence against such influence for teens (ages 12–18 years).

A rather large number of results in the systematic evidence review measured everyday television viewing as a means of assessing exposure to food and beverage advertising on television. This was a deliberate measurement choice by many of the researchers who conducted the studies included in the systematic evidence review for the relationship of marketing to precursors of diet and for the relationship of marketing to diet. In cases reviewing the relationship of marketing to diet-related health, researchers generally did not use television viewing to measure exposure to televised advertising. In such studies, television viewing was treated as a measure of several different possible variables, of a sedentary lifestyle, of time away from physical activity, and the like. Nonetheless, the research design, methods, and analyses were essentially the same as those in many studies testing marketing's influence on precursors of diet and on diet. For this reason, the committee included all such research in the systematic evidence review, whether or not the researchers intended their work to be about television advertising.

The committee's decision to accept that measures of television viewing could be interpreted as assessing young people's advertising exposure had two important ramifications. First, studies that relied on estimates of time spent watching television as an indicator of advertising exposure could not fare very well in terms of the rated measurement quality. This stems from several factors, including the possibility that part of any person's total television time was devoted to viewing mostly noncommercial programming (e.g., public broadcasting) or that some people may leave the room during commercials, successfully avoiding exposure to the ads. Despite these possibilities, broad-based estimates of time spent watching television function reasonably well to identify an individual's relative exposure to commercial messages, as advertising permeates the large majority of television viewed by most individuals, in particular young people.

A second important ramification of having included these studies in the systematic evidence review is that the committee must accept the burden of carefully considering alternative explanations for any association found between television advertising, measured by television viewing, and precursors of diet, diet, or diet-related health. This burden increases as one moves from precursors such as requests for foods known to be advertised on programming popular with children, to aspects of diet such as short-term choices for snacks known to be advertised on television, to health issues related to the quality of a young person's usual diet.

To arrive at findings when television viewing was the measure of exposure to televised food and beverage advertising, plausible alternative explanations had to be generated for each outcome variable and the possibility of ruling out these alternatives examined. This was easier when the same relationship was studied with experimental methods as well as cross-sectional methods. Longitudinal methods were also informative. In addition, research that included methodological and statistical controls for alternative explanations was useful. In the absence of very well-controlled studies or a body of research that includes experimental as well as correlational methods, however, it was hard to draw many findings from research using television viewing as the measure of exposure to television advertising.

Finally, in interpreting the results, the committee kept in mind that diet and diet-related health are complex and multiply determined. There was no expectation that marketing would be the only influence on diet or diet-related health, nor did it seem likely that marketing would be the major determinant of diet or diet-related health. Moreover, people are forgetful and changeable enough that any limited marketing experience was not expected to have more than a limited influence. With these realities in mind, the committee looked for all possible effects, including powerful and long-lasting effects on diet and diet-related health, but it also considered small effects and short-term effects both reasonable and meaningful.

Overall, the research results included in the systematic evidence review were of sufficient quality, diversity, and scope to support certain findings about the influence of marketing, including the overall finding that food and beverage marketing influences the preferences and purchase requests of children, influences consumption at least in the short term, is a likely contributor to less healthful diets, and may contribute to negative diet-related health outcomes and risks.

Presentation of the Systematic Evidence Review Analysis

The next three sections review in detail the evidence related to each of the three specific relationships. They have a similar structure. To begin, the evidentiary base for the relationship between marketing and the relevant outcome (precursors, then diet, then diet-related health) is considered in terms of the descriptive and evaluative characteristics of all significant and nonsignificant results for that relationship. Because the evidence for all three relationships is almost entirely about one form of marketing—advertising distributed via television and cable television—and a limited set of outcomes, any result about a different form of marketing or an infrequently studied outcome is then removed from the evidentiary base, and the main analysis of the results proceeds. This analysis takes into account the age of the research participants, the kind of outcome, and the causal inference validity for each significant and nonsignificant result. Each section ends with a summary of the important findings drawn from the available research about the target relationship.

In presenting the results of the systematic evidence review for the three relationships, the committee has sought to meet the likely interests of readers with varying levels of expertise in social science research. Many data tables are presented. The main points to be drawn from the tables are also described in terms that should be meaningful to all readers. Examples from the research are offered to bring life to the work. The text, particularly the introduction and findings for each of the three sections, should be useful for every reader. For some, the middle sections, the data tables, the summary evidence table (available in Appendix F-2), and references should provide enough of the analytic methods and results to support an independent assessment of the committee's work.

SYSTEMATIC EVIDENCE REVIEW OF THE RELATIONSHIP BETWEEN MARKETING AND PRECURSORS OF DIET

This section considers the evidence relevant to the effect of marketing on precursors of diet. In order for food and beverage marketing to influence young people's diets, one or more of several things need to occur as the result of marketing. Young people need to become aware of the product or brand or service. They need to develop some sense that consuming the food or beverage is desirable, perhaps because they expect it will taste good, give them energy, cost just a little, be easy to acquire or consume, be fun to handle, be sold in a fun environment, have a toy in the package, help them fit in with their peers, promote strong bones and teeth, please their parents, or provide some other benefit. They may need to influence their parents, older siblings or friends, or caretakers to purchase the product or brand or to go to the restaurant. In the five-element causal framework (see Figure 5-1), these relationships between marketing and the precursors of diet initiate the path from marketing to diet and diet-related health, the primary outcomes of interest to the committee.

Evidentiary Base

For the systematic evidence review of the relationship between marketing and precursors of diet, the evidence table includes 45 results from 42 different published research reports. The earliest study was published in 1974 and the latest in 2005. Table 5-3 summarizes the descriptive characteristics of those studies that reported a statistically significant relationship between any form of marketing and any mediator or precursor, and of those that reported a nonsignificant relationship. All significant results show that more exposure to marketing is associated with greater preference or more purchase requests for what was advertised or more beliefs like that presented via marketing. Virtually all studies in the systematic evidence review focused on marketing of high-calorie and low-nutrient foods and beverages, either due to researcher selection for an experiment or due to the predominant marketing of such products in naturalistic studies. Thus, most of the systematic evidence review focuses on the effects of marketing high-calorie and low-nutrient foods and beverages. No information is included that demonstrates whether the findings would apply to the marketing of more healthful foods and beverages (see Chapter 6 for a discussion of social marketing campaigns).

All but four of the results involved television advertising, occasionally using commercials the researchers had made, often using commercials taken off the air, and sometimes using a measure of likely exposure to commercials as a result of everyday television viewing. For more recent studies, television might include material available via cable television rather than

TABLE 5-3 Descriptive Characteristics of Research on the Influence of Commercial Marketing on the Precursors, or Mediators to Young People's Diets

Characteristic	Significant Results	Nonsignificant Results
Total Results*	35	10
Decade Published		
1970	5	1
1980	13	8
1990	9	1
2000	8	0
Research Design		
Experimental	18	7
Natural experiment	1	0
Longitudinal	2	0
Cross-sectional	14	3
Age Group*		
Younger children (2–5)	17	6
Older children (6–11)	21	7
Teens (12–18)	6	0
Sample Size		
0–49	7	1
50–99	7	3
100–499	18	6
500–999	1	0
1,000 or more	2	0
Type of Marketing		
TV ads: experimental treatment	18	6
TV ads: TV viewing only	12	3
TV ads: TV campaign	2	0
Print ads	0	1
Radio ads	1	0
Multimedia campaign	1	0
Price and promotion	1	0
Type of Precursor*		
Preferences	19	8
Purchase requests	13	1
Beliefs	10	3
Intent and credibility of advertising	1	0

*One result in the evidence table could be about more than one age group or type of precursor. For these two characteristics the column totals can be more than the number of results.

broadcast systems. The remaining four results addressed the influence of print advertising (Macklin, 1990), radio advertising (Bao and Shao, 2002), a multimedia advertising campaign (Bao and Shao, 2002), and price and promotion (Norton et al., 2000). Twenty-three of the results were about younger children (ages 2–5), 28 about older children (ages 6–11), and 6 about teens (ages 12–18).

Twenty-seven of the results examined the effects of food and beverage marketing on young people's preferences. Most were experiments; some were cross-sectional designs. As an example of an experiment, Borzekowski and Robinson (2001) showed two short cartoons to preschoolers, half of whom also saw about 2.5 minutes of educational material between the two cartoons and the other half of whom saw 2.5 minutes of ads. All material had been broadcast previously on television. The advertisements were for juice, sandwich bread, donuts, candy, a fast food chicken entrée, snack cakes, breakfast cereal, peanut butter, and a toy. Immediately after viewing, children who saw the advertisements preferred the advertised brand over an alternate similar product with similar packaging, even if the advertised brand (of donut) was unfamiliar and the alternate was a local favorite. Advertisements varied in effectiveness, and advertisements run twice were more effective. The advertising effects were the same for boys and girls, children whose home language was English or Spanish, and children with varying levels of access to media. Parents also reported that television advertising influenced their children's preferences and purchase requests.

Fourteen of the results examined the effects of food and beverage marketing on young people's purchase requests. Somewhat more than half were cross-sectional designs; the rest were experiments. As an example of a cross-sectional design, Isler et al. (1987) had mothers of 250 children between ages 3 and 11 years keep detailed diaries for 4 weeks. Weekly in-person or telephone checks were made. For younger and older children, there were small, statistically significant relationships between the amount of television watched and the total number of requests and between the amount of television watched and the number of requests for cereal and candy; relationships were not significant for fast foods and snack foods, nor for foods such as fruits and vegetables that are advertised infrequently on television. In an experimental study, Stoneman and Brody (1982) had young children view a 20-minute television cartoon with or without advertisements for two candy bars, one chocolate drink mix, one brand of grape jelly, and two salty snack chips. Mothers separately viewed the cartoons without advertisements and did not know whether their children were seeing advertisements with the cartoons. Mothers and children then participated in a "separate study" of family shopping for weekly groceries in a mini-grocery store. A "clerk," who was unaware of the nature of the research, surreptitiously recorded what happened. Children who had seen the commercials more often asked for products, whether or not advertised, pointed to them, grabbed them off the shelf, or put them into the grocery cart; they also did so more often for the advertised products. Mothers of these children also more often said no, put items back, and offered alternatives to children's requests. The article does not say whether children who had seen the commercials ultimately took home more requested products themselves.

Thirteen of the results examined the effects of food and beverage marketing on young people's beliefs about foods and beverages. The majority was experiments, a few were cross-sectional designs, and one was a longitudinal panel study. As an example of a cross-sectional study, Signorielli and Staples (1997) administered questionnaires to about 400 fourth and fifth graders. Children who viewed more television knew less about which foods and beverages were healthier, and the significant relationship remained when the effects of gender, race/ethnicity, reading level, parents' education, and parents' occupation were all also taken into account. More recently, Harrison (2005) carried out a similar study except that children were measured twice, 6 weeks apart, for beliefs about healthier food choices offered as pairs. There were two diet food items (fat-free ice cream versus *cottage cheese* and Diet Coke versus *orange juice*, with the italicized choice being healthier) and four nondiet food items (celery versus *carrots*, rice cakes versus *wheat bread*, jelly versus *peanut butter*, and lettuce versus *spinach*). Taking into account at time 1, grade, and gender, the more children watched television at time 1 the less accurate their choices at time 2 for diet foods (both pairs have items likely to be advertised on television) but not for nondiet foods (only one of four pairs has items likely to be advertised on television).

Table 5-4 summarizes the evaluative characteristics of the 45 results included in the evidentiary base for the relationship between marketing and precursors of diet. Measurement quality was high for 5 results, medium for 27, and low for 13. Eleven of 45 were of high relevance to inferring a causal connection from marketing to the precursors of diet, 20 were of medium relevance, and 14 were of low relevance. The ability to generalize from these studies (ecological validity) was generally good. Thirteen studies were of high ecological validity, 19 medium, and 13 low. A closer examination of the distribution of significant and nonsignificant results according to the relevance of the research, specifically the ability to make a clear causal inference and the ecological validity, also revealed no difference in relevance between the studies reporting significant results and those reporting nonsignificant results (see Table 5-5). As the relevance of the research increased (high or medium ratings compared to low), the proportion of significant results remained high, providing further confidence in evidence-based findings for the influence of marketing on young people's preferences for, purchase requests of, and beliefs about foods and beverages.

TABLE 5-4 Evaluative Characteristics of Research on the Influence of Commercial Marketing on the Precursors, or Mediators, of Young People's Diets

Characteristic	Significant Results	Nonsignificant Results
Total Results	35	10
Quality of Measures		
High	5	0
Medium	21	6
Low	9	4
Causal Inference Validity		
High	9	2
Medium	15	5
Low	11	3
Ecological Validity		
High	11	2
Medium	14	5
Low	10	3

TABLE 5-5 Relevance Ratings of Research on the Influence of Commercial Marketing on Precursors, or Mediators, to Young People's Diets

Causal Inference Validity	Ecological Validity	Significant Results	Nonsignificant Results
Total Results		35	10
High	High	0	0
	Medium	5	1
	Low	4	1
Medium	High	4	0
	Medium	5	3
	Low	6	2
Low	High	7	2
	Medium	4	1
	Low	0	0

Relationships Between Television Advertising and Precursors of Diet

Given the descriptive characteristics of research about the relationship of marketing to the precursors of diet, any findings about this relationship must be findings about the relationship of television advertising to food and beverage preferences, purchase requests, and beliefs among children and teens. To create a dataset that only examined these relationships, four

TABLE 5-6 Distribution of Significant and Nonsignificant Results by Causal Inference Validity for the Relationship of Television Advertising to the Food and Beverage Preferences of Younger Children, Older Children, and Teens

Causal Inference Validity	Younger Children (2–5 years)		Older Children (6–11 years)		Teens (12–18 years)	
	Significant Results	Non-significant Results	Significant Results	Non-significant Results	Significant Results	Non-significant Results
Total Results	7	4	12	5	2	0
High	2	1	6	2	0	0
Medium	5	2	6	2	2	0
Low	0	1	0	1	0	0

results (from three articles: Bao and Shao, 2002; Macklin, 1990; Norton et al., 2000) were removed. The overall patterns of descriptive and evaluative characteristics and relevance ratings of the remaining 41 results did not change when results involving marketing other than television advertising and precursors other than preferences, requests, and beliefs were removed.

Tables 5-6, 5-7, and 5-8 present the distribution of significant and nonsignificant findings for the relationships of television advertising to food and beverage preferences, purchase requests, and beliefs, respectively. For each outcome, the distribution is examined according to the age of the

TABLE 5-7 Distribution of Significant and Nonsignificant Results by Causal Inference Validity for the Relationship of Television Advertising to the Food and Beverage Purchase Requests of Younger Children, Older Children, and Teens

Causal Inference Validity	Younger Children (2–5 years)		Older Children (6–11 years)		Teens (12–18 years)	
	Significant Results	Non-significant Results	Significant Results	Non-significant Results	Significant Results	Non-significant Results
Total Results	9	0	6	0	1	0
High	2	0	0	0	0	0
Medium	2	0	2	0	0	0
Low	5	0	4	0	1	0

TABLE 5-8 Distribution of Significant and Nonsignificant Results by Causal Inference Validity for the Relationship of Television Advertising to the Food and Beverage Beliefs of Younger Children, Older Children, and Teens

Causal Inference Validity	Younger Children (2–5 years)		Older Children (6–11 years)		Teens (12–18 years)	
	Significant Results	Non-significant Results	Significant Results	Non-significant Results	Significant Results	Non-significant Results
Total Results	4	1	9	2	1	0
High	0	0	1	0	0	0
Medium	4	1	8	1	1	0
Low	0	0	0	1	0	0

participants and the causal inference validity. Because a single result in the evidence base could apply to more than one age group, when results are characterized by age group, the total number of results may be more than the total number in the evidence table.

Television Advertising and Food and Beverage Preferences

In the research, preferences are measured in a variety of ways and include both which brand is preferred and which type of product is preferred. Examples from the research include which type of food Cub Scouts choose as a snack at their meetings (one of the types of choices had been advertised), which brand of food or beverage product is preferred when choosing between pairs of images of similar products and packaging (one of the pair had been advertised), preference for salty food or nonsalty alternatives when choosing between pairs of slides (one of the types had been advertised), and eating preference for a healthful or less healthful food or beverage product when pairs are presented (amount of television viewing used to indicate amount of exposure to advertising for the less healthful product type).

For younger and older children, the evidence clearly supports the finding that television advertising influences their food and beverage preferences (see Table 5-6). The number of significant results is about twice the number of nonsignificant results. Overall, the causal inference validity is high and medium, and the causal inference validity of the significant results is at least as good as it is for the nonsignficant results. Among the significant results are studies measuring the immediate influence of television advertising on preferences and studies measuring longer term influence, as well as studies indicating that more exposure to advertising is associated with greater influence and that affected preferences are for product types as well as specific brands. Although the results for teens are like those for children, the total number is insufficient to support any finding.

Finding: There is strong evidence that television advertising influences the food and beverage preferences of children ages 2–11 years. There is insufficient evidence about its influence on the preferences of teens ages 12–18 years.

Television Advertising and Food and Beverage Purchase Requests

In the research, purchase requests are measured in a variety of ways and include both which brand is requested and which type of product is requested. Examples from the research include unobtrusive observations of mothers and children in a real or simulated grocery store and the children asking for a product type or putting it into the grocery cart, children's reports of whether they would ask their mothers to buy the advertised brand of cereal, parents' reports in interviews or questionnaires of children's purchase requests, and a 4-week diary by the mother of her child's product requests.

For younger and older children, the evidence clearly supports the finding that television advertising influences their food and beverage purchase requests (see Table 5-7). There are only significant results in the evidentiary base. The causal inference validity for younger children is high, medium, and low; for older children, medium and low. Among the significant results are studies measuring the immediate influence of television advertising on purchase requests and studies measuring longer term influence, as well as studies indicating that more exposure to advertising is associated with greater influence and that affected purchase requests are for product types as well as specific brands.

Finding: There is strong evidence that television advertising influences the food and beverage purchase requests of children ages 2–11 years. There is insufficient evidence about its influence on the purchase requests of teens ages 12–18 years.

Television Advertising and Food and Beverage Beliefs

In the research, food and beverage beliefs is measured in a variety of ways. Examples include judgments of the fruit content of six cereals and six beverages, rankings of three cereals according to how good they are for children, expectations of the taste of advertised food products, judgments about the healthfulness of various foods and beverages, nutritional reasoning, knowledge of the variety of flavors for a product, descriptions of a healthful breakfast, and identification of healthful breakfasts from a range of options. In most of these studies the beliefs measured are those conveyed by advertisements for products such as breakfast cereals (what constitutes a healthful breakfast) and sugared fruit drinks (how much fruit juice is in the drink). In many cases, but certainly not all, the knowledge gained may be inaccurate or misleading in the view of nutrition experts. For this reason, the term beliefs rather than knowledge is used for this precursor of diet.

For younger and older children, the evidence clearly supports the finding that television advertising influences their belief about food and beverage composition, the healthfulness of different foods and beverages, and other aspects of nutrition (see Table 5-8). The number of significant results is much greater than the number of nonsignificant results. Overall, the causal inference validity is medium for all results except one that is high and one that is low, and the causal inference validity of the significant results is at least as good as it is for the nonsignificant results. Among the significant results are studies measuring the immediate influence of television advertising on beliefs and studies measuring longer-term influence. The one result for teens is like those for children, but insufficient to support any finding.

Finding: There is moderate evidence that television advertising influences the food and beverage beliefs of children ages 2–11 years. There is insufficient evidence about its influence on the beliefs of teens ages 12–18 years.

Television Advertising and Preferences, Requests, and Beliefs

The committee's findings about the influence of television advertising on food and beverage preferences, purchase requests, and beliefs are supported (1) in research involving short-term exposure to television advertising and immediate subsequent testing of the dependent variable and (2) in research involving intermediate-term exposure and intermediate lengths (e.g., 1 week) of subsequent testing of the dependent variable. The research involving long-term exposure does so by measuring television viewing outside the research setting. The great majority of the results when television viewing was the measure of exposure to television advertising report a positive relationship between viewing and preferences, purchase requests, or beliefs, the same type of relationship found in studies using other more direct (often experimental) but short-term measures of exposure to television advertising. When exposure to television advertising is measured by reported viewing outside the research context, the measurement appropriately segregates television viewing from video game playing and computer use; not enough is known about their advertising and what is known suggests that it is different from television advertising. If cable television viewing is included, that is reasonable given that nearly everything a child or teen would view on cable would also have advertising like that found on television. The consistency of results from a combination of experimental and correlational designs and from researcher-controlled, short-term exposure to advertising and naturally occurring, long-term exposure from home viewing provides a strong case for concluding that television advertising influences children's food and beverage preferences, purchase requests, and beliefs. The very small amount of evidence for teens is consistent with these findings.

What, then, are the implications of these results for diet? The little available research indicates that nutritional beliefs do not have much influence on the preferences or behavior of children and teens (e.g., Murphy et al., 1995; Signorielli and Lears, 1992; Signorielli and Staples, 1997). However, there is good evidence that purchase requests exert some influence on parental purchases, bringing the requested product into the home (e.g., Galst and White, 1976; Taras et al., 1989, 2000; Ward and Wackman, 1972). It is reasonable to believe that the young person then consumes the product at least once. If the product itself or the brand is not liked, then repeat purchase is unlikely. If it is liked, then repeat purchase is possible. If the product continues to be advertised, then the young person will have repeat opportunities to be influenced to request the product. As reviewed elsewhere in the committee's report (see Chapter 3), preferences influence diet. Preferences include biologically based preferences for sweet, salty, and fatty foods and beverages as well as preferences developed from exposure, repetitive consumption, and association with pleasant circumstances, admired models, and the like. In the systematic evidence review, preference is measured in many ways. Other research indicates that the more distal measurement methods (e.g., preference expressed on a smiley-face rating scale) are reasonable indicators of preferences expressed more directly (e.g., choosing the food or beverage to eat) (e.g., Fisher and Birch, 1995). Thus, it is likely that the influence that television advertising has on children's and teens' preferences and purchase requests would lead to some influence on their diets. Given the nutritional characteristics of the foods and beverages advertised on television (see Chapter 4), their diets would be adversely impacted to some degree. What would happen if healthier foods and beverages were advertised instead is an open question.

Finding: Given the findings from the systematic evidence review of the influence of marketing on the precursors of diet, and given the evidence from content analyses that the preponderance of television food and bever-

age advertising relevant to children and youth promotes high-calorie and low-nutrient products, it can be concluded that television advertising influences children to prefer and request high-calorie and low-nutrient foods and beverages.

SYSTEMATIC EVIDENCE REVIEW OF THE RELATIONSHIP BETWEEN MARKETING AND DIET

This section considers the evidence relevant to the influence of marketing on diet. In the previous section, results in which the outcome variable was a precursor to diet (e.g., food and beverage preferences, food and beverage purchase requests, or food and beverage beliefs) were considered. This section considers results in which the outcome is some dietary *behavior*. The difference is important because the causal connection from the precursors of diet discussed in the previous section and dietary behavior is sometimes unclear. For example, several of the results discussed in the previous section measure food or beverage preferences by asking participants[5] to choose between photographs of two foods or beverages. Other results measure food or beverage purchase requests by asking young people what they will request their mother to purchase during the next visit to the supermarket. In either case, differences between individuals on these measurements might or might not translate into differences in actual food or beverage consumption or differences in diet. Self-reported intentions about future behavior are not generally reliable. In some cases, however, research has been carried out on the effect of a precursor to diet on diet itself. For example, Galst and White (1976) studied the effect of attentiveness to television on food and beverage purchase requests, and they also studied the proportion of food and beverage purchase requests acceded to by parents in the supermarket.

Evidentiary Base

The committee categorized a result on the effect of marketing on diet as relevant if it reported on a quantitative relationship between some exposure to marketing and some dietary behavior. There were 36 such results from 33 different published reports, and Table 5-9 breaks down their characteristics by several dimensions. Research has been active in this area from the 1980s through the present, involving a variety of study designs, age groups, and sample sizes. Twelve results focused on younger children (ages 2–

---

[5]The term "participant" is used throughout this chapter to describe subjects participating in research studies.

TABLE 5-9 Descriptive Characteristics of Research on the Influence of Commercial Marketing on Young People's Diet

Characteristic	Significant Results	Nonsignificant Results
Total Results*	30	6
Decade Published		
1970 or earlier	0	0
1980	8	2
1990	10	3
2000	12	1
Research Design		
Experimental	7	3
Natural experiment	2	1
Longitudinal	2	0
Cross-sectional	19	2
Age Group		
Younger children (2–5)	12	0
Older children (6–11)	18	4
Teens (12–18)	7	3
Sample Size		
0–49	4	0
50–99	6	0
100–499	13	3
500–999	1	1
1,000 or more	6	2
Type of Marketing		
TV ads: experimental treatment	6	3
TV ads: TV viewing only	29	3
TV ads: TV campaign	1	0
TV ads: TV viewing and other media use	2	0
Product placement in film	1	0
Price and promotion	1	0
Type of Diet Outcome		
Short-term consumption	7	2
Usual dietary intake	23	4

*One result in the evidence table could be about more than one age group or type of diet outcome. For these two characteristics the column totals can be more than the number of results.

5 years), 22 on older children (ages 6–11 years), and 10 on teens (ages 12–18 years). As it turns out, the results vary with age, so the discussion below first presents gross findings and then separate the results according to age.

Clearly the dominant type of marketing studied involves television. Only 2 of the 36 results did not involve television: one by Auty and Lewis

(2004) on the effects of product placement in films, and one by French et al. (2001a) on the effect of vending machine prices on the consumption of low-fat snacks.

Nine of the 36 results describe experiments that probe the short-term effects of exposure to different forms of television advertising by measuring a choice involving consumption shortly after exposure. For example, in Galst (1980), over a 4-week period children ages 3–6 years were allowed to select a snack each day after, and researchers recorded which and how many sugar-added versus no-sugar-added snacks the child consumed each day. For the last 4 weeks children also watched children's television programs and two factors were varied: (1) whether the television program included commercials for food and beverage products with added sugar content, or included commercials for fruit or milk and pro-nutritional public service announcements (PSAs); and (2) whether a female graduate student made comments (negative comments about products with added sugar when they were advertised or positive comments about healthy foods and beverages and PSAs), or remained silent. An untreated control group was also included. Children in all five groups selected sugared snacks the majority of the time, and the groups were not statistically distinguishable by the end of the experiment (week 6). At intermediate times, it did appear that the graduate student's comments, and less so commercials for healthy food and PSAs, were somewhat effective at reducing sugared snack intake.

The remaining 27 results probe the usual dietary habits of young people along with their usual exposure to marketing. For example, Bolton (1983) asked 262 parent and child pairs to keep 16-day diaries on television exposure from which they calculated exposure to advertising, and 7-day dietary intake diaries from which they calculated snacking frequency and nutrient intake. The study found that exposure to television advertising was associated with an increased number of snacks, but that variations in parental snacking behavior (but not parental supervision) explained much more of the variation in the children's snacking behavior than did variations in television advertising exposure.

Table 5-10 summarizes the evaluative characteristics of the 36 results. Ten of 36 were rated high for measure quality, 14 were of medium quality, and 12 of low quality. Eleven of 36 were of high relevance to inferring a causal connection (mostly the experimental studies), 9 were of medium relevance, and 16 of low relevance (mostly the cross-sectional studies of overall television viewing). The ability to generalize from these results (ecological validity) was generally very good. Twenty-four results were of high ecological validity (the bulk of them cross-sectional studies using overall television viewing as the measure of exposure to advertising), 10 were medium, and 2 were low.

Because all but two of the 36 results were about the influence of televi-

TABLE 5-10 Evaluative Characteristics of Research on the Influence of Commercial Marketing on Young People's Diet

Characteristic	Significant Results	Nonsignificant Results
Total Results	30	6
Quality of Measures		
High	8	2
Medium	11	3
Low	11	1
Causal Inference Validity		
High	8	3
Medium	7	2
Low	15	1
Ecological Validity		
High	20	4
Medium	8	2
Low	2	0

sion advertising, the remaining assessment of the evidence was carried out with those two results (Auty and Lewis, 2004; French et al., 2001a) removed. These 34 results were then divided into (1) those concerned with the influence on short-term consumption and (2) those concerned with the influence on usual dietary intake.

TABLE 5-11 Relevance Ratings of Research on the Influence of Television Advertising on Young People's Short-Term Consumption

Causal Inference Validity	Ecological Validity	Significant Results	Nonsignificant Results
Total Results		6	2
High	High	1	0
	Medium	4	1
	Low	1	0
Medium	High	0	0
	Medium	0	1
	Low	0	0
Low	High	0	0
	Medium	0	0
	Low	0	0

Influence of Television Advertising on Short-Term Consumption

The evidence on the overall influence of television advertising on short-term consumption is summarized in Table 5-11. Seven of the eight results are of high causal inference validity, with six having a significant influence. As we discussed in previous sections, for each causal relationship under consideration, the committee categorized the research reviewed as providing either: (1) strong, moderate, or weak evidence in favor of the existence of a causal relationship, (2) no evidence either way, or (3) strong, moderate, or weak evidence in favor of the *lack of* (nonexistence of) a causal relationship.

Influence of Television Advertising on Usual Dietary Intake

The evidence on the overall influence of television advertising on usual dietary intake is summarized in Table 5-12. Among the results with high causal inference validity, none showed a significant effect and two showed no effect. Conversely, among the results rated medium on the ability to infer causation, seven of eight found a significant effect. Although 15 of 16 results with low causal inference validity found a significant statistical association between exposure to television advertising and usual dietary intake these results provide little support for interpreting the association as causal. The great bulk of them are from cross-sectional studies in which television viewing and dietary habits are measured by diary or survey, both of which involve measurement difficulties, and in most of these studies little effort

TABLE 5-12 Relevance Ratings of Research on the Influence of Television Advertising on Young People's Usual Dietary Intake

Causal Inference Validity	Ecological Validity	Significant Results	Nonsignificant Results
Total Results		22	4
High	High	0	2
	Medium	0	0
	Low	0	0
Medium	High	5	1
	Medium	2	0
	Low	0	0
Low	High	13	1
	Medium	1	0
	Low	1	0

was exerted to rule out alternative explanations of the observed association between diet and television viewing (as the measure of exposure to television advertising).

These are gross-level findings, and a slightly more detailed analysis reveals that, not surprisingly, things are more complicated. Stratifying the 34 results that involve television advertising by the age of the research participants is illuminating.

Influence by Age

Short-Term Consumption

The systematic evidence review recorded the age of research participants for each result as younger children ages 2–5 years, older children ages 6–11 years, or teens ages 12–18 years. Table 5-13 summarizes the significance of the influence of television advertising on short-term consumption broken down by age.

Among younger children, all four results find a significant effect and are rated high on causal inference. Among older children, five results are strong on causal inference and among these, four find an effect. In contrast there are no results on the influence of television advertising on short-term consumption for teens.

Finding: There is strong evidence that television advertising influences the short-term consumption of children ages 2–11 years. There is insufficient

TABLE 5-13 Distribution of Significant and Nonsignificant Results by Causal Inference Validity for the Relationship of Television Advertising to the Short-Term Consumption of Younger Children, Older Children, and Teens

Causal Inference Validity	Younger Children (2–5 years)		Older Children (6–11 years)		Teens (12–18 years)	
	Significant Results	Non-significant Results	Significant Results	Non-significant Results	Significant Results	Non-significant Results
Total Results	4	0	4	2	0	0
High	4	0	4	1	0	0
Medium	0	0	0	1	0	0
Low	0	0	0	0	0	0

evidence about its influence on the short-term consumption of teens ages 12–18 years.

These studies all consider the effect of television advertising, and there are enough results to support some findings. The one study on the influence of product placement will simply be described, because it is pertinent to the committee's concerns and well done. In an experiment in which children ages 6–7 years and 11–12 years saw clips from a popular Hollywood movie, Auty and Lewis (2004) found, consistent with the television results, that product placement of a branded carbonated soft drink had a short-term effect on the children's choice of beverage for refreshment during a later interview.

Usual Dietary Intake

A review of the evidence also considered differences in usual dietary intake by age and by how exposure to television advertising was measured. Some studies measured exposure to television advertising solely by measuring overall television viewing, the assumption being in these circumstances that exposure to television advertising and overall television viewing are highly correlated. Other studies also employed some explicit measure related to advertising, in some cases particular advertisements. For example, in Boynton-Jarrett et al. (2003), only overall television viewing was measured and its relationship to fruit and vegetable intake was assessed. In contrast, Hitchings and Moynihan (1998) measured the relationship between recall of advertisements for seven targeted food groups and items

TABLE 5-14 Distribution of Significant and Nonsignificant Results by Causal Inference Validity for the Relationship of Television Advertising to the Usual Dietary Intake of Younger Children, Older Children, and Teens Where a Direct Measure of Television Advertising Was Included

Causal Inference Validity	Younger Children (2–5 years)		Older Children (6–11 years)		Teens (12–18 years)	
	Significant Results	Non-significant Results	Significant Results	Non-significant Results	Significant Results	Non-significant Results
Total Results	3	0	4	1	0	2
High	0	0	0	1	0	1
Medium	1	0	2	0	0	0
Low	2	0	2	0	0	1

TABLE 5-15 Distribution of Significant and Nonsignificant Results by Causal Inference Validity for the Relationship of Television Advertising to the Usual Dietary Intake of Younger Children, Older Children, and Teens Where Television Advertising Was Measured Only by Television Viewing

Causal Inference Validity	Younger Children (2–5 years)		Older Children (6–11 years)		Teens (12–18 years)	
	Significant Results	Non-significant Results	Significant Results	Non-significant Results	Significant Results	Non-significant Results
Total Results	5	0	9	1	6	1
High	0	0	0	0	0	0
Medium	2	0	3	1	1	1
Low	3	0	6	0	5	0

eaten as recorded by a 3-day diary. Twenty-two of such results used only overall television viewing as a measure of advertising exposure. In 10 other results, exposure to television advertising was measured in some more explicit way. Given the difference in how directly advertising exposure is measured, the two sets of studies will be examined separately. Both are informative about the influence of exposure to television advertising on usual dietary intake.

Tables 5-14 and 5-15 present the results on usual dietary intake, broken down by age. Table 5-14 presents the results that involve a direct measure of television advertising, and Table 5-15 presents results in which exposure to advertising was measured solely by overall television viewing.

For younger children, the evidence from both Tables 5-14 and 5-15 is entirely consistent. All results show a significant influence, but none are rated high on causal inference. The committee interpreted this to indicate that there is moderate evidence that television advertising influences the usual dietary intake of younger children ages 2–5 years.

For older children, the evidence is not entirely consistent, but seems to favor an effect. Evidence for the lack of an effect is strongest from Robinson (1999), the only result in this group rated high on causal inference. Robinson staged a large interventional study in which the treatment group was exposed to classes and time management aids aimed at reducing television, video, and video game usage among third and fourth graders. Participants in the intervention group did reduce media use and had substantially lower BMIs by the end of the study, but their consumption of highly advertised foods and beverages was indistinguishable from that of the untreated control groups. In this case, the effect through media may have been not through television, but rather through the reduction in video and video game use, both of which are likely to involve much less exposure to food and beverage advertising. The Robinson study notwithstanding, the committee interprets these results collectively to indicate that there is weak evidence that television advertising influences the usual dietary intake of older children ages 6–11 years. It is worth noting that among all of the studies with medium causal inference validity (including with both younger and older children, as just described), the usual diet measures were generally either brand choice or snacking frequency.

The results for the influence of television advertising on the usual dietary intake of teens ages 12–18 years are much less compelling. First, of the two results that involve a more direct measure of television advertising (Table 5-14), both found no effect. Second, of the three results rated either high or medium on causal inference validity in Tables 5-14 and 5-15, one found an effect and two did not.

Finally, although the five remaining results found a significant effect, they are all rated low on causal inference validity because they are from correlational studies that failed to rule out alternative explanations. Furthermore, they all reported very small effects, and often include substantial caveats or limitations. For example, Crespo et al. (2001) found no effect for boys. French et al. (2001b) found that the television viewing measure was associated with fast food consumption, which the committee counted as a significant effect, but they also found that fast food consumption among teens was independent of BMI. Gracey et al. (1996) found no association between television watching and food variety score or BMI. On balance, the committee interprets these studies to indicate that there is weak evidence that television advertising does not influence the usual dietary intake of teens ages 12–18 years. This is not to say that marketing has no influence on teens. Although the evidence reviewed is limited, from the committee's review and from other evidence it seems plausible that food and beverage marketing has a greater influence on the diet of teens through price than through advertising, whereas the opposite is true for younger children.

It should be noted that the finding for teens refers only to the influence of television advertising. It does not include the interventional study by French et al. (2001a) which found a significant effect of vending machine prices and a very small effect of product packaging on teens' purchase of low-fat snacks. This study on the effects of price is persuasive and methodologically sound, and rates high on causal inference validity. However, it is the only study in the systematic evidence review that examines the effect of price on diet, and the committee was unwilling to come to any finding based on a single study. It is worth noting, however, that other research on the influence of price on teen consumption of alcohol and tobacco supports the hypothesis that price may be a major determinant of teen behavior (Harwood et al., 2003; Ross and Chaloupka, 2003; Waller et al., 2003a).

Finding: There is moderate evidence that television advertising influences the usual dietary intake of younger children ages 2–5 years and weak evidence that it influences the usual dietary intake of older children ages 6–11 years. There is also weak evidence that it does not influence the usual dietary intake of teens ages 12–18 years.

If marketing influences the diets and diet-related health of children and youth, it will do so through children's and teens' preferences for specific foods and beverages, requests made to their parents to purchase foods or to visit restaurants, and their beliefs, attitudes, and values about foods. The committee's systematic evidence review found strong evidence that food and beverage marketing does influence the preferences and purchase requests of children. Of 22 results on the effect of marketing on food or beverage preferences, 15 found an effect. Of 17 results on the effect of marketing on food or beverage purchase requests, 15 found an effect, and of the 8 studies on the effect of marketing on food or beverage beliefs, 5 found an effect.

The committee found evidence that purchase requests are also often successful. For example, Galst and White (1976) found that, overall, children observed in the grocery store with their parents were successful in causing purchases 45 percent of the time. Taras et al. (2000) found a significant correlation between highly advertised food or beverage products (as determined from advertising data) and parental recall of a young child's request for food or beverage purchases and a parent's yielding to those purchase requests. In earlier work (Taras et al., 1989) they similarly found strong agreement between the relative proportion of foods or beverages purchased by mothers and those requested by children ages 3–8 years. Other studies (e.g., Borzekowski and Poussaint, 1998; Brody et al., 1981; Donkin et al., 1993) agree that food or beverage purchase requests are often successful; thus there is evidence for a causal link from marketing through purchase requests to diet.

As reviewed elsewhere in this report (Chapter 3), food and beverage preferences—along with availability and accessibility—are among the strongest predictors of children's and teens' dietary intake. For example, children ages 3–5 years who indicated strong preferences for high-fat foods (for foods served at lunch) had high total fat intake; these children's fat preferences were associated with parental adiposity (Fisher and Birch, 1995). In a study of one group of American Indians children ages 4–9 years, food preferences were the strongest predictor of food behavior (as assessed by questionnaire) and explained 71 percent of the variation in the behavior score (Harvey-Berino et al., 1997). Preference for and frequency of consumption of 64 foods and beverages as self-reported by African American girls, ages 8–10 years, were moderately correlated; however, correlations with BMI were not significant (Sherwood et al., 2003). In children ages 8–13 years, preference for the taste of carbonated soft drinks was the strongest predictor of carbonated soft drink consumption (both measures self-reported), with those who reported the strongest taste preference 4.5 times more likely to consume carbonated soft drinks five or more times per week than those with a lower taste preference (Grimm et al., 2004). Carbonated soft drink consumption also was related to the frequency of consumption by parents.

The strongest correlates of fruit and vegetable intake among adolescents, mean age 14.9 years, were taste preferences and home availability (Neumark-Sztainer et al., 2003). Interestingly, even when taste preferences for fruits and vegetables were low, intake increased if they were available. Similarly, in fourth through sixth graders, for children with high preferences for fruit, fruit juice, and vegetables, availability was the only significant predictor of intake, whereas availability and accessibility were significantly related to consumption for children with low preferences (Cullen et al., 2003).

Although it is clear that preference influences diet, measures of preference in studies on the relationship between preference and consumption may not be the same as measures of preference in studies on the influence of marketing on preference. In those studies, it is hard to separate recall and recognition effects prompted by advertising from real preference. In Greenberg and Brand (1993), for example, marketing had a demonstrable effect on measured preference for a product, but no effect on typical consumption. That caveat aside, the evidence indicates that there is a link from marketing through preference to diet.

Nutritional beliefs do not appear to have a strong or consistent association with the preferences or diets of children and teens (as reviewed in Chapter 3). For example, focus group interviews with kindergarten students revealed they understood the general relationships among food choices, exercise, body fat, and health (Murphy et al., 1995). They were also able to name foods high in salt, fat, and sugar and thought consumption of sugar should be limited, but their self-reported food and beverage preferences were not consistent with dietary recommendations to moderate foods high in these nutrients. In the study cited of American Indian children, nutrition beliefs explained 40 percent of the variance in dietary behavior; however, although beliefs scores increased with age, they did not translate into changes in eating behavior and nutrient intakes (Harvey-Berino et al., 1997). Conversely, among another group of adolescents, health and nutrition attitudes were associated with taste preferences for fruits and vegetables, and preferences in turn were associated with fruit/vegetable intake (Neumark-Sztainer et al., 2003).

SYSTEMATIC EVIDENCE REVIEW OF THE RELATIONSHIP BETWEEN MARKETING AND DIET-RELATED HEALTH

This section considers the evidence relevant to the influence of marketing on diet-related health. For marketing to influence young people's diet-related health, it must influence their diet, as depicted in the five-element causal framework (see Figure 5-1) that guided the systematic evidence review. Elsewhere in this report (see Chapter 2 and Appendix D), evidence that links diet to health has been presented. Here, consonant with the committee's charge, research that includes marketing as a possible causal factor and diet-related health as an outcome is reviewed and assessed. Such research could address any of the four major marketing elements (product, place, price, and promotion) as an influence on juvenile health outcomes such as weight, obesity, cholesterol, and type 2 diabetes. In point of fact, some research has included marketing as a consideration, but little research has intentionally focused on any aspect of the relationship of marketing to diet-related health. As noted previously, the committee acknowledges that various factors in addition to food and beverage marketing might affect this relationship, but these are not the direct subject of the committee's inquiry and therefore the focus here is on the specific relationship of marketing to diet-related health.

The committee identified a substantial body of research that is relevant to understanding the relationship of marketing to diet-related health. These studies examined the relationship between television viewing and diet-related health, almost always juvenile adiposity. Sixty-five articles that examined this relationship were identified and included in the systematic evidence review. All but one study (Robinson, 1999) employed a correlational design, gathering data at either one or two points in time to examine the relationship between amount of television viewing and diet-related health. One study (Wong et al., 1992) examined cholesterol levels; one study (Guillaume et al., 1997) examined cardiovascular fitness and adiposity; all the rest examined adiposity. Most studies also measured some possible moderating variables such as age, race/ethnicity, or socioeconomic status or some possible alternative explanatory variables such as activity level or snacking while viewing television. Nearly all employed various statistical controls to better elucidate the underlying causal mechanisms accounting for any significant association of television viewing and diet-related health.

After careful consideration, the committee judged that it was reasonable to include these studies in the systematic evidence review for the relationship of marketing to diet-related health. Studies that intentionally used television viewing as a measure of exposure to marketing (advertising) and employed similar correlational designs had already been included in the systematic evidence review for the relationship of marketing to precursors of diet and for the relationship of marketing to diet. Moreover, television viewing is well related to exposure to food and beverage advertising because, as explicated in Chapter 4, food and beverage marketing messages are common across the television landscape, particularly in programming with the highest concentrations of youth in the audience. For this reason, any correlation reported between young people's time watching television and precursors of diet, diet, or diet-related health may be caused by exposure during television viewing time to commercial messages for food and beverage products, which are likely to be high in calories and low in nutrients.

It becomes more difficult to infer causality in an individual study and to arrive at findings about causality from a group of studies as the outcome moves from precursor to diet to health. The increasing difficulty arises from two conditions. First, due to the decreasing proportion of experimental studies in the evidence for precursor, diet, and health outcomes, respectively, the ability to use the correlational studies to confirm results from experimental studies and arrive at findings about causality decreases from precursor to diet to health outcomes. Second, as one moves from precursor to diet to health outcomes, there is a substantial increase in the number of plausible alternative explanations for any correlation between the outcome and advertising exposure as measured by television viewing. Accordingly, for any given study that employs television viewing as a measure of exposure to television advertising, as one moves from precursor to diet to health it becomes increasingly difficult to infer causality.

In drawing on the available research to assess the influence of exposure to television advertising on adiposity, as measured by television viewing, three challenges were paramount, given the fact that all but one of the studies were correlational. One challenge is the fact that television viewing may represent or be highly associated with several other factors that could influence adiposity. In addition to exposure to commercial food and beverage advertising, a measure of television viewing may indicate or be closely associated with physical activity, snacking, propensity to engage in other sedentary activities (e.g., reading, videogaming), reduced metabolic rate, exposure to food and beverage consumption within programs, and blunting of physiological cues to satiety. A second challenge, given the correlational design of these studies, is the possibility of reverse causation. Perhaps heavier young people watch more television because it demands less of them physically. A third challenge is the possibility that television viewing and weight status are unrelated to each other, but well related to a third variable that influences each of them independently. For example, adiposity and television viewing each vary to some degree according to socioeconomic status and racial/ethnic group, and these two independent relationships could underlie an apparent relationship between adiposity and television viewing.

As it turned out, there was a fourth challenge as well. Many studies measured a wide variety of variables that could have been included in the analyses. Reporting, however, was not always explicit enough to know which were actually included in the analyses. For example, the statement "demographic variables were entered first into the regression model" and the statistical reporting were not always sufficient to explain whether all or some, and if some, which, of the measured demographic variables were entered. Because the ability to draw causal inferences from correlational data depends heavily on the ability to rule out alternative explanations, difficulties in determining which alternative explanations had been tested limited the utility of some research.

There are several implications in the committee's decision to accept that measures of television viewing can be used as an indication of young people's exposure to advertising. First, because exposure to television advertising is not measured directly, measurement strength will always be rated low or medium, even for exceptionally good measurement of television viewing per se. As a corollary, in the relevance rating system, causal inference validity will always be rated medium or low due to the relatively weak measurement of exposure to advertising, the target causal variable in this systematic evidence review. Finally, in assessing the evidence, there is a substantial burden to consider alternative explanations, and strong findings about causality are unlikely.

Evidentiary Base

Sixty-five articles with relevant empirical data were identified and included in the systematic evidence review, yielding 74 distinct results (see Table 5-16). These studies began to appear in the 1980s, became more frequent in the 1990s, and have continued to accelerate in volume since 2000, with 45 results published in the literature in roughly the past 5 years.

Older children (ages 6–11 years) were most often the focus of study (58 results), with teens (ages 11–18 years, 33 results) and younger children (ages 2–5 years, 17 results) also receiving some attention. Just one result involved infants and toddlers (under age 2 years) as part of the research sample of children, and it is the only such result in the entire systematic evidence review. The use of large data sets was common, with nearly half of all results derived from samples of 1,000 or more children or teens. Much of the research relied on secondary analyses of nationally representative survey data from ongoing studies such as the National Health and Nutrition Examination Survey (NHANES).

TABLE 5-16 Descriptive Characteristics of Research on the Influence of Commercial Marketing on Young People's Diet-Related Health

Characteristic	Significant Results	Nonsignificant Results
Total Results*	51	23
Decade Published		
1980	3	1
1990	14	11
2000	34	11
Research Design		
Experimental	1	0
Natural experimental	0	0
Longitudinal	12	5
Cross-sectional	38	18
Age Group*		
Infants and toddlers (under 2)	0	1
Younger children (2–5)	11	6
Older children (6–11)	44	14
Teens (12–18)	23	10
Sample Size		
0–49	0	1
50–99	4	2
100–499	13	8
500–999	6	5
1,000 or more	28	7
Type of Marketing		
TV ads: observed in natural setting	0	2
TV ads: TV viewing only	41	15
TV ads: TV viewing and other media use	10	6
Type of Diet-Related Health Outcome*		
Adiposity	50	23
Other	2	0

NOTE: The two "Other" outcomes were cholesterol levels and cardiovascular fitness.

*One result in the evidence table could be about more than one age group or type of diet-related health outcome. For these two characteristics the column totals can be more than the number of results.

This body of research almost exclusively provides evidence about the relationship of television advertising exposure to adiposity. Seventy-three of the 74 results assessed adiposity as the diet-related health outcome; one (Guillaume et al., 1997) also assessed cardiovascular fitness, and one only assessed cholesterol levels (Wong et al., 1992). Typically, adiposity was measured by BMI, but skinfold thickness measures and designations such as obese or super obese were also used. In some of the longitudinal studies, change in BMI or other adiposity measures was assessed. All 74 results involved viewing of television advertising as the putative causal variable; 58 involved television advertising alone (or with other media measured separately), and the remaining 16 involved television advertising and some other media use—videos, music videos, video games, computer games, and computers—combined with television use such that it could not be separately assessed. This was particularly common in studies in which researchers sought to test hypotheses about the relationship between adiposity and television viewing as a form of sedentary activity. For all 74 results, exposure to television advertising was measured by overall television viewing in young people's daily lives outside of school, either television viewing by itself or combined with time spent with other media and technology. All but two results involved self-report and/or parent-report of media use; for the other two, children's everyday behavior was directly observed.

For the committee's purposes, among all the media and technology that young people use, only engagement with television can reasonably serve as an indication of exposure to food and beverage marketing. Although marketing is frequently part of all media and technology, only for television is there enough good evidence about the nature and extent of food and beverage marketing to instill confidence that amount of television viewing is a reasonable measure of exposure to advertising for foods and beverages, the majority of which promote high-calorie and low-nutrient products (see Chapter 4). For this reason, in those studies that measured use of other media in addition to measuring television viewing, the committee's focus was on the evidence about a relationship between television viewing and adiposity.

The studies that combined television use with other media use, without reporting them separately, were included in the systematic evidence review. This is because research on out-of-school use of media and technology has repeatedly demonstrated that, on average, young people spend much more time with television than with any other medium or technology. The Kaiser Family Foundation report on media use by a national sample of 8- to 18-year-olds found that, on a combined basis, just over 3 hours a day were spent on television viewing (broadcast, cable, and prerecorded), almost 1 hour a day watching videos/DVDs, and about 0.75 hours a day playing console and hand-held video games (Roberts et al., 2005). At times, media use overlapped; total media time could be less than the sum for each medium separately. The average usage times included all research participants. In fact, most (81 percent) watched television on a typical day, and fewer watched videos/DVDs (42 percent) or played console video games (41 percent) or hand-held video games (35 percent). There were some differences in media use by age, gender, and race/ethnicity, but the general findings do

TABLE 5-17 Evaluative Characteristics of Research on the Influence of Commercial Marketing on Young People's Diet-Related Health

Characteristic	Significant Results	Nonsignificant Results
Total Results	51	23
Quality of Measures		
High	0	0
Medium	23	9
Low	28	14
Causal Inference Validity		
High	1	0
Medium	13	5
Low	37	18
Ecological Validity		
High	44	19
Medium	6	3
Low	1	1

not differ. Thus, even results measuring television viewing and other media use combined are likely to be largely reflective of television viewing time. For this reason, they were included in the systematic evidence review.

Table 5-17 presents the evaluative characteristics of the 74 results, and Table 5-18 identifies the relevance of the results to the committee's goals when both causal inference validity and ecological validity are considered

TABLE 5-18 Relevance Ratings of Research on the Influence of Commercial Marketing on Young People's Diet-Related Health

Causal Inference Validity	Ecological Validity	Significant Results	Nonsignificant Results
Total Results		51	23
High	High	1	0
	Medium	0	0
	Low	0	0
Medium	High	12	4
	Medium	1	1
	Low	0	0
Low	High	31	15
	Medium	5	2
	Low	1	1

together. As anticipated given the research methods and the use of television viewing as a measure of exposure to advertising, the quality of the measures was medium or low, never high, and, with the one experiment as an exception, causal inference validity was never high and most often was low. On the other hand, with two exceptions, ecological validity was never low and was most often high because the research methods and measures permitted assessment of everyday life phenomena. Also as anticipated, ecological validity tended to be higher when causal inference validity was lower (see Table 5-18). The results for the relationship of marketing to diet-related health do support generalization to everyday life, but do not make it easy to determine cause and effect.

The preponderance of results (51 of 74, 69 percent) reported a significant association between marketing and diet-related health. Examination of the data in Tables 5-16, 5-17, and 5-18 indicated that there is no apparent difference in the characteristics of the research producing significant and nonsignificant results. Further exploration of possible differences based on breakdowns using multiple variables did not change this finding. Moreover, the two relevance ratings (see Table 5-17) indicated that the significant results were from research that was at least as relevant as the research that produced the nonsignificant results: For causal inference validity, 28 percent of the significant results were rated medium (one was high) compared to 22 percent of the nonsignificant results, and for ecological validity, 86 percent of the significant results were rated high compared to 83 percent of the nonsignificant results. This general pattern did not change when causal inference validity and ecological validity were considered together (see Table 5-18).

Relationship Between Television Advertising and Adiposity

As Table 5-16 shows, available evidence about the relationship of marketing and diet-related health is almost entirely evidence about the relationship of television advertising exposure and adiposity among children and teens. In contrast to the evidence about the relationship of marketing to precursors of diet, or to diet itself, in which two or three different types of outcomes have been studied, there is only one outcome that has been studied to any degree: adiposity. Also, only one type of marketing has been studied: exposure to television advertising. To determine what can be concluded about the relationship of television advertising exposure to adiposity in children and teens, one result (Wong et al., 1992) that was not about adiposity was omitted from further consideration. Of the 73 results remaining in the evidence table, the infant/toddler sample in the Vandewater et al. (2004) study and the cardiovascular fitness outcome in the Guillaume et al. (1997) result were both removed from further consideration.

TABLE 5-19 Distribution of Significant and Nonsignificant Results by Measure of Exposure to Advertising for the Relationship of Television Advertising to the Adiposity of Younger Children, Older Children, and Teens (For Each Cell, Number of Results with Medium Causal Inference Validity Is Indicated in Parentheses)

Measure of Advertising Exposure	Younger Children (2–5 years)		Older Children (6–11 years)		Teens (12–18 years)	
	Significant Results	Non-significant Results	Significant Results	Non-significant Results	Significant Results	Non-significant Results
Total Results	11 (4)	6 (2)	44 (14*)	14 (3)	23 (7)	10 (3)
TV ads: observed in natural setting	0 (0)	2 (0)	0 (0)	1 (0)	0 (0)	0 (0)
TV ads: TV viewing only	11 (4)	4 (2)	35 (11*)	8 (3)	18 (5)	8 (3)
TV ads: TV viewing and other media use	0 (0)	0 (0)	9 (3)	5 (0)	5 (2)	2 (0)

*One causal inference validity rating is high, not medium.

Clearly, the descriptive and evaluative characteristics of the evidence base about the relationship between television advertising exposure and adiposity remain nearly the same as for the entire sample. Further examination of this evidence, considering the age of the participants (see Table 5-19), indicated that the preponderance of significant associations is about the same (around 75 percent) for younger children, older children, and teens, regardless of the way in which exposure to advertising was measured. Moreover, the causal inference validity status of the significant and nonsignificant results did not change from that for the whole sample and does not seem to vary by age.

Finding: Statistically, there is strong evidence that exposure to television advertising is associated with adiposity in children ages 2–11 years and teens ages 12–18 years.

As discussed elsewhere, evidence of association is not evidence of causation, and the committee's interest is in causation and relevance to everyday life. To assess the likelihood that the positive association between exposure to television advertising and adiposity reflected a causal influence from advertising to adiposity, the committee examined three issues: (1) whether the association could be explained by adiposity affecting exposure to television advertising; (2) whether the association could be explained by other variables that the advertising exposure measure (television viewing) could also represent; and (3) whether the association could be explained by a third variable that influenced both the advertising exposure measure and adiposity.

Whether Advertising Exposure Predicts Adiposity or Vice Versa

If the significant association found between advertising exposure and adiposity represents a causal relationship, then the question becomes which influences the other. Because advertising exposure was measured by television viewing, the obtained association could logically be explained as "adiposity influences exposure to television advertising (as measured by television viewing)" or "exposure to television advertising (as measured by television viewing) influences adiposity." Of the 73 results that examined the relationship between children's and teens' exposure to television advertising and their adiposity, 1 was experimental and the remaining 72 were correlational; 17 of these 72 correlational studies employed a longitudinal design (all panel studies). The experimental and longitudinal studies provide the best evidence as to the direction of any causal relationship that might exist between advertising exposure and adiposity.

The one experimental study (Robinson, 1999) was a well-conceived and well-conducted randomized controlled trial intervention. Nearly 200 third and fourth graders and their teachers and parents participated. Over a period of 6 months, children in the experimental intervention engaged in an 18-lesson classroom curriculum to reduce television, videotape, and video game use. The intervention effort was concentrated into the first 2 months, and part of the intervention sought to bring parents into the process. The analytic framework compared the intervention and control groups on a variety of outcome measures, while covarying on age, gender, and pretest score for the specific outcome measure. As compared to the control group, the intervention group had significantly less increase in BMI and in three of four other measures of adiposity. Also, for both child and parent measures, for the intervention group compared to the control group, there was a highly significant reduction (4–6 hours a week) in television viewing and a significant reduction (about one a week) in meals eaten in front of the television set. In addition, children in the intervention group compared to the control group reported relative reductions in servings of high-fat foods, although the differences were not significant (p = 0.12). There were no group differences in frequency of snacking while viewing, servings of highly advertised foods, other sedentary behaviors, and various measures of physical activity. Clearly the variety of findings for the intervention group compared to the control group offer interpretive challenges as to what variables are influencing adiposity and how they work together in everyday life. However, if a causal claim were to be made with respect to the link between adiposity and television advertising, the direction of influence would be from television advertising (as measured by television viewing) to adiposity.

The longitudinal studies also provided a good test of the direction of any causal relationship when they assessed advertising exposure before assessing adiposity or related prior exposure to change in adiposity. Logically, if a statistically significant association is found between advertising exposure at one time and adiposity at a later time, then any causal relationship that might exist would be described as "advertising exposure at time 1 influences adiposity at time 2" not as "adiposity at time 2 influences advertising exposure at time 1." Two of the 17 longitudinal studies measured exposure to television advertising at the time of the last measure of adiposity and then related exposure to some aspect of the longitudinal course of adiposity. Among the 15 longitudinal studies in which advertising exposure was measured prior to adiposity, the evidence for an association between advertising exposure and adiposity is strong, with 12 (80 percent) reporting a significant relationship.

Based on the 1 result of the experimental study and the 15 results of the longitudinal studies, it is unlikely that any causal relationship that might be found between advertising exposure, as measured by television viewing, and adiposity would be explained primarily by the fact that heavier young people watch more television. The committee interprets the evidence as ruling out any reverse causation explanation. The evidence is strong and favors the finding that, if the relationship between television advertising and adiposity were causal, the direction would be that exposure to television advertising predicts adiposity rather than that adiposity predicts exposure to television advertising.

Whether Alternative Explanations Account for the Positive Association Between Exposure to Television Advertising and Adiposity

To conclude that the significant association found between television advertising exposure and adiposity reflects a causal relationship, plausible alternative explanations must be examined and, to a convincing degree, must be shown *not* to account for the significant positive association. To examine alternative explanations, the evidentiary base was restricted to correlational studies with a medium rather than a low causal inference validity rating (recall that there was only one experimental study in the entire body of evidence and that was the only result with a high causal inference validity rating). A higher causal inference validity rating for correlational studies indicates more likelihood of being able to rule out various alternative explanations of findings. Consequently, studies rated medium are likely to provide information pertinent to deciding whether exposure to television advertising influences adiposity over and above, or instead of, plausible alternative explanations. There were 16 different correlational studies rated medium on causal inference validity; they yielded 17 different results.

Of the 17 results, 12 (71 percent) reported a significant relationship between exposure to television advertising, as measured by television viewing, and adiposity. The descriptive characteristics of the 12 significant and 5 nonsignificant results are presented in Table 5-20 and the evaluative characteristics are in Table 5-21. Overall, the characteristics are similar to

TABLE 5-20 Descriptive Characteristics of Cross-Sectional and Longitudinal Research on the Influence of Exposure to Television Advertising on Young People's Adiposity, for Results with Medium Causal Inference Validity

Characteristic	Significant Results	Nonsignificant Results
Total Results*	12	5
Decade Published		
1980	1	0
1990	2	1
2000	9	4
Research Design		
Longitudinal	8	3
Cross-Sectional	4	2
Age Group*		
Younger children (2–5)	3	2
Older children (6–11)	12	3
Teens (12–18)	6	3
Sample Size		
100–499	2	1
500–999	2	1
1,000 or more	8	3
Type of Marketing		
TV ads: TV viewing only	9	5
TV ads: TV viewing and other media use	3	0

*One result in the evidence table could be about more than one age group, and so the column total can be more than the number of results.

TABLE 5-21 Evaluative Characteristics of Cross-Sectional and Longitudinal Research on the Influence of Exposure to Television Advertising on Young People's Adiposity, for Results with Medium Causal Inference Validity

Characteristic	Significant Results	Nonsignificant Results
Total Results	12	5
Quality of Measures		
High	0	0
Medium	9	3
Low	3	2
Ecological Validity		
High	11	4
Medium	1	1
Low	0	0

those of the full set of evidence (74 results, see Tables 5-16 and 5-17), and they too provide no indication of any consistent difference that would explain why some results were significant and some were not. Moreover, additional exploration, such as by age group, produced no indication of any consistent difference. Because these 17 results are exclusively from studies in which the methods and statistical analyses provide a medium degree of ability to infer causality and because 71 percent of the results favor a relationship, it is possible that the positive association reflects a causal relationship, but more analysis is needed before any finding could be drawn.

To pursue further the question of whether television advertising influences adiposity, the variables other than television viewing that were included in the 16 studies (17 results) with medium causal inference validity were identified. These variables could be roughly categorized as (1) *television-related nonadvertising variables* that the advertising measure, television viewing, could be assessing, (2) *third variables* that would account independently for both television viewing and adiposity, or (3) *other adiposity-related variables*. The 16 studies (17 results) varied considerably in which variables were included, and authors were only sometimes explicit about how they thought these variables functioned in assessing the factors influencing juvenile adiposity. For this reason, results will be examined simultaneously for all three types of variables (television-related nonadvertising, third, and other adiposity-related).

In addition to exposure to television advertising, several variables could be indexed by television viewing and are suspected of influencing, or known to influence, adiposity directly or indirectly, and might explain the positive association between viewing and adiposity. Only the last is the committee's focus.

- Television viewing might take up time that otherwise would be given to greater physical activity, and more physical activity could lead to higher calorie expenditure, which could lead to lesser adiposity.
- Television viewing might be an indicator of a preference for a more sedentary lifestyle, and more sedentary activity could lead to lower energy expenditure, which could lead to greater adiposity.
- Television viewing might be a context for snacking, and more snacking could lead to higher calorie intake, which could lead to greater adiposity.
- Television viewing might blunt one's sensitivity to satiety cues, and greater insensitivity to satiety cues could lead to greater calorie intake when eating during viewing, which could lead to greater adiposity.
- Television viewing might reduce one's metabolic level, and a lower metabolic level could lead to less efficient processing of calorie intake, which could lead to greater adiposity.
- Television viewing might be an indicator of exposure to depictions of eating and drinking within the program (either scripted or product placement), and more exposure to these depictions could increase preferences, purchase requests, and other precursors of diet which then increase calorie intake and could lead to greater adiposity.
- Television viewing might be an indicator of exposure to food and beverage advertising, and more exposure to this advertising could increase preferences, purchase requests, and other precursors of diet, which then increase dietary intake and could lead to greater adiposity.

Realistically, several of these variables and pathways may operate simultaneously to influence adiposity. The question for the committee is whether exposure to television advertising is among them, not whether exposure to television advertising is the sole influence or the most important influence. None of the 17 results that tested enough variables to receive a medium causal inference validity rating covered all seven plausible explanations using measures other than television viewing. Not one included direct measures of satiety cues, metabolic rate, consumption depictions, or television advertising. For each of the other plausible explanations, at least one study tested one or more of them using measures other than television viewing.

In addition to examining what happens to television advertising as a potential causal variable when measures of television-related nonadvertising variables are included in the analysis, the possibility that the apparent relationship is due to a third variable, independently related both to advertising exposure (as measured by viewing) and to adiposity, also must be examined. The most likely third variables are age, gender, race/ethnicity, and socioeconomic status. Each has been shown to have some relationship to television viewing, and hence to exposure to advertising, and each has been shown to have some relationship to adiposity. For example, television viewing tends to be inversely related to socioeconomic status and adiposity also tends to be inversely related to socioeconomic status. Socioeconomic status, then, could account for the obtained positive association between television viewing and adiposity. If so, when socioeconomic status is included as a variable, the positive association between the advertising measure (television viewing) and adiposity should disappear or markedly diminish. Existing evidence about the relationship of age, gender, race/ethnicity, and socioeconomic status to television viewing and to adiposity suggests that only some of the four are likely third variables. Nonetheless, they should each be examined in order to see whether the positive association between television viewing and adiposity exists when potential third variable explanations have been taken into account. If the association remains, the claim that television advertising influences adiposity cannot be rejected on the basis of existing evidence about that third variable explanation.

To examine further whether exposure to television advertising was causally connected to adiposity, each of the 17 results with medium causal inference validity was reexamined. Using the statistical analysis that included television viewing (the measure of exposure to television advertising) and the largest possible number of television-related nonadvertising, third, and other adiposity-related variables, such variables that were included in that analysis were identified. Also recorded was whether television advertising was significant in this analysis.

These counts were used in two different ways. First (see Table 5-22), for each of the five television-related nonadvertising variables and four third variables found to be included in the analyses, a comparison was made of the number of results in which television viewing was a significant predictor, and the number in which it was not a significant predictor, when that variable was included with television viewing in the statistical analysis with the largest possible number of variables in it. The same was done for two other adiposity-related variables—parental adiposity and initial child adiposity—that were included in enough of the statistical analyses to make comparisons possible. Second (see Table 5-23), a count was made of the total number of television-related nonadvertising variables, of third variables, and of other adiposity-related variables included in the statistical analysis with the largest possible number of variables in it. Also counted was the total number of variables of any type in this statistical analysis. The

TABLE 5-22 Television-Related Nonadvertising, Third, and Other Adiposity-Related Variables Included in Statistical Tests of the Relationship of Television Advertising, Measured by Television Viewing, and Adiposity, for Cross-Sectional and Longitudinal Studies with Medium Causal Inference Validity Ratings (Cell Entries Are Number of Results with That Variable Included in the Statistical Analysis with Television Viewing)

Variables	Cross-Sectional Methods		Longitudinal Methods		Total for Both Methods	
	Significant Results (n = 4)	Non-significant Results (n = 2)	Significant Results (n = 8)	Non-significant Results (n = 3)	Significant Results (n = 12)	Non-significant Results (n = 5)
Television-Related Nonadvertising Variables						
Physical activity	3	1	4	2	7	3
Mild or sedentary activity	0	0	3	0	3	0
Other media use	1	0	1	1	2	1
Snacking context	1	0	1	0	2	0
Diet	3	1	4	1	7	2
Third Variables						
Age	4	2	4	3	8	5
Gender	4*	2	7*	3*	11	5
Race/ethnicity	3	2	6**	2	9	4
Statuses	4	2	7	2	11	4
Other Adiposity-Related Variables						
Parent adiposity	0	0	5	1	5	1
Initial adiposity	n/a	n/a	6	2	n/a	n/a
1–10 other variables*	3	1	7	3	10	4

*One result is from a study of girls only.
**One result is from a study of non-Hispanic Caucasians only.

287

TABLE 5-23 Number of Variables Total and by Type Included in Statistical Tests of the Relationship of Television Advertising, Measured by Television Viewing, and Adiposity, for Cross-Sectional and Longitudinal Studies with Medium Causal Inference Validity Ratings (Cell Entries Are Number of Results with the Indicated Number of Variables [Left Column] Included in the Statistical Analysis with Television Viewing)

Variables	Cross-Sectional Methods		Longitudinal Methods		Total for Both Methods	
	Significant Results (n = 4)	Non-significant Results (n = 2)	Significant Results (n = 8)	Non-significant Results (n = 3)	Significant Results (n = 12)	Non-significant Results (n = 5)
Television-Related Nonadvertising Variables in Test (5 maximum)						
0	0	1	2	1	2	2
1	1	0	1	1	2	1
2	2	1	3	0	5	1
3	1	0	2	1	3	1
Third Variables in Test (4 maximum)						
1	0	0	0	0	0	0
2	0	0	1	0	1	0
3	1	0	6	2	7	2
4	3	2	1	1	4	3
Other Adiposity-Related Variables in Test						
0	4	2	1	1	5	3
1 (maximum cross-sectional)	0	0	3	1	3	1
2 (maximum longitudinal)	n/a	n/a	4	1	n/a	n/a
Total Variables in Test (21 maximum)						
3–4	0	1	0	0	0	1
5–6	1	0	0	1	1	1
7–8	2	1	2	1	4	2
9–10	0	0	3	0	3	0
11–12	1	0	2	0	3	0
14	0	0	0	1	0	1
21	0	0	1	0	1	0

number of results for which television advertising was significant and non-significant was compared as the number of television-related nonadvertising, third, other adiposity-related, and all variables in the analysis increased.

In each approach, if television viewing is significant in the preponderance of the results, then the claim that television advertising influences adiposity cannot be rejected. This is so because the statistical analyses tested whether the positive association between the television advertising measure and adiposity was explained by the television-related nonadvertising, third, and other adiposity-related variables. If the association were explained by any one or number of these variables (and assuming the variables were well measured), then there would be no significant association between the advertising measure (television viewing) and adiposity when the explanatory variables were included with television viewing in the analysis predicting adiposity.

The evidence presented in Table 5-22 indicates the extent to which the statistically significant positive association between exposure to television advertising, as measured by television viewing, and adiposity is accounted for by a television-related nonadvertising, third, or other adiposity-related variable. For alternative interpretations of what television viewing measures (nonadvertising variables in the table), there are either no results (for satiety cues, metabolic rate, and consumption depictions) or too few results (mild or sedentary activity and snacking context) to directly address the question. For physical activity and diet, when each was measured by something other than television viewing and included in the statistical analysis, the positive, statistically significant association between the television viewing measure and adiposity remained for 54 percent and 78 percent of the results, respectively. As described earlier, depending on how diet is measured it could be an indicator of snacking frequency and context, sensitivity to satiety cues, exposure to consumption depictions, or exposure to television advertising. The diet measures used in the 17 studies are sufficiently varied that their meaning and the implications of findings involving different measures cannot be further unraveled. For other media use, which could indicate mild or sedentary activity preference, time taken away from physical activity, or exposure to some uncertain amount of food and beverage marketing or consumption depiction, the association between television viewing and adiposity was significant for 67 percent of the results. Overall, then, for the television-related nonadvertising variable interpretations of the television viewing measure that can be assessed, there is some evidence that the positive association between advertising exposure, as measured by television viewing, and adiposity remains when these alternatives are taken into account. Thus, the claim that television advertising influences adiposity cannot be rejected on the basis of current evidence about nonadvertising interpretations of the television viewing measure.

It should be noted that the evidence presented here does not offer any indication as to whether the plausible television-related nonadvertising variables do, indeed, explain the positive association between television viewing and adiposity. Table 5-22 only shows how the advertising exposure interpretation holds up when these plausible alternative explanations are considered simultaneously. If any television-related nonadvertising variable (which it is argued is measured by television viewing) were to be considered causal, then there would need to be evidence that the television-related nonadvertising variable is well correlated with television viewing, that it influences adiposity, and that it does so when advertising, other television-related nonadvertising, third, and other adiposity-related variables are simultaneously taken into account. None of that evidence is assessed here. A general review of the research literature and of the analyses conducted in the 16 articles analyzed here suggested there is limited evidence, and it is not highly supportive of a claim that any of the television-related nonadvertising variables both is indexed by television viewing and also independently influences adiposity. By the same token, because the measurement of many of the key variables is problematic, the inability to find a relationship does not rule out its existence.

The same points can be made for the third variable explanations, which are described next. For third variable explanations of the positive association between television advertising, as measured by television viewing, and adiposity, the evidence is clear (see Table 5-22). Neither age nor gender nor race/ethnicity nor socioeconomic status explains the association. These variables were included in most analyses. When they were, the positive association between exposure to television advertising, as measured by television viewing, and adiposity was statistically significant in the great majority of the results.

For most other adiposity-related variables that might explain the positive association between television advertising exposure and adiposity, or produce meaningful variations in the association, in general there is not enough evidence to assess any role they might play. Among the 16 studies (17 results), the number of these other adiposity-related variables included in analyses with television viewing ranged from 1 to 10. Examples are region, population density, parental smoking, maternal marital status, maternal diabetes, child's birth weight, and child's initial adiposity.

Two other adiposity-related variables were included in enough analyses that it is possible to assess whether the television advertising–adiposity relationship exists when they are taken into account. For parental adiposity, which is known to be associated with child adiposity, the number of significant results for the television viewing measure of advertising exposure is still large compared to the number of nonsignificant results. The same is true for the child's initial adiposity, which could only be included in analyses in longitudinal studies. Prior adiposity is probably the strongest predictor of current or future adiposity. Nonetheless, when early adiposity is taken into account, the positive association between television viewing and adiposity is statistically significant. Because television viewing is significantly associated with adiposity when a variety of other adiposity-related variables, including parental and initial child adiposity, are included in the analyses, the claim that television advertising influences adiposity cannot be rejected on the basis of the current evidence.

The second approach to testing the claim is presented in Table 5-23. Here the number of results for which television advertising was significant and nonsignificant is compared as the number of television-related nonadvertising, third, other adiposity-related, and all variables in the analysis increased. Again, the counts are taken from the statistical analysis that predicted adiposity, included television viewing (the measure of advertising exposure) as a predictor, and had the largest number of television-related nonadvertising, third, and other adiposity-related variables in the analysis. For the television-related nonadvertising variables, as more variables of that type were included, from none to three, the percentage of significant results tended to increase. For third variables, as the number of variables increased from one to four, the percentage of significant results decreased from 100 percent to 57 percent with all four third variables included in the analysis. For other adiposity-related variables, as the number of variables increased from none to two, the percentage of significant results increased somewhat. For the total number of variables, no matter what type, except for the two studies with the largest number of variables (14, 21) in which television viewing was respectively not significantly and significantly associated with adiposity, as the number of variables in the analysis increased from 3 to 12, the percentage of significant results also increased. Overall, then, because in most cases television viewing remained significantly associated with adiposity for the majority of results when more variables were included in the analyses, the claim that television advertising influences adiposity cannot be rejected on the basis of the evidence at hand.

In summary, the 17 results from cross-sectional and longitudinal studies with medium causal inference validity provided useful—but not conclusive—information about the likelihood that the positive association reflected a causal relationship of exposure to television advertising on adiposity. The majority of studies that provided evidence about plausible alternative explanations of the statistically significant positive association between exposure to television advertising and adiposity did not convincingly demonstrate that this association *was* explained by these alternative variables and *not* explained by exposure to television advertising. However, it is an unwarranted inference that alternative explanations can therefore be ruled out. This is partly due to the difficulty of exhaustively including all plausible alternative explanations in any given study and partly due to the difficulty of accurately and precisely measuring each alternative.

If, for example, television viewing had a causal influence on adiposity solely through decreasing physical activity, and no third factor or other alternative variable mattered—including exposure to television advertising—then television viewing and adiposity would be associated, but this association would disappear after statistically controlling for physical activity. If physical activity were measured with error, however, then the association between television viewing and adiposity would *not* disappear after controlling for physical activity using the imprecise measure of it. It is difficult to measure dietary intake, physical activity, and other factors that are plausible alternative explanations for the connection between television viewing and adiposity, and such measurement is rarely done with high validity, precision, and reliability. Thus, even though the association between exposure to television advertising and adiposity continued to be significant in the majority of studies that statistically adjusted for alternative or third variables, it is still possible that this is due to measurement error and not due to the association reflecting a causal influence of television advertising on adiposity.

Although current evidence does not allow a definite finding on this matter, it does suggest that any causal relationship that might exist would constitute a relatively small influence of exposure to television advertising on young people's adiposity. Two types of evidence support this inference. One is that the research examined typically explained a small rather than large amount of the overall variability in adiposity among the young people being studied. For example, Storey et al. (2003) examined multivariate models of the relationship between demographic and lifestyle variables and adiposity using data from two national surveys. For data from the Continuing Survey of Food Intake for Individuals (CSFII) 1994–1996 and 1998, analyses that took into account diet, age, gender, race/ethnicity, socioeconomic status, and two other adiposity-related variables, in addition to television viewing, accounted for 8.5 percent of the variability in children's adiposity and 11.4 percent of the variability in teens' adiposity. For data from the NHANES III, analyses that took into account physical activity, diet, age, gender, race/ethnicity, socioeconomic status, and two other adiposity-related variables accounted for just about the same amount of variability in children's and teens' adiposity. Other research in the evidence base provided varying estimates, but none indicated that all the variables studied together accounted for most of the variability in young people's adiposity. Better prediction might come about through the inclusion of more of the influential variables and better measurement of them, but current evidence indicates that the explanatory variables at hand, including exposure to television advertising, altogether do not account for a substantial amount of the variability in juvenile adiposity.

Given that exposure to television advertising is just one of the likely influences on adiposity that is included in these analyses, if this exposure has a direct causal and independent influence on adiposity, it will be smaller still than the influence of all variables together. In fact, those studies that have provided estimates of that influence suggest that it would be small. For example, Storey et al. (2003) estimated that for every additional hour of daily television viewing, children's and teens' BMI could increase by about 0.2, and Dietz and Gortmaker (1985) estimated that the prevalence of teenage obesity could increase by about 2 percent of teens. Although any causal influence of television advertising on adiposity is likely to be very small, it is not necessarily inconsequential. In a national population of about 75 million young people under age 18 years (U.S. Census Bureau, 2005), 2 percent is 1.5 million young people. With these factors in mind, if exposure to television advertising directly influences childhood adiposity, the influence would be consequential when aggregated over the entire population of American children and teens.

In summary, as was the case when examining the influence of marketing on precursors of diet and on diet itself, most of the research relevant to marketing's influence on diet-related health is about the effects of television advertising of foods and beverages. The one diet-related health outcome that has been studied to any degree is adiposity. Most of the research about television advertising and adiposity has not focused explicitly on exposure to television advertising as the causal variable, but it is amenable to use for the committee's purposes because it measures television viewing, which is well correlated with exposure to television advertising (Chapter 4).

Finding: The association between adiposity and exposure to television advertising remains after taking alternative explanations into account, but the research does not convincingly rule out other possible explanations for the association; therefore, current evidence is not sufficient to arrive at any finding about a causal relationship from television advertising to adiposity among children and youth. It is important to note that even a small influence, aggregated over the entire population of American children and youth, would be consequential in impact.

This finding is based entirely on the available research that permits examination of the relationship between exposure to television advertising and adiposity. When this research is considered in the context of the research reviewed earlier on the relationship of television advertising to precursors of diet and to diet itself, there is some basis for concluding that there may be a causal connection. Moreover, as depicted in the analytic framework (see Figure 5-1) and assessed in earlier parts of this chapter, there is reason to believe that marketing influences the precursors of diet, and these precursors are associated to some degree with diet. The relationships between dietary deficiencies and excesses and adverse health outcomes are summarized in Chapter 2 and Appendix D.

MODERATORS OF MARKETING INFLUENCE

The systematic evidence review indicates that television advertising is related to the precursors of diet (e.g., food preferences), diet, and diet-related health (particularly adiposity). The question addressed in this section is whether these relationships are moderated by age, gender, race/ethnicity, or socioeconomic status. The systematic evidence review compared the pattern of results between different age groups across different studies. In this section, a narrative review considers the comparisons that were made within each study.

Statistically speaking, a moderator effect occurs when a relationship between two variables differs according to levels of a third variable in which case that third variable is a moderator of the relationship between the first two variables. As an example, suppose that food advertising influenced food preference in younger children (ages 2 to 5 years), but not in older children and teens. In this hypothetical example, age would be a moderator of the effect of advertising on food preference.

Each study in the systematic evidence review was examined for moderator effects. In many studies, however, investigators did not test for moderator effects. For example, a study might test the relationship between the amount of television viewing and adiposity in Hispanic/Latino and white children. Finding that Hispanic/Latino children had greater adiposity than white children, the study might enter race/ethnicity as a statistical control variable, examining the relationship between television viewing and adiposity after adjusting for the relationship between race/ethnicity and adiposity. Such an approach does not explicitly test whether race/ethnicity is a moderator variable, that is, whether the strength of the relationship between television viewing and adiposity differs between white and Hispanic/Latino children. To test for a moderator effect, the study must, in one way or another, determine whether the statistical relationships differ at different levels of the moderator variable.

In the review of moderators, if a study explicitly tested interaction effects, or if the study explicitly determined whether subgroups of the larger sample did or did not show differing effects, the study was considered as testing for moderator effects. The variables reviewed as potential moderators were age, gender, race/ethnicity, and socioeconomic status. Because moderator effects were not subjected to the same stringent analyses done for the effects described earlier in this chapter as part of the systematic evidence review, the following should be considered a narrative review of moderator effects.

Age

The systematic evidence review examined whether, across studies, there were age group differences in the influence of television food and beverage advertising. It found that there were no differences in effects on young and older children and that in both age groups, there were relationships between food and beverage advertising and precursors of diet, diet, and diet-related health. Findings with respect to teens were not as clear because of lack of evidence or, in the case of diet, lack of effect. In the present section, studies are reviewed that analyzed for moderating effects of age.

Eight studies tested the relationship between advertising and precursors of diet from younger to older children, with six finding that age did not moderate the influence of television advertising. Of the two studies that found an effect of age as a moderator, one (Faber et al., 1984) found that younger children were more likely to recall a health message that was based on fear than were older children and teens. The other study (Kunkel, 1988) found that younger children were more influenced by cereal commercials than were older children, although this difference disappeared when the advertisements were presented in a host-selling format (use of the same characters in commercials as are featured in the adjacent program content), a tactic that is prohibited on broadcast television by the U.S. Federal Communications Commission (FCC, 1974). Overall, age has not been found to be a consistent moderator of advertising effects on precursors of diet. This finding is consistent with that of the systematic evidence review.

A review of the studies on the influence of advertising on diet leads to a similar finding. Of four studies that tested age as a moderator from younger to older children and that involved experimental use of television advertising or product placement, none found that age was a significant moderator, although all found the advertising and product placement to influence food and beverage choices. Two studies examined diet in relation to amount of television viewing as a measure of advertising exposure, one using teens and one using older children. Neither found age differences in effects within the teen years or within the older children. Again, there is no evidence that age is a consistent moderator of the effects of television advertising and again, there is little evidence with respect to teens, especially in comparison to younger ages.

When the relationship of adiposity and television viewing as a measure of advertising exposure was considered, it was found that seven studies tested age as a moderator. Of these, five found age to be a nonsignificant moderator, one found a larger relationship of television viewing to adiposity in children ages 9 to 18 years than in children ages 5 to 8 years (Gray and Smith, 2003), and one found a larger relationship in 8-year-olds than in 12-year-olds (Maffeis et al., 1998). In other words, although there is a consistent relationship indicating that advertising exposure, as measured by amount of television viewing, is associated with adiposity in children, there is no evidence that this relationship is consistently moderated by age. This conclusion is consistent with that of the systematic evidence review.

In nearly all the studies considered above, tests of age as a moderator have not been theoretically motivated. In particular, none of the studies have considered the possibility that understanding of the persuasive intent behind advertising may be important. In general, of course, such understanding would be less in younger children. As discussed below, the most appropriate comparisons would consider children younger and older than age 8 years in order to test the premise that understanding of persuasive intent may be an important moderator of advertising effects.

Persuasive Intent

Related to the moderator of age, but worthy of separate mention is the issue of the understanding of persuasive intent. This topic has been a part of public policy discussions about the legitimacy of advertising to children. At what point do children perceive advertising as a message category that is separate and distinct from television programming? When do they begin to apply a degree of skepticism to their understanding of advertising claims and appeals? Researchers have examined age-related developmental differences in children's comprehension of the nature and purpose of television advertising quite extensively, affording strong confidence in the conclusions that can be drawn across studies.

Children must acquire two basic information processing skills to achieve mature comprehension of advertising messages: capacity to discriminate commercial from noncommercial content and ability to attribute persuasive intent to advertising, adjusting their interpretation of commercial messages accordingly (Gunter et al., 2005; John, 1999; Kunkel, 2001; Young, 1990). Each of these capabilities develops over time, as a result of cognitive growth and development more than the accumulation of exposure to media content (Kunkel, 2001).

Program/Commercial Discrimination

Estimates of the age at which children can consistently discriminate advertisements as separate and distinct from adjacent programming range from as young as age 3 years to as old as age 6 years (Gunter et al., 2005). The variability depends on the nature of the measurement strategy used by the researcher as well as the difficulty of the particular task, which can be affected by the advertising and programming selected for testing. For example, when both programs and advertisements employ similar animation formats, drawing perceptual distinctions may be more challenging than when one format is animated and another uses live action. In general, most reviews of research agree that children can discriminate perceptually between television programming and advertising consistently by the ages of 4 to 5 years (John, 1999; Kunkel, 2001; Kunkel et al., 2004).

No studies could be located that examined development of skills to identifying advertising in print media. Presumably this is because there would be little variance at such a task by the time children's literacy skills had matured to the point where they would likely encounter print advertising in their natural environment. As was noted in Chapter 4, advertising to children is growing substantially on the Internet. In this context, however, researchers have yet to evaluate children's ability to recognize commercial content. Given widespread recognition that the boundaries between commercial and noncommercial content are more blurred on the Internet than in traditional print, radio, or television media, there is some reason to expect a delay in the development of children's ability to recognize advertising on the Internet as compared to other media. This is an issue that should be addressed by future research.

Comprehension of Advertising's Persuasive Intent

Television advertising intends to persuade. Older children and adults recognize this concept and often use it to "discount" self-interested claims and appeals included in commercial messages. In contrast, young children do not yet comprehend the persuasive intent of advertising and hence may be more susceptible to its influence. It is important to consider the age at which children develop the ability to attribute persuasive intent to advertising, because such knowledge should logically moderate the effects of commercial persuasion.

The most rudimentary aspect of children's comprehension of persuasive intent in advertising is the recognition that a commercial wants the viewer to buy the product. In fact, however, merely understanding that an advertisement "intends to sell" does not represent all or even most elements of mature comprehension of persuasive intent. The best explication of mature comprehension of the persuasive intent of advertising was offered by Roberts (1983). Roberts posited four key elements that must be understood: (1) The source of the message has other interests and perspectives than the receiver; (2) the source intends to persuade; (3) persuasive messages are biased; and (4) biased messages demand different interpretive strategies than unbiased messages. In summary, children who have developed a mature ability to recognize persuasive intent in advertising recognize the inherent bias, exaggeration, and self-interest of commercial messages, and can apply that knowledge in shaping their reactions to advertising.

The ability to recognize persuasive intent in advertising clearly requires the child to take the perspective of another into account. Young children tend to be highly egocentric, and to have difficulty considering the perspective of another person (Flavell, 1977; Kurdek and Rodgon, 1975; Selman, 1971). Accordingly, children's ability to produce persuasive messages that reflect sensitivity to a listener's perspective is highly constrained in the preschool and early elementary years (Kline and Clinton, 1998; Weiss and Sachs, 1991). It is not surprising, then, to find that young children under the ages of approximately 7–8 years also have great difficulty recognizing the persuasive intent that necessarily underlies all television advertising.

Numerous empirical studies (e.g., Blosser and Roberts, 1985; Donohue et al., 1978; Robertson and Rossiter, 1974; Ward et al., 1977) indicate that at least half or more of children under the ages of 7–8 years are generally unable to recognize the persuasive intent of television advertising, even when this skill is measured in only its most rudimentary form of selling intent (i.e., a commercial intends to sell a product). Although much of this research was conducted several decades ago in response to Federal Trade Commission concern with the issue, more recent studies of the topic (Bjurstrom, 1994; Gunter et al., 2005; Oates et al., 2002; Chapter 1) corroborate the identical patterns identified in the earlier research.

In summary, the ability to recognize persuasive intent in television advertising begins to appear in its most basic form at approximately ages 7–8 years, but it is not consolidated and consistently applied until later years. Indeed, several studies have demonstrated that even when older children and adolescents possess mature knowledge about advertising's persuasive intent, such understanding is not consistently applied to effectively defend against commercial claims, appeals, and persuasive outcomes (Brucks et al., 1988; Derbaix and Bree, 1997; Linn et al., 1982). Moreover, although the age at which children understand persuasive intent in advertising has been well established for television, the issue has not yet been scrutinized on the Internet. Given the greater overall blurring of boundaries between commercial and noncommercial messages on the Internet, there is reason to expect that such ability may be delayed in surfacing as compared to the developmental patterns established as normative for television. This is a topic that should be addressed by future research.

*Finding: Most children ages 8 years and under do not effectively compre-
hend the persuasive intent of marketing messages, and most children ages
4 years and under cannot consistently discriminate between television advertising and programming. The evidence is currently insufficient to determine whether or not this meaningfully alters the ways in which food and
beverage marketing messages influence children.*

Gender

Unlike age, there are no general theoretical reasons to suppose that
boys may be differentially affected by food and beverage advertising as
compared to girls. Eight studies that examined television advertising and
precursors of diet tested gender as a potential statistical moderator. Of
these, six studies found that gender was not significant as a moderator.
Of the two finding that gender was a significant moderator, both (Miller
and Busch, 1979; Pine and Nash, 2003) found that girls' product preference
was more influenced by advertising than was boys'. Five studies used
amount of television viewing to measure advertising exposure and tested
gender as a moderator of precursors of diet: four found no significant
differences, and one (Signorielli and Lears, 1992) found that boys were
more influenced by television in eating intention than were girls.

One study tested gender differences in the influence of television advertising on young children's food consumption (Jeffrey et al., 1982). It found
that boys were more influenced by advertising for low-nutrition products
than were girls. When amount of television viewing was the measure of
advertising exposure in relation to diet, six studies tested gender effects.
Two found gender to be not significant as a moderator, two found effects to
be larger in boys, and two found effects to be larger in girls.

Twenty-five studies that examined the amount of television viewing (as
a measure of exposure to advertising) in relation to adiposity tested gender
moderator effects. Of these, 14 found gender to be not significant as a
moderator, and 8 found that girls showed larger effects than did boys.
Three studies showed larger effects in boys than girls.

Although the majority of studies found that gender was not significant
as a moderator, there was some slight trend for greater effects in girls than
in boys. This was particularly true for the relationship between when advertising exposure was measured by amount of television viewing and adiposity was the outcome variable. Because adiposity was nearly always measured as BMI, some caution is needed in interpreting this relationship.
There is some evidence that BMI may be a more appropriate measure of
adiposity in girls, especially adolescents, than in boys (Sardinha et al., 1999).

Nevertheless, girls may be more vulnerable than are boys to the health-related effects of television advertising (as measured by television viewing).

Race and Ethnicity

Overall, only a few studies have examined whether race and ethnicity moderates the effects of television advertising. None of these studies have employed products or advertising that were identified as targeting a particular racial or ethnic group. Three studies tested race and ethnicity as a moderator of the influence of advertising on precursors of diet. Two (Miller and Busch, 1979; Stoneman and Brody, 1981) found that white children were more influenced by advertising than were African American children. One (Barry and Hansen, 1973) found that African American children were more influenced than were white children. One study (Borzekowski and Robinson, 2001) found no difference between home English and Spanish speakers in the influence of advertising.

Two studies examined race and ethnicity in considering television advertising, measured by amount of television viewing, in relation to precursors of diet. One (Signorielli and Lears, 1992) found that minorities (African American, Hispanic/Latino) were more influenced than were whites. Another study found no race differences (Carruth et al., 1991).

Three studies tested moderating influences of race and ethnicity on the influence of television advertising on diet. Robinson (1999) found ethnicity to be nonsignificant, Robinson and Killen (1995) found that African American and white girls were less influenced by television advertising than were Hispanic/Latina girls and all boys, and Signorielli and Lears (1992) found that minorities were more influenced than were whites. Two studies examined home language as a moderator, with one finding no significant effect among English- and Spanish-speaking Hispanic/Latino Americans (Borzekowski and Poussaint, 1998), and another finding that in Quebec, English speakers were more influenced by American commercial television than French speakers were (Goldberg, 1990).

With respect to the relationship between amount of television advertising exposure, as measured by overall television viewing, and adiposity, seven studies examined race and ethnicity with two finding nonsignificant moderator effects. One study found greater effects in whites than in minorities, one found greater effects in whites than in American Indians, one found greater effects in African Americans and in American Indians than in whites, and one found greater effects in African Americans than whites.

Overall, when tested, moderator effects of race/ethnicity, or home language were frequently found, but they were not consistent across studies. In particular, there is no consistent evidence that whites are more or less affected by food and beverage advertising than are minorities.

Socioeconomic Status

Although studies frequently reported the socioeconomic status of their research participants, and frequently used it as a control variable in analyses, only a few studies examined socioeconomic status as a moderator of effects. One study tested amount of exposure to television advertising, measured by overall viewing, in relation to precursors of diet, with no significant socioeconomic status moderator effect (Reid et al., 1980). Two studies examined amount of advertising exposure, with a television viewing measure in relation to diet, with one study of young children finding socioeconomic status to be a nonsignificant moderator (Borzekowski and Poussaint, 1998) and another finding that low-income older children were more influenced by television than were high-income older children (Goldberg, 1990). With respect to adiposity and television advertising exposure (measured by viewing), one study (Muller et al., 1999) found that low-socioeconomic-status children showed a greater effect than did middle- and high-socioeconomic-status children. In sum, there is no consistent effect of socioeconomic status in moderating the influence of food and beverage advertising on television. That said, few studies have tested the moderating effect of socioeconomic status.

Summary of Moderator Effects

Moderator effects have not been tested frequently, and when they have, the most frequent finding is that they are not significant. When differences occur, there appears to be a somewhat greater influence of television advertising on girls than on boys. Age is rarely a significant moderator, and when it is, the effects are not consistent across studies. A theoretically important moderator, understanding of the persuasive intent of advertising, has not been studied in relation to advertising influence on precursors of diet, diet, or diet-related health, although before certain ages children are not able to discriminate between television advertising and programming or to comprehend the persuasive intent of marketing messages. Overall, the evidence concerning moderator effects is insufficient to come to any findings on age, race/ethnicity, or socioeconomic status as moderators of the effects of television food and beverage advertising.

RELATIONSHIP TO OTHER RECENT ASSESSMENTS

In addition to the U.S. attention to this topic, several related reviews of research on food and beverage marketing and childhood obesity have been produced in recent years in other countries and through international organizations. Among these are a systematic evidence review sponsored by the United Kingdom's Food Standards Agency (Hastings et al., 2003); a narrative research review conducted by the United Kingdom's Office of Communications (Ofcom), the new regulator for the UK communications industries (Ofcom, 2004); a collaborative analysis of research from 20 European countries sponsored by the European Commission and administered through the European Heart Network (Matthews et al., 2005); and a series of related reports published by the World Health Organization (WHO) examining the possible linkages between marketing and childhood obesity (WHO and FAO, 2003), as well as the international regulatory environment for addressing such concerns (Hawkes, 2004).

These international reports all concur on a number of fundamental conclusions. First, they all find that advertising directed to children, particularly on television, is heavily populated by commercials for foods that pose adiposity and related health risks for children when consumed in abundance, although each report prefers different language for labeling such commodities. For example, the Ofcom (2004) report terms such food products "high in fat, salt, and sugar" and uses the acronym HFSS in an effort to be sensitive to the argument that there are no less healthful foods, whereas the European Heart Network's report explicitly rejects such argument and uses the term "unhealthy foods" to describe the dominant category of edibles marketed to children (Matthews et al., 2005). Second, all these reports agree that food marketers spend significant resources to advertise to children, and that children consequently have heavy exposure to such advertising. And third, they all agree (ones that address this topic) that children under age 8 years have limited ability to recognize persuasive intent in commercials, leading to the expectation that food advertising to young children may be particularly effective (Hastings et al., 2003; Ofcom, 2004; WHO and FAO, 2003).

On the critical question of the direct evidence linking marketing to children's food consumption and to childhood obesity, the research reviews take somewhat different paths to end up at similar points, reaching conclusions consonant with those established by this committee's own analysis presented earlier in this chapter. Most of the reports employ a traditional narrative approach in which the relevant research is reviewed and evaluated in interpretive fashion. Some, such as the Ofcom (2004) report, buttress their analysis with commissioned literature review papers prepared by media effects experts (Livingstone, 2004; Livingstone and Helsper, 2004).

The key conclusion of the Ofcom report holds that television ". . . advertising has a modest, direct effect on children's food choices" (Ofcom, 2004, P. 23). It notes further that indirect effects are likely to be larger, but that there is insufficient evidence at the present time to determine their size relative to other factors. The WHO and FAO (2003) report concludes that the heavy marketing of high-calorie and low-nutrient foods and fast food outlets represents a probable increased risk for childhood obesity. This report is supported by selected background reviews (Hawkes, 2002; Swinburn et al., 2004), including an international analysis of the marketing activities of food and beverage industries. The European Heart Network report (Matthews et al., 2005) does not directly engage the advertising effects literature, opting instead to conclude that television "advertising of unhealthy food to children should be prohibited" (P. 14) based solely on the evidence of its pervasiveness in the children's advertising environment and implicit assumptions about its efficacy. In its recently published report *Preventing Childhood Obesity*, the British Medical Association (2005) concludes that "marketing is effective in influencing food choices made by children and parents" (P. 27) and similarly recommends an outright ban on food advertising to children because many children lack the capability to "make informed judgments about the advertisements they see" (P. 27).

As noted earlier, the Hastings et al. (2003) study conducted for the United Kingdom Food Standards Agency is the analysis most directly comparable to the investigation this committee has pursued and reported earlier in this chapter. There were some differences between the two, in scope, in depth, and in the nature of the evidence base. For example, our committee chose not to undertake a separate systematic evidence review of the nature and extent of food advertising to children, relying instead on the extensive information and consensus from work done elsewhere. On the other hand, our committee considered a substantially more extensive body of peer-reviewed evidence for its systematic review of the evidence on the influence of food marketing on children. Despite the differences, the findings presented in this chapter are fundamentally similar and certainly complementary to the conclusions derived from the Hastings et al. (2003) systematic evidence review. Our more extensive base of research evidence has afforded us the ability to draw somewhat more detailed conclusions than those of Hastings et al. (2003), reflecting a natural step forward in the progress of science that is a function of the increased accumulation of evidence across studies. Especially clear from any perspective, is the substantial need for further investigation in this area.

RECOMMENDATIONS FOR FUTURE RESEARCH

The systematic evidence review found that there are several important gaps in the existing research relating marketing to diet and diet-related health. First and foremost, the great preponderance of research done to date has narrowly focused on, in marketing, television and television advertising, and in diet-related health, obesity. There has been almost no research on the influence of other forms of food and beverage marketing as they relate to diet and diet-related health. Even within the domain of television, most of the research that relates television viewing to diet and to diet-related health does not distinguish exposure to food and beverage advertising from exposure to television in general. This lack of relevant research severely constrains the findings that can be drawn about the influence of food and beverage marketing on the diet and diet-related health of American children and youth. For example, of the 36 results involving the effect of marketing on diet, only 2 did not involve television: one by Auty and Lewis (2004) on the effects of product placement in films, and one by French et al. (2001a) on the effect of vending machine prices and signage on the consumption of low-fat snacks. Of the 74 results involving the influence of marketing on diet-related health, *all* involved television.

Second, although the research in this area depends crucially on accurately measuring dietary intake, physical activity, family habits, and other factors involved in the relationships among marketing, diet, and diet-related health, commonly used measures are known to be problematic and are seriously impeding the science in this area. Extremely little is known about how much error infects these measures, and being able to reliably tease apart and quantify the different mechanisms by which controllable factors such as marketing, media use, or physical activity might influence diet and diet-related health depends crucially on such knowledge. For example, broad consensus exists that if television viewing affects obesity, then it must be either through physical activity or through dietary intake. Proctor et al. (2003) found a significant association between television viewing and obesity, but they could not eliminate this association even after controlling for both physical activity and diet. The only plausible explanation for this discrepancy is measurement error for either physical activity or diet or both. Similarly, Robinson (1999) found that an intervention that reduced the amount of television viewing, video watching, and game playing resulted in a significant decrease in obesity, but he also found that, as measured, there was no decrease in high-fat food intake, moderate to vigorous physical activity, consumption of highly advertised foods, or cardio respiratory fitness. Likewise, data on dietary intake trends for children over the past 30 years are inconsistent, yielding different findings from different measures and yielding findings that are often difficult to interpret (see Chapter 2). As discussed above in the finding to the consideration of studies relating marketing to diet-related health, eliminating alternative explanations of an association in cross-sectional studies requires accurate measurement of alternative mechanisms.

New Forms of Research

The committee therefore recommends that resources be made available to support new research on food marketing and its influence on diet and diet-related health and research on improving measurement strategies for factors involved centrally in this research. Much of this research must be interdisciplinary and fairly large scale in nature, although some highly focused small-scale research is also desirable. More specifically, the committee suggests several specific forms of research that would improve our knowledge in this area.

Broader Research

- **Marketing other than television** There should be extensive experimental and observational investigations of the influence of food marketing practices other than television advertising. These include print advertising, billboard advertising, Internet advertising, advergaming, contests and sweepstakes, kids' clubs, product placement in movies and computer games, and product placement strategies at points of purchase.
- **Health other than obesity** There should be more research focused on food marketing in relationship to overall diet as well as health outcomes, in addition to obesity, including blood lipid profiles, blood pressure, blood sugar, vitamin and mineral status, and others in addition to adiposity.

Measurement

- **Improved measurement** There should be research focused on understanding, reducing, and quantifying measurement error for dietary intake, physical activity, exposure to marketing, and other factors crucial to this research.

Intervention Research

- **Healthful diet promotion** Research should be conducted on intervention strategies promoting healthful diets that incorporate the most effective and powerful techniques employed by food and beverage marketers. Research should evaluate these strategies in the context of less healthy food and beverage choices and advertising for less healthy foods and beverages that remain available to young people.

Longitudinal Research

- **The National Children's Study** The proposed, longitudinal study of 100,000 American children from prenatal development to age 21 years should include measures of exposure to food and beverage marketing, diet, energy expenditure, and diet-related health. More than any other panel study, the National Children's Study has the potential to determine the relative importance of food and beverage marketing, as compared to other factors in children's lives, to diet-related health.

Separating Mechanisms

- **Marketing compared to media use** There is now evidence that reducing television, video games, and video watching reduces BMI. If marketing has an influence, then reducing television viewing should have more of an influence than reducing video game playing or video watching, as the latter involve less marketing and often no marketing of foods and beverages. More research is needed on teasing apart effects from just participating in media and effects from the marketing occurring in that media.

- **Snacking and marketing** There is some evidence that snacking while watching television may play a role in obesity. Detailed observational and experimental research should study this phenomenon. For example, is snacking stimulated by food advertising or depictions of eating and drinking during television programming? Do people consume more while watching television because they are distracted from monitoring internal satiety signals? Or does engagement in other kinds of activities than television viewing distract people from internal hunger signals?

- **Parents of young children** Food preferences and eating habits are to a substantial extent established in early childhood. Research is needed on parents' knowledge of healthful nutrition for children and on feeding practices during infancy and the preschool years. A special focus should be put on first-time parents and the degree to which their feeding practices are shaped by food and beverage marketing.

- **Persuasive intent** Children's understanding of the persuasive intent of television advertising has been suggested as a likely moderator of effects, but no systematic research has yet been pursued to elucidate this relationship. Such investigation is warranted to better understand whether the developing child's ability to comprehend the inherent bias and exaggeration of advertising is important in helping children to defend more effectively against commercial persuasion. Given the migration of child-directed food and beverage to other forms of marketing across a diverse range of new media and advertising contexts, it may be equally valuable to investigate the possible moderating effect of persuasive intent attribution in media contexts other than television. Such evidence may be particularly important because many of these new forms of marketing are less transparent and regulated than is television advertising. Given the greater blurring of boundaries between commercial and noncommercial content on new media such as the Internet (Chapter 4), the age of effective comprehension of persuasive intent of these new forms may be considerably older than that for television advertising.

Family Studies

• **Modern family life** In-depth family studies should be undertaken to understand how marketing influences food and beverage purchases, food and beverage availability in the home, meal preparation, and snacks. These studies should take into account the time and financial pressures on the modern American family.

In the process of carrying out the systematic evidence review, the committee identified several areas in which additional research was needed in order to address various elements of the committee's charge. It also realized that changes to research methods could increase the relevance of the research to the committee's purposes. These areas and changes have been described in this section.

Finding: New research is needed on food and beverage marketing and its impact on diet and diet-related health and on improving measurement strategies for factors involved centrally in this research. Much of this research must be interdisciplinary and fairly large-scale in nature, although some highly-focused small-scale research is also desirable. Among the specific research needed are studies of newer promotion techniques, newer venues, and healthier products and portion sizes.

SUMMARY

This chapter has focused on the identification and assessment of the research evidence about the influence of food and beverage marketing on the diets and diet-related health of children and youth. The committee conducted a wide search, including online databases, literature reviews, and outreach to experts, to identify a set of relevant and important research evidence. An explicit selection process identified studies to be included in the review. Using a causal framework and a systematic evidence review process, the committee assessed the available evidence on the influence of food and beverage marketing on young people's diets and diet-related health.

The committee found a large body of peer-reviewed, published research (155 results from 123 studies). The research spans more than three decades, from the 1970s to the present. Results from earlier research are broadly consistent with more recent research in the same area. All three main research designs—experimental, cross-sectional, and longitudinal—were employed, such that the usual limitations associated with a particular approach are counterbalanced by other approaches. All but 6 of the 155 results had television advertising as the marketing variable.

In general, quality ratings were reasonably good across the spectrum of categories included in the systematic evidence review; with one exception, the numbers of high- and medium-quality ratings were equal to or greater than the numbers of low ratings for measure quality, causal inference validity, and ecological validity. As anticipated, many results from cross-sectional observational and longitudinal studies were rated low on causal inference validity, and many results from experiments were rated low on ecological validity—typical for the respective designs employed. The research results included in the systematic evidence review were of sufficient quality, diversity, and scope to support several findings about the influence of marketing. The overall finding from the research was that food and beverage marketing influences the preferences and purchase requests of children, influences consumption at least in the short term, is a likely contributor to less healthful diets, and may contribute to negative diet-related health outcomes and risks. The overall finding is drawn from a systematic evidence review of research in three areas, and the findings from these three areas provide more specific information in support of the general finding.

With respect to the specific influence of food and beverage marketing on the precursors (e.g., food preferences and purchase requests) of young people's diet, a systematic evidence review supported the following findings:

- There is strong evidence that television advertising influences the food and beverage preferences of children ages 2–11 years. There is insufficient evidence about its influence on the preferences of teens ages 12–18 years.

- There is strong evidence that television advertising influences the food and beverage purchase requests of children ages 2–11 years. There is insufficient evidence about its influence on the purchase requests of teens ages 12–18 years.

- There is moderate evidence that television advertising influences the food and beverage beliefs of children ages 2–11 years. There is insufficient evidence about its influence on the beliefs of teens ages 12–18 years.

- Given the findings from the systematic evidence review of the influence of marketing on the precursors of diet, and given the evidence from content analyses that the preponderance of television food and beverage advertising relevant to children and youth promotes high-calorie and low-nutrient products, it can be concluded that television advertising influences children to prefer and request high-calorie and low-nutrient foods and beverages.

With respect to the specific influence of food and beverage marketing on young people's diets, a systematic evidence review supported the following findings:

- There is strong evidence that television advertising influences the short-term consumption of children ages 2–11 years. There is insufficient evidence about its influence on the short-term consumption of teens ages 12–18 years.
- There is moderate evidence that television advertising influences the usual dietary intake of younger children ages 2–5 years and weak evidence that it influences the usual dietary intake of older children ages 6–11 years. There is also weak evidence that it does not influence the usual dietary intake of teens ages 12–18 years.

With respect to the specific influence of food and beverage marketing on young people's diet-related health, a systematic evidence review relied on research investigating the relation between amount of television viewing, among other variables, and diet-related health. Amount of television viewing is highly correlated with amount of exposure to television advertising and is frequently used as a measure of advertising exposure. The committee's purposes are served by reviewing research about television viewing and diet-related health, but findings about advertising effects are difficult because of measurement quality, alternative explanations of findings, and other factors. With these caveats noted, the systematic evidence review supported the following findings:

- Statistically, there is strong evidence that exposure to television advertising is associated with adiposity in children ages 2–11 years and teens ages 12–18 years.
- The association between adiposity and exposure to television advertising remains after taking alternative explanations into account, but the research does not convincingly rule out other possible explanations for the association; therefore, current evidence is not sufficient to arrive at any finding about a causal relationship from television advertising to adiposity. It is important to note that even a small influence, aggregated over the entire population of American children and youth, would be consequential in impact.

In addition to conducting a systematic evidence review of the research examining the relationships of marketing to the precursors of diet, to diet, and to diet-related health, the committee conducted a narrative review of this research and other relevant research in order to understand the role of moderators in altering the marketing relationships. The committee found the literature too small altogether and too varied in topic to support any conclusions about the ways in which differences in age, gender, race/ethnicity (including home language), and socioeconomic status may alter (moderate) the influence of marketing on these precursors. However, with respect to age, the committee found that:

• Most children ages 8 years and under do not effectively comprehend the persuasive intent of marketing messages, and most children ages 4 years and under cannot consistently discriminate between television advertising and programming. The evidence is currently insufficient to determine whether or not this meaningfully alters the ways in which food and beverage marketing messages influence children.

Finally, both the systematic evidence review and the narrative review revealed areas in which new research is needed, as well as the characteristics of research that is most likely to be helpful to committees addressing charges such as ours. Specific recommendations for future research are offered in a preceding section. The committee's overall finding is as follows:

• New research is needed on food and beverage marketing and its impact on diet and diet-related health and on improving measurement strategies for factors involved centrally in this research. Much of this research must be interdisciplinary and fairly large-scale in nature, although some highly-focused small-scale research is also desirable. Among the specific research needed are studies of newer promotion techniques, newer venues, and healthier products and portion sizes.

REFERENCES

*Andersen RE, Crespo CJ, Bartlett SJ, Cheskin LJ, Pratt M. 1998. Relationship of physical activity and television watching with body weight and level of fatness among children: Results from the Third National Health and Nutrition Examination Survey. *J Am Med Assoc* 279(12):938–942.

*Anderson DR, Huston AC, Schmitt KL, Linebarger DL, Wright JC. 2001. Early childhood television viewing and adolescent behavior: The recontact study. *Mon Soc Res Child Dev* 66(1):I–VIII, 1–147.

*Armstrong CA, Sallis JF, Alcaraz JE, Kolody B, McKenzie TL, Hovell MF. 1998. Children's television viewing, body fat, and physical fitness. *Am J Health Promot* 12(6):363–368.

ATSDR (Agency for Toxic Substances and Disease Registry). 2002. *Analytical Methods.* [Online]. Available at: http://www.atsdr.cdc.gov/toxprofiles/tp13-c6.pdf [accessed October 14, 2005].

---

*These references are studies included in the systematic evidence review.

*Auty S, Lewis C. 2004. Exploring children's choice: The reminder effect of product placement. *Psychol Market* 21(9):697–713.

*Bao Y, Shao AT. 2002. Nonconformity advertising to teens. *J Ad Res* 42(3):56–65.

*Barry TE, Gunst RF. 1982. Children's advertising: The differential impact of appeal strategy. *Current Issues Res Ad* 5:113–125.

Barry TE, Hansen RW. 1973. How race affects children's TV commercials. *J Ad Res* 13(5): 63–67.

*Berkey CS, Rockett HR, Field AE, Gillman MW, Frazier AL, Camargo CA Jr, Colditz GA. 2000. Activity, dietary intake, and weight changes in a longitudinal study of preadolescent and adolescent boys and girls. *Pediatrics* 105(4):E56.

*Berkey CS, Rockett HR, Gillman MW, Colditz GA. 2003. One-year changes in activity and in inactivity among 10- to 15-year-old boys and girls: Relationship to change in body mass index. *Pediatrics* 111(4 Pt 1):836–843.

Bjurstrom E. 1994. *Children and Television Advertising*. Report No. 1994/95:8. Stockholm, Sweden: Swedish Consumer Agency.

Blosser BJ, Roberts DF. 1985. Age differences in children's perceptions of message intent. Responses to TV news, commercials, educational spots, and public service announcements. *Commun Res* 12(4):455–484.

*Bogaert N, Steinbeck KS, Baur LA, Brock K, Bermingham MA. 2003. Food, activity and family—environmental vs. biochemical predictors of weight gain in children. *Eur J Clin Nutr* 57(10):1242–1249.

*Bolton RN. 1983. Modeling the impact of television food advertising on children's diets. *Current Issues and Research in Advertising* 6(1):173–199.

*Borzekowski DLG, Poussaint AF. 1998. *Latino American Preschoolers and the Media*. Philadelphia, PA: Annenberg Public Policy Center of the University of Pennsylvania.

*Borzekowski DL, Robinson TN. 2001. The 30-second effect: An experiment revealing the impact of television commercials on food preferences of preschoolers. *J Am Diet Assoc* 101(1):42–46.

*Boynton-Jarrett R, Thomas TN, Peterson KE, Wiecha J, Sobol AM, Gortmaker SL. 2003. Impact of television viewing patterns on fruit and vegetable consumption among adolescents. *Pediatrics* 112(6 Pt 1):1321–1326.

British Medical Association. 2005. *Preventing Childhood Obesity*. London, UK: British Medical Association.

*Brody GH, Stoneman Z, Lane TS, Sanders AK. 1981. Television food commercials aimed at children, family grocery shopping, and mother–children interactions. *Family Relations* 30:435–439.

Brucks M, Armstrong GM, Goldberg ME. 1988. Children's use of cognitive defenses against television advertising: A cognitive response approach. *J Consum Res* 14:471–482.

*Burke V, Beilin LJ, Simmer K, Oddy WH, Blake KV, Doherty D, Kendall GE, Newnham JP, Landau LI, Stanley FJ. 2005. Predictors of body mass index and associations with cardiovascular risk factors in Australian children: A prospective cohort study. *Int J Obes Relat Metab Disord* 29(1):15–23.

*Cantor J. 1981. Modifying children's eating habits through television ads: Effects of humorous appeals in a field setting. *J Broadcasting* 23(1):37–47.

*Carruth BR, Goldberg DL, Skinner JD. 1991. Do parents and peers mediate the influence of television advertising on food-related purchases? *J Adolesc Res* 6(2):253–271.

*Christenson PG. 1982. Children's perceptions of TV commercials and products. The effects of PSAs. *Commun Res* 9(4):491–524.

*Clancy-Hepburn K, Hickey AA, Nevill G. 1974. Children's behavior responses to TV food advertisements. *J Nutr Ed* 6(3):93–96.

*Clarke TK. 1984. Situational factors affecting preschoolers' responses to advertising. *J Acad Marketing Sci* 12(4):25–40.

*Coon KA, Goldberg J, Rogers BL, Tucker KL. 2001. Relationships between use of television during meals and children's food consumption patterns. *Pediatrics* 107(1):e7.

*Crespo CJ, Smit E, Troiano RP, Bartlett SJ, Macera CA, Andersen RE. 2001. Television watching, energy intake, and obesity in US children: Results from the third National Health and Nutrition Examination Survey, 1988–1994. *Arch Pediatr Adolesc Med* 155(3):360–365.

*Crooks DL. 2000. Food consumption, activity, and overweight among elementary school children in an Appalachian Kentucky community. *Am J Phys Anthropol* 112(2):159–170.

Cullen KW, Baranowski T, Owens E, Marsh T, Rittenberry L, de Moor C. 2003. Availability, accessibility, and preferences for fruit, 100% fruit juice, and vegetables influence children's dietary behavior. *Health Ed Behav* 30(5):615–626.

*Dawson BL, Jeffrey DB, Walsh JA. 1988. Television food commercials' effect on children's resistance to temptation. *J Appl Soc Psychol* 18(16):1353–1360.

*Deheeger M, Rolland-Cachera MF, Fontvieille AM. 1997. Physical activity and body composition in 10 year old French children: Linkages with nutritional intake? *Int J Obes Relat Metab Disord* 21(5):372–379.

*Dennison BA, Erb TA, Jenkins PL. 2002. Television viewing and television in bedroom associated with overweight risk among low-income preschool children. *Pediatrics* 109(6):1028–1035.

Derbaix C, Bree J. 1997. The impact of children's affective reactions elicited by commercials on attitudes toward the advertisement and the brand. *Int J Res Marketing* 14:207–229.

*Dietz WH Jr, Gortmaker SL. 1985. Do we fatten our children at the television set? Obesity and television viewing in children and adolescents. *Pediatrics* 75(5):807–812.

*Donkin AJM, Neale RJ, Tilston C. 1993. Children's food purchase requests. *Appetite* 21(3):291–294.

*Donohue TR. 1975. Effect of commercials on black children. *J Advertising Res* 15(6):41–47.

Donohue TR, Meyer TP, Henke LL. 1978. Black and white children: Perceptions of TV commercials. *J Marketing* 42(4):34–40.

*Dowda M, Ainsworth BE, Addy CL, Saunders R, Riner W. 2001. Environmental influences, physical activity, and weight status in 8- to 16-year-olds. *Arch Pediatr Adolesc Med* 155(6):711–717.

*duRant RH, Baranowski T, Johnson M, Thompson WO. 1994. The relationship among television watching, physical activity, and body composition of young children. *Pediatrics* 94(4 Pt 1):449–455.

*duRant RH, Thompson WO, Johnson M, Baranowski T. 1996. The relationship among television watching, physical activity, and body composition of 5- or 6-year-old children. *Pediatric Exerc Sci* 8:15–26.

*Dwyer JT, Stone EJ, Yang M, Feldman H, Webber LS, Must A, Perry CL, Nader PR, Parcel GS. 1998. Predictors of overweight and overfatness in a multiethnic pediatric population. Child and Adolescent Trial for Cardiovascular Health Collaborative Research Group. *Am J Clin Nutr* 67(4):602–610.

*Eisenmann JC, Bartee RT, Wang MQ. 2002. Physical activity, TV viewing, and weight in U.S. youth: 1999 Youth Risk Behavior Survey. *Obes Res* 10(5):379–385.

*Faber RJ, Meyer TP, Miller MM. 1984. The effectiveness of health disclosures within children's television commercials. *J Broadcasting* 28(4):463–476.

FCC (U.S. Federal Communications Commission). 1974. Children's television programs: Report and policy statement. *Federal Register* 39:39396–39409.

Fisher JO, Birch LL. 1995. Fat preferences and fat consumption of 3-year-old to 5-year-old children are related to parental adiposity. *J Am Diet Assoc* 95(7):759–764.

Flavell JH. 1977. *Cognitive Development*. Englewood Cliffs, NJ: Prentice-Hall.

*Fontvieille AM, Kriska A, Ravussin E. 1993. Decreased physical activity in Pima Indian compared with Caucasian children. *Int J Obes Relat Metab Disord* 17(8):445–452.

*Francis LA, Lee Y, Birch LL. 2003. Parental weight status and girls' television viewing, snacking, and body mass indexes. *Obes Res* 11(1):143–151.

*French SA, Jeffery RW, Story M, Breitlow KK, Baxter JS, Hannan P, Snyder MP. 2001a. Pricing and promotion effects on low-fat vending snack purchases: The CHIPS Study. *Am J Public Health* 91(1):112–117.

*French SA, Story M, Neumark-Sztainer D, Fulkerson JA, Hannan P. 2001b. Fast food restaurant use among adolescents: Associations with nutrient intake, food choices and behavioral and psychosocial variables. *Int J Obes Relat Metab Disord* 25(12): 1823–1833.

*Galst JP. 1980. Television food commercials and pro-nutritional public service announcements as determinants of young children's snack choices. *Child Dev* 51:935–938.

*Galst JP, White MA. 1976. The unhealthy persuader: The reinforcing value of television and children's purchase-influencing attempts at the supermarket. *Child Dev* 47:1089–1096.

*Giammattei J, Blix G, Marshak HH, Wollitzer AO, Pettitt DJ. 2003. Television watching and soft drink consumption: Associations with obesity in 11- to 13-year-old schoolchildren. *Arch Pediatr Adolesc Med* 157(9):882–886.

Glymour CN, Cooper GF. 1999. *Causation, Computation, and Discovery*. Menlo Park, CA: AAAI Press.

*Goldberg ME. 1990. A quasi-experiment assessing the effectiveness of TV advertising directed to children. *J Marketing Res* 27(4):445–454.

*Goldberg ME, Gorn GJ, Gibson W. 1978. TV messages for snack and breakfast foods: Do they influence children's preferences? *J Consum Res* 5:73–81.

*Gordon-Larsen P, Adair LS, Popkin BM. 2002. Ethnic differences in physical activity and inactivity patterns and overweight status. *Obes Res* 10(3):141–149.

*Gorn GJ, Florsheim R. 1985. The effects of commercials for adult products on children. *J Consumer Res* 11(4):962–967.

*Gorn GJ, Goldberg ME. 1980. Children's responses to repetitive television commercials. *J Consum Res* 6:421–424.

*Gorn GJ, Goldberg ME. 1982. Behavioral evidence of the effects of televised food messages on children. *J Consum Res* 9:200–205.

*Gortmaker SL, Must A, Sobol AM, Peterson K, Colditz GA, Dietz WH. 1996. Television viewing as a cause of increasing obesity among children in the United States, 1986–1990. *Arch Pediatr Adolesc Med* 150(4):356–362.

*Gracey D, Stanley N, Burke V, Corti B, Beilin LJ. 1996. Nutritional knowledge, beliefs, and behaviours in teenage school students. *Health Ed Res* 11(2):187–204.

*Graf C, Koch B, Dordel S, Schindler-Marlow S, Icks A, Schuller A, Bjarnason-Wehrens B, Tokarski W, Predel HG. 2004. Physical activity, leisure habits and obesity in first-grade children. *Eur J Cardiovasc Prev Rehabil* 11(4):284–290.

*Gray A, Smith C. 2003. Fitness, dietary intake, and body mass index in urban Native American youth. *J Am Diet Assoc* 103(9):1187–1191.

*Greenberg BS, Brand JE. 1993. Television news and advertising in schools: The *Channel One* controversy. *J Commun* 43(1):143–151.

Grimm GC, Harnack L, Story M. 2004. Factors associated with soft drink consumption in school-aged children. *J Am Diet Assoc* 104(8):1244–1249.

*Grund A, Dilba B, Forberger K, Krause H, Siewers M, Rieckert H, Muller MJ. 2000. Relationships between physical activity, physical fitness, muscle strength and nutritional state in 5- to 11-year-old children. *Eur J Appl Physiol* 82(5-6):425–438.

*Guillaume M, Lapidus L, Bjorntorp P, Lambert A. 1997. Physical activity, obesity, and cardiovascular risk factors in children. The Belgian Luxembourg Child Study II. *Obes Res* 5(6):549–556.

Gunter B, Oates C, Blades M. 2005. *Advertising to Children on TV. Content, Impact, and Regulation.* Mahwah, NJ: Lawrence Erlbaum Associates.

*Halford JC, Gillespie J, Brown V, Pontin EE, Dovey TM. 2004. Effect of television advertisements for foods on food consumption in children. *Appetite* 42(2):221–225.

*Harrison K. 2005. Is 'fat free' good for me? A panel study of television viewing and children's nutritional knowledge and reasoning. *Health Commun* 17(2):117–132.

Harvey-Berino J, Hood V, Rourke J, Terrance T, Dorwaldt A, Secker-Walker R. 1997. Food preferences predict eating behavior of very young Mohawk children. *J Am Diet Assoc* 97(7):750–753.

Harwood EM, Erickson DJ, Fabian LE, Jones-Webb R, Slater S, Chaloupka FJ. 2003. Effects of communities, neighborhoods and stores on retail pricing and promotion of beer. *J Stud Alcohol* 64(5):720–726.

Hastings G, Stead M, McDermott L, Forsyth A, MacKintosh A, Rayner M, Godfrey C, Caraher M, Angus K. 2003. *Review of Research on the Effects of Food Promotion to Children.* Glasgow, UK: Center for Social Marketing, University of Strathclyde.

Hawkes C. 2002. Marketing activities of global soft drink and fast food companies in emerging markets: A review. In: Uusitalo U, ed. *Globalization, Diets, and Non-Communicable Diseases.* Geneva: World Health Organization.

Hawkes C. 2004. *Marketing Food to Children: The Global Regulatory Environment.* Geneva: World Health Organization.

*Hernandez B, Gortmaker SL, Colditz GA, Peterson KE, Laird NM, Parra-Cabrera S. 1999. Association of obesity with physical activity, television programs and other forms of video viewing among children in Mexico City. *Int J Obes Relat Metab Disord* 23(8): 845–854.

*Heslop LA, Ryans AB. 1980. A second look at children and the advertising of premiums. *J Consumer Res* 6(4):414–420.

*Hitchings E, Moynihan PJ. 1998. The relationship between television food advertisements recalled and actual foods consumed by children. *J Hum Nutr Diet* 11:511–517.

Holland P. 1986. Statistics and Causal Inference. *J Am Statistical Assoc* 81:945–970.

*Horn OK, Paradis G, Potvin L, Macaulay AC, Desrosiers S. 2001. Correlates and predictors of adiposity among Mohawk children. *Prev Med* 33(4):274–281.

*Hoy MG, Young CE, Mowen JC. 1986. Animated host-selling advertisements: Their impact on young children's recognition, attitudes, and behavior. *J Pub Policy Marketing* 5: 171–184.

*Isler L, Popper ET, Ward S. 1987. Children's purchase requests and parental responses: Results from a diary study. *J Advert Res* 27(5):28–39.

*Janz KF, Levy SM, Burns TL, Torner JC, Willing MC, Warren JJ. 2002. Fatness, physical activity, and television viewing in children during the adiposity rebound period: the Iowa Bone Development Study. *Prev Med* 35(6):563–571.

*Jeffrey DB, McLellarn RW, Fox DT. 1982. The development of children's eating habits: The role of television commercials. *Health Ed Q* 9(2 suppl 3):174–189.

John D. 1999. Consumer socialization of children: A retrospective look at twenty-five years of research. *J Consumer Res* 26(3):183–213.

*Kant AK, Graubard BI. 2003. Predictors of reported consumption of low-nutrient-density foods in a 24-h recall by 8–16 year old US children and adolescents. *Appetite* 41(2): 175–180.

*Katzmarzyk PT, Malina RM, Song TM, Bouchard C. 1998. Television viewing, physical activity, and health-related fitness of youth in the Quebec Family Study. *J Adolesc Health* 23(5):318–325.

*Kaur H, Choi WS, Mayo MS, Harris KJ. 2003. Duration of television watching is associated with increased body mass index. *J Pediatr* 143(4):506–511.

*Klein-Platat C, Oujaa M, Wagner A, Haan MC, Arveiler D, Schlienger JL, Simon C. 2005. Physical activity is inversely related to waist circumference in 12-y-old French adolescents. *Int J Obes Relat Metab Disord* 29(1):9–14.

Kline SL, Clinton BL. 1998. Developments in children's persuasive message practices. *Commun Ed* 47(April):120–136.

*Krassas GE, Tzotzas T, Tsametis C, Konstantinidis T. 2001. Determinants of body mass index in Greek children and adolescents. *J Pediatr Endocrinol Metab* 14(suppl 5): 1327–1333.

*Kunkel D. 1988. Children and host-selling television commercials. *Commun Res* 15(1): 71–92.

Kunkel D. 2001. Children and television advertising. In: Singer DG, Singer JL, eds. *Handbook of Children and the Media*. Thousand Oaks, CA: Sage Publications. Pp. 375–393.

Kunkel D, Wilcox BL, Cantor J, Palmer E, Linn S, Dowrick P. 2004. *Report of The APA Task Force on Advertising and Children. Section: Psychological Issues in the Increasing Commercialization of Childhood*. [Online]. Available at: http://www.apa.org/releases/childrenads.pdf [accessed September 3, 2004].

Kurdek LA, Rodgon MM. 1975. Perceptual, cognitive, and affective perspective taking in kindergarten through sixth-grade children. *Dev Psychol* 11(5):643–650.

*Levin S, Martin MW, Riner WF. 2004. TV viewing habits and body mass index among South Carolina Head Start children. *Ethn Dis* 14(3):336–339.

*Lewis MK, Hill AJ. 1998. Food advertising on British children's television: A content analysis and experimental study with nine-year olds. *Int J Obes Relat Metab Disord* 22(3): 206–214.

*Lin BH, Huang CL, French SA. 2004. Factors associated with women's and children's body mass indices by income status. *Int J Obes Relat Metab Disord* 28(4):536–542.

Linn MC, de Benedictis T, Delucchi K. 1982. Adolescent reasoning about advertisements: Preliminary investigations. *Child Dev* 53:1599–1613.

Livingstone S. 2004. Appendix 1. A commentary on the research evidence regarding the effects of food promotion on children. In: Office of Communications (Ofcom). *Childhood Obesity—Food Advertising in Context. Children's Food Choices, Parents' Understanding and Influence, and the Role of Food Promotion*. London, UK: Ofcom.

Livingstone S, Helsper E. 2004. Appendix 2. Advertising foods to children: Understanding promotion in the context of children's daily lives. In: Office of Communications (Ofcom). *Childhood Obesity—Food Advertising in Context. Children's Food Choices, Parents' Understanding and Influence, and the Role of Food Promotion*. London, UK: Ofcom.

*Locard E, Mamelle N, Billette A, Miginiac M, Munoz F, Rey S. 1992. Risk factors of obesity in a five year old population. Parental versus environmental factors. *Int J Obes Relat Metab Disord* 16(10):721–729.

*Macklin MC. 1990. The influence of model age on children's reactions to advertising stimuli. *Psychol Marketing* 7(4):295–310.

*Macklin MC. 1994. The effects of an advertising retrieval cue on young children's memory and brand evaluations. *Psychol Marketing* 11(3):291–311.

*Maffeis C, Talamini G, Tato L. 1998. Influence of diet, physical activity and parents' obesity on children's adiposity: A four-year longitudinal study. *Int J Obes Relat Metab Disord* 22(8):758–764.

*Manios Y, Yiannakouris N, Papoutsakis C, Moschonis G, Magkos F, Skenderi K, Zampelas A. 2004. Behavioral and physiological indices related to BMI in a cohort of primary schoolchildren in Greece. *Am J Hum Biol* 16(6):639–647.

*Matheson DM, Killen JD, Wang Y, Varady A, Robinson TN. 2004. Children's food consumption during television viewing. *Am J Clin Nutr* 79(6):1088–1094.

Matthews A, Cowburn G, Rayner M, Longfield J, Powell C. 2005. *The Marketing of Unhealthy Food to Children in Europe. A Report of Phase 1 of 'The Children, Obesity and Associated Avoidable Chronic Diseases' Project*. Brussels: European Heart Network.

*McMurray RG, Harrell JS, Deng S, Bradley CB, Cox LM, Bangdiwala SI. 2000. The influence of physical activity, socioeconomic status, and ethnicity on the weight status of adolescents. *Obes Res* 8(2):130–139.

*Miller JH, Busch P. 1979. Host selling vs. premium TV commercials: An experimental evaluation of their influence on children. *J Market Res* 16(3):323–332.

*Morton HN. 1990. A survey of the television viewing habits, food behaviours, and perception of food advertisements among south Australian year 8 high school students. *J Home Econ Assoc Australia* 22(2):34–36.

*Muller MJ, Koertzinger I, Mast M, Langnase K, Grund A. 1999. Physical activity and diet in 5 to 7 years old children. *Pub Health Nutr* 2(3A):443–444.

Murphy AS, Youatt JP, Hoerr SL, Sawyer CA, Andrews SL. 1995. Kindergarten students' food preferences are not consistent with their knowledge of the Dietary Guidelines. *J Am Diet Assoc* 95(2):219–223.

Neumark-Sztainer D, Wall M, Perry C, Story M. 2003. Correlates of fruit and vegetable intake among adolescents. Findings from Project EAT. *Prev Med* 37(3):198–208.

*Norton PA, Falciglia GA, Ricketts C. 2000. Motivational determinants of food preferences in adolescents and pre-adolescents. *Ecology Food Nutr* 39(3):169–182.

Oates C, Blades M, Gunter B. 2002. Children and television advertising: When do they understand persuasive intent? *J Consum Behav* 1(3):238–245.

*Obarzanek E, Schreiber GB, Crawford PB, Goldman SR, Barrier PM, Frederick MM, Lakatos E. 1994. Energy intake and physical activity in relation to indexes of body fat: The National Heart, Lung, and Blood Institute Growth and Health Study. *Am J Clin Nutr* 60(1):15–22.

Ofcom (Office of Communications). 2004. *Childhood Obesity—Food Advertising in Context. Children's Food Choices, Parents' Understanding and Influence, and the Role of Food Promotion.* London, UK: Ofcom.

*O'Loughlin J, Gray-Donald K, Paradis G, Meshefedjian G. 2000. One- and two-year predictors of excess weight gain among elementary schoolchildren in multiethnic, low-income, inner-city neighborhoods. *Am J Epidemiol* 152(8):739–746.

*Palmer EL, McDowell CN. 1981. Children's understanding of nutritional information presented in breakfast cereal commercials. *J Broadcasting* 25(3):295–301.

*Pate RR, Ross JG. 1987. Factors associated with health-related fitness. The National Children and Youth Fitness Study II. *J Physical Ed Recreat Dance* 58:93–95.

Pearl J. 2000. *Causality: Models, Reasoning, and Inference.* New York: Cambridge University Press.

*Peterson PE, Jeffrey DB, Bridgwater CA, Dawson B. 1984. How pronutrition television programming affects children's dietary habits. *Dev Psychol* 20(1):55–63.

Petticrew M. 2001. Systematic reviews from astronomy to zoology: Myths and misconceptions. *Br Med J* 322(7278):98–101.

*Pine KJ, Nash A. 2003. Barbie or Betty? Preschool children's preference for branded products and evidence for gender-linked differences. *Dev Behav Pediatr* 24(4):219–224.

*Proctor MH, Moore LL, Gao D, Cupples LA, Bradlee ML, Hood MY, Ellison RC. 2003. Television viewing and change in body fat from preschool to early adolescence: The Framingham Children's Study. *Int J Obes Relat Metab Disord* 27(7):827–833.

*Reid LN, Bearden WO, Teel JE. 1980. Family income, TV viewing and children's cereal ratings. *Journalism Q* 57(2):327–330.

*Reilly JJ, Armstrong J, Dorosty AR, Emmett PM, Ness A, Rogers I, Steer C, Sherriff A. 2005. Early life risk factors for obesity in childhood: Cohort study. *Br Med J* 330(7504): 1357–1364.

*Resnik A, Stern BL. 1977. Children's television advertising and brand choice: A laboratory experiment. *J Advertisng* 6:11–17.

*Ritchey N, Olson C. 1983. Relationships between family variables and children's preference for and consumption of sweet foods. *Ecology Food Nutr* 13:257–266.

Roberts DF, Foehr UG, Rideout V. 2005. *Generation M: Media in the Lives of 8–18 Year Olds.* Menlo Park, CA: Henry J. Kaiser Family Foundation.

Roberts P. 1983. Children and commercials: Issues, evidence, interventions. *Prevention Hum Services* 2:19–35.

Robertson TS, Rossiter JR. 1974. Children and commercial persuasion: An attribution theory analysis. *J Consumer Res* 1(1):13–20.

Robins JM. 1988. Confidence intervals for causal parameters. *Stat Med* 7(7):773–785.

*Robinson TN. 1999. Reducing children's television viewing to prevent obesity. A randomized controlled trial. *J Am Med Assoc* 282(16):1561–1567.

*Robinson TN, Killen JD. 1995. Ethnic and gender differences in the relationships between television viewing and obesity, physical activity, and dietary fat intake. *J Health Educ* 26(2):S91–S98.

*Robinson TN, Hammer LD, Killen JD, Kraemer HC, Wilson DM, Hayward C, Taylor CB. 1993. Does television viewing increase obesity and reduce physical activity? Cross-sectional and longitudinal analyses among adolescent girls. *Pediatrics* 91(2):273–280.

Rosenbaum PR. 2002. *Observational Studies.* 2nd ed. New York: Springer.

Ross H, Chaloupka FJ. 2003. The effect of cigarette prices on youth smoking. *Health Econ* 12(3):217–230.

*Ross RP, Campbell T, Huston-Stein A, Wright JC. 1981. Nutritional misinformation of children: A developmental and experimental analysis of the effects of televised food commercials. *J Appl Dev Psychol* 1:329–347.

Rubin D. 1974. Estimating causal effects of treatments in randomized and nonrandomized studies. *J Ed Psychol* 66:688–701.

Sardinha LB, Going SB, Teixeira PJ, Lohman TG. 1999. Receiver operating characteristic analysis of body mass index, triceps skinfold thickness, and arm girth for obesity screening in children and adolescents. *Am J Clin Nutr* 70(6):1090–1095.

Selman R. 1971. Taking another's perspective: Role taking development in early childhood. *Child Dev* 42:1721–1734.

*Shannon B, Peacock J, Brown MJ. 1991. Body fatness, television viewing and calorie-intake of a sample of Pennsylvania sixth grade children. *J Nutr Educ* 23(6):262–268.

*Sherwood NE, Story M, Neumark-Sztainer D, Adkins S, Davis M. 2003. Development and implementation of a visual card-sorting technique for assessing food and activity preferences and patterns in African American girls. *J Am Diet Assoc* 103(11):1473–1479.

*Signorielli N, Lears M. 1992. Television and children's conceptions of nutrition: Unhealthy messages. *Health Commun* 4(4):245–257.

*Signorielli N, Staples J. 1997. Television and children's conceptions of nutrition. *Health Commun* 9(4):289–301.

Sobel ME. 1996. An introduction to causal inference. *Sociol Methods Res* 24(3):353–379.

Spirtes P, Glymour CN, Scheines R. 2000. *Causation, Prediction, and Search.* 2nd ed. Cambridge, MA: MIT Press.

Spirtes P, Scheines R, Glymour C, Richardson T, Meek C. 2004. Causal inference. In: Kaplan D, ed. *The Sage Handbook of Quantitative Methodology in the Social Sciences.* Thousand Oaks, CA: Sage Publications. Pp. 445–475.

*Stettler N, Signer TM, Suter PM. 2004. Electronic games and environmental factors associated with childhood obesity in Switzerland. *Obes Res* 12(6):896–903.

*Stoneman Z, Brody GH. 1981. Peers as mediators of television food advertisements aimed at children. *Dev Psychol* 17(6):853–858.

*Stoneman Z, Brody GH. 1982. The indirect impact of child-oriented advertisements on mother–child interactions. *J Appl Dev Psychol* 2:369–376.

*Storey ML, Forshee RA, Weaver AR, Sansalone WR. 2003. Demographic and lifestyle factors associated with body mass index among children and adolescents. *Int J Food Sci Nutr* 54(6):491–503.

Story M, French SA, Resnick MD, Blum RW. 1995. Ethnic/racial and socioeconomic differences in dieting behaviors and body image perceptions in adolescents. *Int J Eat Disord* 18(2):173–179.

*Sugimori H, Yoshida K, Izuno T, Miyakawa M, Suka M, Sekine M, Yamagami T, Kagamimori S. 2004. Analysis of factors that influence body mass index from ages 3 to 6 years: A study based on the Toyama cohort study. *Pediatr Int* 46(3):302–310.

Swinburn BA, Caterson I, Seidell JC, James WP. 2004. Diet, nutrition and the prevention of excess weight gain and obesity. *Pub Health Nutr* 7(1A):123–146.

*Tanasescu M, Ferris AM, Himmelgreen DA, Rodriguez N, Perez-Escamilla R. 2000. Biobehavioral factors are associated with obesity in Puerto Rican children. *J Nutr* 130(7): 1734–1742.

*Taras HL, Sallis JF, Patterson TL, Nader PR, Nelson JA. 1989. Television's influence on children's diet and physical activity. *Dev Behav Pediatr* 10(4):176–180.

*Taras H, Zive M, Nader P, Berry CC, Hoy T, Boyd C. 2000. Television advertising and classes of food products consumed in a paediatric population. *Int J Ad* 19:487–493.

*Toyran M, Ozmert E, Yurdakok K. 2002. Television viewing and its effect on physical health of schoolage children. *Turk J Pediatr* 44(3):194–203.

*Tremblay MS, Willms JD. 2003. Is the Canadian childhood obesity epidemic related to physical inactivity? *Int J Obes Relat Metab Disord* 27(9):1100–1105.

*Trost SG, Kerr LM, Ward DS, Pate RR. 2001. Physical activity and determinants of physical activity in obese and non-obese children. *Int J Obes Relat Metab Disord* 25(6):822–829.

*Tucker LA. 1986. The relationship of television viewing to physical fitness and obesity. *Adolescence* 21(84):797–806.

U.S. Census Bureau. 2005. *Table 2: Annual Estimates of the Population by Selected Age Groups and Sex for the United States: April 1, 2000 to July 1, 2004 (NC-EST2004-02).* [Online]. Available at: http://www.census.gov/popest/national/asrh/NC-EST2004/NC-EST2004-02.xls [accessed October 21, 2005].

*Utter J, Neumark-Sztainer D, Jeffery R, Story M. 2003. Couch potatoes or French fries: Are sedentary behaviors associated with body mass index, physical activity, and dietary behaviors among adolescents? *J Am Diet Assoc* 103(10):1298–1305.

*Vandewater EA, Shim MS, Caplovitz AG. 2004. Linking obesity and activity level with children's television and video game use. *J Adolesc* 27(1):71–85.

*Wake M, Hesketh K, Waters E. 2003. Television, computer use and body mass index in Australian primary school children. *J Paediatr Child Health* 39(2):130–134.

Waller BJ, Cohen JE, Ferrence R, Bull S, Adlaf EM. 2003a. The early 1990s cigarette price decrease and trends in youth smoking in Ontario. *Can J Public Health* 94(1):31–35.

*Waller CE, Du S, Popkin BM. 2003b. Patterns of overweight, inactivity, and snacking in Chinese children. *Obes Res* 11(8):957–961.

Ward S, Wackman D. 1972. Television advertising and intrafamily influence: Children's purchase influence attempts and parental yielding. In: Rubinstein EA, Comstock GA, Murray JP, eds. *Television and Social Behavior, vol IV: Television in Day-to-Day Life: Patterns of Use.* Washington DC: National Institute of Mental Health. Pp. 516–525.

Ward S, Wackman DB, Wartella E. 1977. *How Children Learn to Buy: The Development of Consumer Information-Processing Skills.* Beverly Hills, CA: Sage Publications.

Wasserman L. 2004. *All of Statistics. A Concise Course in Statistical Inference.* New York: Springer.

Weiss DM, Sachs J. 1991. Persuasive strategies used by preschool children. *Discourse Processes* 14:55–72.

WHO and FAO (World Health Organization and Food and Agriculture Organization). 2003. *Diet, Nutrition, and the Prevention of Chronic Diseases.* WHO Technical Report Series No. 916. Geneva, Switzerland: WHO.

*Wolf AM, Gortmaker SL, Cheung L, Gray HM, Herzog DB, Colditz GA. 1993. Activity, inactivity, and obesity: Racial, ethnic, and age differences among schoolgirls. *Am J Public Health* 83(11):1625–1627.

*Wong ND, Hei TK, Qaqundah PY, Davidson DM, Bassin SL, Gold KV. 1992. Television viewing and pediatric hypercholesterolemia. *Pediatrics* 90(1):75–79.

*Woodward DR, Cumming FJ, Ball PJ, Williams HM, Hornsby H, Boon JA. 1997. Does television affect teenagers' food choices? *J Human Nutr Diet* 10:229–235.

*Yavas U, Abdul-Gader A. 1993. Impact of TV commercials on Saudi children's purchase behaviour. *Marketing Intelligence Planning* 11(2):37–43.

Young BM. 1990. *Television Advertising and Children.* Oxford, UK: Clarendon Press.

*Zive MM, Frank-Spohrer GC, Sallis JF, McKenzie TL, Elder JP, Berry CC, Broyles SL, Nader PR. 1998. Determinants of dietary intake in a sample of white and Mexican-American children. *J Am Diet Assoc* 98(11):1282–1289.

6

Public Policy Issues in Food and Beverage Marketing to Children and Youth*

INTRODUCTION

Public policies at the federal, state, and local levels are central to the promotion, protection, and enhancement of the diets and health of U.S. children and youth. Public policy and activities that shape dietary guidance, nutrition education, food labeling, regulation of food marketing, food services, and food production and distribution, are all important determinants of the nutritional environments of children and youth. This chapter begins with an overview of education and information-related policies, including dietary guidelines, nutrition education programs and campaigns, and food labeling to guide healthful choices for children, youth, and their families. It then reviews several of the policies related to the role of schools in children's diets, and follows with the description of the experience to date with social marketing campaigns to improve health-related behaviors. The chapter devotes substantial attention to legal considerations in regulation of advertising and marketing, including the constitutional protection of commercial free speech in the United States. The chapter also examines other potential legislative actions that may create industry incentives or support agricultural subsidies to produce and market more healthful foods, as well as taxation to reduce the demand for less healthful foods. The chapter con-

---

*Endnotes for Chapter 6 can be found on page 478–480 in Appendix G.

cludes with a review of the international policy environment for policies relevant to food and beverage marketing to children and youth.

EDUCATION AND INFORMATION PROGRAMS AND POLICIES

Numerous education and information programs and policies are sponsored by government at every level and in many venues. At the federal level, these efforts are anchored in the principles set out in the Dietary Guidelines for Americans, previously introduced in Chapter 2. This section describes several nutrition education and promotion efforts offered through the U.S. Department of Agriculture (USDA), Department of Education, and the Department of Health and Human Services (DHHS). It also describes federal nutrition labeling policies designed to facilitate healthful food choices at the point of purchase.

Dietary Guidelines for Americans and *MyPyramid*

The policy touchstones for federal education and information programs on nutrition are the Dietary Guidelines for Americans and its graphic representation, *MyPyramid*. Jointly developed by the DHHS and USDA, the Guidelines were designed to move federal nutrition policy to a more explicit focus on chronic disease prevention. They are now legislatively mandated, revised every 5 years, and draw from the recommendations of a nonfederal Dietary Guidelines Advisory Committee, constituted to review the most current scientific evidence and medical knowledge. The sixth edition of the Dietary Guidelines for Americans was released in 2005 and provide specific recommendations for physical activity, consumption of food groups, fats, carbohydrates, sodium and potassium, alcoholic beverages, and food safety (DHHS and USDA, 2005). Described in Chapter 2, the Dietary Guidelines provide the basis for the educational components of all 15 federal nutrition programs administered by the USDA. The USDA introduced the Food Guide Pyramid in 1992, in cooperation with the DHHS, as a graphic representation of selected Dietary Guidelines to help consumers better understand and select a balanced diet that promoted health and prevented chronic diseases. In 2005, the USDA took an additional step to personalize the guidance through an interactive food guidance system, *MyPyramid*, released to replace the existing Food Guide Pyramid (USDA, 2005f). *MyPyramid* offers recommendations tailored to the age and needs of the individual. This initiative includes an online educational tool to obtain information on an individual's diet quality, related nutrition messages, and links to nutrition information (USDA, 2005f). A child-friendly version of *MyPyramid* was released to reach children ages 6–11 years with targeted messages about the importance of healthful eating and physical activity, and an interactive computer game to apply these messages (USDA, 2005e; Chapter 2). *MyPyramid* is described in more detail in Chapter 2.

Federal Nutrition Education and Promotion Programs

A number of federal programs include important efforts to educate consumers of various ages about improving nutritional practices. Many target children, youth, or their care providers about the importance of a nutritionally balanced diet and regular physical activity. They can be found in agencies ranging from the DHHS and USDA, to the Departments of Education, Defense, and Interior. Some examples are described here.

The federal government's largest nutrition education work is sponsored by the USDA, which embeds education throughout its various food programs, and overall, devoted approximately $715 million to nutrition education and promotion in FY2005 (personal communication, Sid Clemens, Office of Budget and Program Analysis, USDA, November 1, 2005). The USDA Center for Nutrition Policy and Promotion is the focal point for leadership within the USDA on nutrition policy and dietary guidance in programs throughout the agency. The USDA administers 15 nutrition assistance programs that totaled $46 billion in 2004, including the Food Stamp Program (FSP), the Special Supplemental Program for Women, Infants, and Children (WIC), and the Child Nutrition Programs (USDA, 2005i). All have nutrition education components. For example, the WIC program, serving 8 million participants, provides both individualized and group nutrition education. Many state WIC agencies include nutrition education classes, fact sheets, newsletters, individual counseling guides, and lesson plans for schools (IOM, 2005c).

The FSP also offers a nutrition education component through selected states, although it operates on a smaller scale and reaches fewer low-income audiences than the WIC program. The activities of the Food Stamp Nutrition Education Program vary by state and provide practical nutrition information to low-income families and children. Some of these programs are developed and implemented in cooperative relationships between local FSP and state land-grant universities or nonprofit organizations (USDA, 2005d). The USDA Expanded Food and Nutrition Education Program (EFNEP) works collaboratively with county services and other local agencies to reach low-income families, children, and youth (Cooperative State Research, Education, and Extension Service, 2005). Additionally, the USDA Food and Nutrition Service has developed the Eat Smart, Play Hard™ Campaign that provides practical suggestions based on the Dietary Guidelines for Americans to motivate children and their care providers to eat healthful foods and be physically active every day (USDA, 2005a).

There are several federal partnerships that promote nutrition and healthful diets. In 2004, the USDA Food and Nutrition Service partnered with the Department of Education to launch the *HealthierUS* School Challenge that encourages schools and parents to promote healthful lifestyles for children. The school challenge is an extension of the DHHS-coordinated *Steps to a HealthierUS* initiative, and is designed to build upon and expand the USDA Team Nutrition program that provides schools with nutrition education materials for children and families; technical assistance for school food service directors, managers, and staff; and materials to build community-based support for healthful eating and physical activity. The initiative also enhances the USDA's effort to improve the nutritional quality of school food service through the School Meals Initiative that establishes nutritional requirements for federally reimbursed school meals (USDA, 2004a).

The national *Steps to a HealthierUS* initiative focuses on lowering the incidence of obesity and type 2 diabetes in disproportionately affected at-risk populations, especially African Americans, Hispanics/Latinos, American Indians, Alaska Natives, Asian Americans, and Pacific Islanders (DHHS, 2005e). As a component of this initiative, the DHHS partnered with the Ad Council to create *Small Step* (DHHS, 2005c) and *Small Step Kids!* (DHHS, 2005d), which target parents, teens, and children and include public service announcements (PSAs), a public relations campaign, a health care provider's toolkit, and consumer materials. The child-targeted component includes games and activities, television advertisements, and links to other materials.

The DHHS Centers for Disease Control and Prevention (CDC), through its Division of Nutrition and Physical Activity (DNPA), currently sponsors the national *5 a Day for Better Health* program (previously administered by the National Cancer Institute [NCI]) (DHHS, NIH, NCI, 2005), which encourages consumers to eat a variety of fruits and vegetables every day (CDC, 2005a). The DNPA also sponsors the national *Powerful Bones, Powerful Girls*™ Campaign to promote awareness of bone health (CDC, 2005e), and the national Youth Media Campaign, *VERB*™, a social marketing effort to encourage tweens, ages 9–13 years, to be physically active every day (CDC, 2005g). In 2005, CDC created a National Center for Health Marketing to provide national leadership in health marketing science and its application for public health improvement (CDC, 2005b).

Also in the DHHS, the National Institute of Child Health and Human Development (NICHD) sponsors the Milk Matters Calcium Education Campaign targeted to tweens and teens ages 11–15 years to promote the daily consumption of low-fat or fat-free milk along with calcium-rich foods (NIH, 2005a). Other institutes of the National Institutes of Health (NIH) also partner with national organizations and local communities in the national education initiative, *We Can!* (Ways to Enhance Children's Activity

& Nutrition), which is a collaboration among four institutes: the National Heart, Lung, Blood Institute; the National Institute of Diabetes and Digestive and Kidney Diseases; the NICHD; and the NCI. *We Can!* is designed to prevent obesity in children and tweens, ages 8–13 years, by providing resources and community-based programs to parents, caregivers, children, and youth that encourage healthful dietary choices, increasing physical activity, and reducing sedentary behaviors (NIH, 2005b).

Other nutrition-related education programs at the DHHS include work of the Surgeon General and of the Head Start program. The Surgeon General has launched an initiative called, Children and Healthy Choices—50 Schools in 50 States, taking him to at least one school in each of the 50 states, the District of Columbia, and Puerto Rico to discuss the benefits of healthy choices with school-aged students, including the importance of a nutritious diet and regular physical activity (DHHS, 2005b). In addition, through the Administration for Children and Families, the Head Start program grantees deliver a range of services related to comprehensive nutrition and nutrition education that foster healthy development and school readiness in low-income preschool children, ages 3–5 years, across the nation (DHHS, 2005a).

Nutrition Labeling

An important means of conveying nutrition information—and of educating about nutrition—is the food label itself. Both the USDA and DHHS have responsibilities for food labeling, but most of the food supply is overseen by the DHHS's Food and Drug Administration (FDA). Information on the food label is intended to enable consumers to compare products and make informed choices about foods and beverages that best meet their nutritional needs. Standards for the implementation of the labeling guidelines were established by the Nutrition Labeling and Education Act of 1990 (NLEA) (P.L. 101–535, 1990), which mandated that labeling information should be communicated so that consumers could readily observe and comprehend such information and understand its relative significance in the context of a total daily diet (FDA, 1993). The NLEA requires nutritional information to be displayed on nearly all packaged foods as to serving size, the number of servings per container, the total number of calories derived from any source and derived from fat, and the amount of total fat, saturated fat, cholesterol, sodium, total carbohydrates, complex carbohydrates, sugars, dietary fiber, total protein, vitamins A, C, E, and iron per serving (21 U.S.C. 343(q)(1)(A)-(E), 2004).

Full serve and quick serve restaurants are currently exempt from the general nutritional labeling standards and requirements of the NLEA (FDA, 1993; 21 U.S.C 343 (q)(5)(A)(i), 2004). However, they are required to meet some nutritional labeling requirements if they identify an item on their menu as "healthy" (Food Labeling Rule, 21 C.F.R. § 101.65, 2004).

The Nutrition Facts panel was developed to provide a set of consistently formatted information items that are displayed on food product labels to help consumers better understand how various foods could be integrated into a healthful diet (IOM, 2005a). Additionally, the NLEA mandates the FDA to enforce food manufacturers' compliance with established guidelines for nutrient and health claims on a product package indicating that a relationship exists between a food and a protection from a disease or health-related condition (IOM, 2003). The FDA's *Calories Count* campaign is an example of an initiative to encourage better industry use of the food label for nutrition education to consumers. In addition to the *Calories Count* campaign, the FDA is proposing to target the prominence of calories on the product label, address the issue of serving size for products that can be reasonably consumed at one time, update the reference amounts to reflect those that are customarily consumed, and examine approaches for recommending smaller portion sizes. These changes derive from extensive stakeholder consultation and consumer research that are intended to help consumers to purchase foods that may be integrated into a healthful diet and to highlight the importance of total calorie intake as a prime factor of concern (FDA, 2005c).

Research conducted by the FDA and the Food Marketing Institute has shown that about half of U.S. adult consumers use food labels when purchasing a food item for the first time (FMI, 1993, 2001), in particular to assess whether a product is high or low in a nutrient, especially fat, and to determine total calories (IOM, 2003). On the other hand, there is little evidence that the information on food labels, at least as currently structured, has a significant impact overall on eating or food purchasing behaviors (Wansink and Huckabee, 2005; Chapter 3). There are ample prospects for enhancing the utility of the label information as a guide to healthier food choices, including choices made by and for children and youth. In its report on preventing childhood obesity, the Institute of Medicine (IOM) recommended that the FDA and other groups conduct consumer research on the use of the nutrition label, on restaurant menu labeling, and on how to revise the Nutrition Facts panel to better design and display the total calorie content for products such as vending machine items, single-serve snack foods, and ready-to-eat (RTE) foods that are typically consumed at one eating occasion (FDA, 2005a,b; IOM, 2005a).

The importance of integrating and improving strategies for using the food label as an educational tool is underscored by the recent food company initiatives described in Chapter 4 to use proprietary logos or icons that communicate the nutritional qualities of their branded products. While representing an important step to draw attention to more nutritious products, the array of categories, icons, and other graphics, as well as the different standards employed by these companies may introduce some confusion, particularly for young consumers, thereby raising the need for developing and regulating standard and consistent approaches. The FDA has not yet fully explored its potential role for providing leadership and expertise to food companies in order to develop and enforce an industrywide rating system and graphic representation on food labels that is appealing to children and youth to convey the nutritional quality of foods and beverages.

Finding: A number of positive steps have been taken by the Food and Drug Administration to improve food and beverage labeling as a means of conveying helpful information to enable healthier choices, including exploration of ways to expand the provision of such information on menus and packaging in quick serve and full serve family restaurants. Still, the reach and effectiveness of such efforts—by FDA, industry, and the two together— are far short of what they could or should be to provide children, youth, and their parents with the information they need, using consistent standards and graphics that are easily understood and engaging.

NUTRITION IN SCHOOLS

Schools present an important means of reaching the nation's children and youth with programs and approaches for healthier diets. School-based interventions seek to provide the more than 50 million elementary and secondary students in the United States with nutrition education, healthy food services, food environments that support healthy choices, and family involvement for healthier lives. The CDC's Division of Adolescent and School Health collaborates with the Department of Education, the USDA, and other federal and state agencies to provide leadership on school health and environments, including nutrition education (with the CDC DNPA) and the nutrition environment of schools.

Nutrition Education in Schools

A beginning point for addressing nutrition in schools is the way it is engaged in the curriculum. A comprehensive survey conducted by the Department of Education among 1,000 school principals in a nationally representative sample of U.S. public elementary, secondary, and high schools showed that nearly all public schools provide nutrition education in the curriculum, primarily concentrated in the health curriculum (84 percent), science classes (72 percent), and school health programs (68 percent) (NCES, 1996). The topics covered in more than 90 percent of all schools surveyed included the relationship between diet and health, identifying and selecting healthful foods, nutrients and their food sources, the Dietary Guidelines for Americans, and the Food Guide Pyramid. The survey found that 97 percent of schools reported receiving nutrition materials for lesson plans from at least one source outside of the school, most often from a professional or trade association (87 percent) and the food industry (86 percent). Of the materials from sources outside the school, schools reported the highest classroom usage for those received from the food industry or commodity groups, professional or trade associations, the USDA, and state education agencies. The survey also found that the school curriculum focused primarily on increasing students' knowledge about nutrition, with less emphasis on influencing students' motivation, attitudes, and eating behaviors (NCES, 1996).

Although this survey showed that school-based nutrition education has been an active area, the quality of the nutritional messages received by students had not been evaluated (NCES, 1996). One evaluation found that behavior change in students is more likely if a comprehensive approach to nutrition education provides messages by multiple persons through a variety of communication channels, including the classroom, school cafeteria, home, and community (USDA, 2004b). Building on this insight, the Child Nutrition and WIC Reauthorization Act of 2004 (P.L. 108–265), requires school districts participating in the National School Lunch Program (NSLP) or School Breakfast Program (SBP) to establish a local school wellness policy by 2006 (USDA, 2004c,d). USDA's Team Nutrition has developed implementation guidance that emphasizes overall goals designed to promote student wellness for nutrition education, physical activity, and other school-based activities; nutrition guidelines for all foods available on every school campus during the school day; guidelines for reimbursable school meals that are no less restrictive than regulations and guidance issued by the USDA Secretary under the Child Nutrition Act; designation of a responsible person to ensure that school meals meet the local school wellness policy criteria; and broadly involving key stakeholders in the development of the school wellness policy (USDA, 2004c).

Media Literacy in Schools

Education in media literacy is another type of school-based educational initiative with potential to help improve the diets of children and youth. Media literacy refers to the ability of children and youth to develop an informed and critical understanding of the nature, technique, and impact of what they see, hear, and read in print, broadcast, and electronic media including books, newspapers, magazines, television, radio, movies, music, advertising, video games, the Internet, and emerging technologies. The goals of media literacy education are to (1) assist students to be critical media consumers, (2) enhance their media experiences, (3) reduce the potential adverse effects of media, and (4) promote potential benefits of media use (Brown, 2001; Buckingham, 2005; KFF, 2003). One of the challenges to developing a program of media literacy education lies in its timing across the kindergarten through 12 spectrum, as a result of the fact that most children ages 8 years and younger do not effectively comprehend the persuasive intent of marketing messages, and most children ages 4 years and younger cannot consistently discern between television advertising and informational content—hence training in the use of those powers of discernment requires that students have reached a certain developmental stage (Chapter 5).

The first large-scale experimental study measuring the acquisition of media literacy skills in the United States found that incorporating an analysis of media messages into the school curriculum could enhance the development of media literacy skills (Hobbs and Frost, 2003; KFF, 2003). On the other hand, since no national media literacy campaign has yet been implemented through a school-wide curriculum in the United States, systematic evaluations are not currently available to assess the effectiveness of a broad program of media literacy education, including whether media literacy skills learned in the classroom might transfer to media exposure outside the school setting. Additionally, there is a need to incorporate skills that move beyond the critical evaluation of television programming into emerging forms of media such as the Internet and mobile marketing; viral marketing; product placement across print, broadcast, electronic media and music; and marketing venues such as schools (Chapter 4).

School Food Services

Ensuring that school food services, including what is offered in school cafeterias, reflect sound nutrition principles, is key. These services are designed and implemented at the school district level, but many fall within the purview of the federal Child Nutrition Programs. The Child Nutrition Programs, which include the NSLP, SBP, Child and Adult Care Food Program (CACFP), and the Summer Food Programs, target low-income children enrolled in public and nonprofit private schools, child-care institutions, and summer recreation programs (Chapter 3). The NSLP is intended to provide nutritionally balanced, reduced-cost or free meals to nearly 29 million children enrolled in public and nonprivate schools every school day (USDA, 2005b). Nearly half (49 percent) of the school lunches served through the NSLP are provided free to students and another 10 percent are provided at a reduced price (USDA, 2005i). The program also provides reimbursements for snacks given to children in after-school educational and enrichment programs.

Participating school districts, independent schools, and institutions receive cash subsidies and donated commodities from the USDA in exchange for serving reduced-cost or free lunches to eligible children that adhere to the guidelines of the NSLP (7 C.F.R. § 210.10, 2005): no more than 30 percent of calories from fat, no more than 10 percent from saturated fat. Federal regulations also require that school lunches provide one-third of the Recommended Daily Allowance (RDA) for protein, calcium, iron, vitamin A, vitamin C, and calories. While the lunches at participating schools must satisfy these federal requirements, local school authorities have discretion to choose what specific foods are served and how they are prepared (USDA, 2005b). A U.S. General Accountability Office report found that dietary fat accounted for 34 percent of calories in the lunches served in the NSLP during the 1998–1999 school year. Although this represents a 4 percent decline from 1991–1992, it still exceeds the USDA-mandated 30 percent (GAO, 2003). The SBP has similar nutritional requirements as the NSLP. In addition to the limits on calories that must be obtained from fat, the SBP must provide children with one-fourth of the RDA for protein, calcium, iron, vitamin A, vitamin C, and calories (USDA, 2005c).

The CACFP is a federal nutrition program providing meals and snacks to low-income children in child-care centers, Head Start programs, family child-care homes, and after-school programs. Child- and adult-care providers who participate in CACFP are reimbursed at fixed rates for each meal and snack served. The USDA has established minimum requirements for the meals and snacks offered by participating child-care providers, but they are not required to meet specific nutrient-based standards such as those required for the NSLP and SBP (USDA, 2002a; Chapter 3).

USDA has also developed the Child Nutrition Labeling Program (CNLP) which is a voluntary technical assistance program designed to assist schools and institutions participating in the NSLP, SBP, and the CACFP by determining the contribution a commercial product makes toward the meal pattern requirements (USDA, 2005g). The CNLP requires an evaluation of product formulation of those products sold and used in these programs, and in order to carry the Child Nutrition label, it must be produced under federal inspection by the USDA (USDA, 2005g,h).

Promoting Fruits and Vegetables in Schools

Increasing the availability of fruits and vegetables to children in schools has been a priority and an important means of improving the quality of foods served in the federal nutrition assistance programs. Several pilot programs have been developed at the school, district, state, and federal level to explore strategies to increase fruit and vegetable consumption among students in schools. The 2002 Farm Bill provided $6 million for the Fruit and Vegetable Pilot Program to distribute fresh and dried fruits and fresh vegetables to elementary and secondary school children in four states and one Indian reservation (Branaman, 2003; ERS, 2002). One hundred schools in four states (e.g., Indiana, Iowa, Michigan, and Ohio) and seven schools in New Mexico's Zuni Indian Tribal Organization participated in the pilot during the 2002–2003 school year (Buzby et al., 2003). The participating schools could choose when and how to distribute the fresh produce to students, but the program requested that the fruits and vegetables be made available to students outside the regular school meal periods. Quantitative outcome data were not collected, but a qualitative process evaluation suggested satisfaction in many schools and food service staff (Buzby et al., 2003). The recent Child Nutrition and WIC Reauthorization Act expanded the program to four more states and two additional Indian reservations (Committee on Education and the Workforce, 2004; Chapter 3).

The Department of Defense's Fresh Produce Program has been working with schools in several states to provide fresh fruits and vegetables for the school meal programs. Schools have also begun to incorporate produce from school gardens (Morris and Zidenberg-Cherr, 2002), school salad bars (USDA, 2002b), and farmers' markets (Azuma and Fisher, 2001) into the school meals programs in an effort to increase student participation and specifically to increase their fruit and vegetable consumption. Evaluations of these programs are essential to assess the effects of these changes on students' dietary behaviors.

Competitive Foods in Schools

School food services, and special fruit and vegetable programs are not the only food and beverage products available to students. Recent attention has been drawn to other sources of "competitive" foods that are often high calorie and low nutrient and viewed as potentially displacing more healthful foods. Competitive foods include items sold through snack shops, student stores, vending machines, a la carte lines, and school fundraisers.

The sale of competitive foods in schools is often used to support academic or other types of programs. Public schools that are under financial pressure are more likely to make competitive foods available to their students through exclusive "pouring rights" contracts and snack food sales (Anderson and Butcher, 2005). Competitive foods are widely available in schools and generate substantial revenues, especially for middle and high schools throughout the United States (GAO, 2005). In 2003–2004, an estimated 30 percent of high schools generating the most revenue from competitive foods raised more than $125,000 per school (GAO, 2005; Chapter 3). An analysis of a sample of schools in 27 states and 11 large urban areas found that the 80 to 90 percent of secondary schools allowed students to purchase snack foods or beverages from vending machines, snack bars, cafeterias, or school stores (CDC, 2005c).

There are presently no comprehensive federal competitive foods standards to guide the type of products that are available and marketed in U.S. schools and other venues (e.g., child-care settings), and in the FY2005 Consolidated Appropriations, Congress directed the Institute of Medicine to conduct a study that is currently underway to develop comprehensive recommendations for appropriate nutritional standards for competitive foods (Hartwig, 2004; IOM, 2005b). Some foods have been designated foods of minimal nutritional value (FMNV) that are precluded from being sold in cafeterias or food service areas during school meal times. Under the competitive foods regulations, any non-FMNV sold outside of the NSLP may be sold anywhere on the school grounds at any time, although individual local-, district-, and state-level governments can establish their own local policies for competitive foods (USDA, 2002c). Because most competitive foods tend to be lower in nutritional value and higher in calories, fat, salt, and added sugars such as carbonated soft drinks, salty snacks, and candy (GAO, 2005), they are increasingly facing closer scrutiny at the state and local levels.

A variety of legislative initiatives pertaining to the availability, marketing, and sales of foods and beverages in schools have been enacted or proposed at the state, district, and local levels. Examples are numerous. Three large school districts in California (e.g., Berkeley, Oakland, and Los Angeles) have passed statutes for creating nutritional standards. The Los Angeles Unified School District enacted a comprehensive act mandating nonfood fundraising activities, prohibiting the sale of FMNV in vending machines after the end of the school day, and eliminating branded fast food product contracts (Vallianatos, 2005). Statewide legislation was passed in California that will enact several restrictions to raise nutritional standards for competitive foods sold in all California schools by 2007 and ban the sale of carbonated soft drinks on all California school campuses by 2009 (Gledhill, 2005).

Seattle Public Schools in Washington State have created guidelines for competitive food portion sizes and required that all beverages except milk be priced higher than water for the same serving size (Vallianatos, 2005). Other school districts have also enacted statutes calling for the prohibition of candy sales during the school day (Olympia, WA) and prohibiting certain foods during school hours and for fundraising (New York City Department of Education) (Vallianatos, 2005). The Flagstaff Unified School District in Arizona improved school meals in elementary and secondary schools by adding more fruit, vegetables, and salad bars (CSPI, 2003). In the Shrewsbury School District in Massachusetts, high schools now close their snack bars which sell candy and snacks of minimal nutritional value during the lunch periods (CSPI, 2005). More than half of the 10 largest school districts in the United States have policies that are more restrictive toward competitive foods in schools than federal and state regulations (GAO, 2004).

In 2003, only two states (e.g., Arkansas and California) enacted laws regarding vending machines in schools, the following year four additional states (e.g., Colorado, Louisiana, Tennessee, and Washington) followed with their own legislation (NCSL, 2005). As of mid-2005, 19 states had limited the availability of competitive foods beyond federal requirements, 11 states had nutritional standards for competitive foods in schools, and 6 states (e.g., Arkansas, Kentucky, South Carolina, South Dakota, Tennessee, and Texas) had established nutritional standards for school lunches, breakfasts, and snacks that are stricter than the USDA requirements (TFAH, 2005). Most include criteria for nutritional standards for foods and beverages sold on school grounds before, during, or after school hours, and regulations for vending machine sales, competitive foods sales, fundraising food sales, and availability of foods and beverages during school events or activities. Most also restrict the availability of competitive foods by either limiting their access during school meal periods, the entire day, or certain times. Examples of specific provisions include banning carbonated soft drinks from elementary or middle schools; requiring elementary schools to only serve food and beverages that meet certain nutrition standards; requiring middle schools to turn off vending machines not meeting nutritional standards until after the lunch period is over; banning the sales of FMNV in schools; and banning the sale of all competitive foods in elementary schools and limiting them in secondary schools (CSPI, 2003; TFAH, 2005).

In addition to statutes already passed, legislation is pending in other states that would address certain of these provisions, as well as others, including those such as setting standards for portion sizes of foods sold in schools; requiring healthy choices at all school activities; eliminating fried foods from cafeterias; requiring nutritional standards for foods sold at fundraising events; requiring school cafeterias to serve more fresh fruits and vegetables; and financially penalizing schools for each meal lost to competitive food sales.

The prospects for such legislation are uncertain, but the proposals reflect growing public sentiment for action. A Wall Street Journal Online and Harris Interactive (2005) poll found that 84 percent of respondents favored stricter public school regulation of less healthful foods and beverages. Many local school districts seem to prefer to develop their own policies, in advance of state or federal initiatives (RWJF, 2003), encouraged in part, not only by the public concern, but by findings from some sites that many schools have been able to implement healthful food and beverage policies without losing revenue (CSPI, 2005). Traditional competitive foods have been replaced with more healthful and low-calorie choices including water, low-fat milk, 100 percent fruit juices, soy drinks, cereal bars, and yogurt products (GAO, 2004; NCSL, 2005).

In an effort to educate and guide parents, school administrators, and legislators through the policy change and implementation process, the USDA has developed the *Changing the Scene—Improving the School Nutrition Environment* tool kit that seeks to help decision makers take a broad approach, addressing the entire school nutrition environment from a commitment to nutrition and physical activity, pleasant eating experiences, quality school meals, other healthful food options, nutrition education, and marketing the issue to the public (USDA, 2000). Other nonprofit groups have also developed resource materials for school districts and states to assist in the development of child nutrition legislation (CSPI, 2004).

Finding: National standards do not exist for the use or marketing of competitive foods and beverages in school settings or after-school venues such as child-care settings. Cooperative initiatives by the U.S. Department of Agriculture and the Department of Education has been limited in shaping policies and approaches related to healthier food and beverage promotion in schools.

SOCIAL MARKETING

One charge to the committee was assessing the lessons learned from various social marketing efforts that might be applied in the adoption of a social marketing strategy to improve the nutritional status of children and youth. Public health practitioners have used social marketing programs to influence a range of consumer behaviors such as reducing fat intake, increasing fruit and vegetable consumption, increasing physical activity, and promoting breastfeeding (Grier and Bryant, 2005; Ngo, 1993). To assist in this work, the committee commissioned a review of the application of the social marketing approach.

The Concepts

Social marketing applies commercial marketing concepts and techniques—exchange theory, audience segmentation, consumer orientation, competition, and an integrated marketing mix—to promote voluntary behavior change in specific groups or target audiences based on their sociodemographic, behavioral, and psychological characteristics (Grier and Bryant, 2005; Lefebvre, 1992; Lefebvre et al., 1995). The basic elements that influence a commercial marketing strategy include defining the target market, determining the marketing mix to meet the needs of the target market, and assessing the environmental factors that influence the marketing mix and the target market (Boone and Kurtz, 1998; Chapter 4). Social marketing engages a similar approach.

Media can be a key element to increase awareness and motivation in a social mobility effort (Contento et al., 1995), and PSAs offer a good example of the media component of social marketing. The concept of PSAs as a form of advertising was first introduced by The Advertising Council, the nonprofit arm of the advertising industry. The Advertising Council has developed a specific set of criteria for PSAs that has been used in social marketing promotional activities (Ad Council, 2005) including sponsorship by nonprofit organizations or government agencies; noncommercial, nonpartisan, and nondenominational; of national importance; and aired using donated advertising time and space.

But social marketing is more than a communication activity. Effective social marketing programs utilize multiple reinforcing communication channels along with public policy and environmental changes to influence consumer behaviors (Andreasen, 1995). The combined strategies used in social marketing programs include mass media campaigns, school-based interventions, community-based programs, interpersonal communications, and public policy. Such programs encompass a variety of activities including PSAs, posters, pamphlets, promotions, and legislation (Lefebvre et al.,1995).

The notion of "exchange" is important in social marketing, as it is in any marketing effort that seeks to offer a behavior or choice for something that offers more value. Social marketers recognize that consumers have tangible and intangible costs associated with changing behaviors, such as trade-offs with time and inconvenience, and understand that all individuals involved in an exchange must receive valued benefits in return for behavioral changes. Thus, an effective social marketing program identifies the motives or drivers of behavior, structures these motives as part of the benefits offered, and develops choices for consumers that provide a comparative advantage (Andreason, 2002).

Just as commercial marketers distinguish target audiences based on different features such as age and race/ethnicity, social marketing differentiates populations into subgroups, segments, or target audiences of individuals who share lifestyle orientations, desires, behaviors, and values that make them likely to respond similarly to public health interventions. Social marketers also distinguish target audiences based on current behaviors (e.g., dietary, physical activity, sedentary, smoking habits), future intentions, readiness to change, product or brand loyalty, and personal characteristics (Grier and Bryant, 2005).

Commercial marketers regard the competition as products and companies that strive to satisfy similar desires and needs among consumers in the marketplace (Chapter 4). Social marketers view competition as the behavioral options that compete with public health recommendations, messages, and services. A commercial marketing framework explores how the benefits of a product compare with the product of other companies; whereas a social marketing framework offers a trade-off that characterizes advantage in terms of better health, wellness, productivity, and psychological outlook (Grier and Bryant, 2005).

Marketing mix is another central concept used by social marketers that is adapted from commercial marketing practices. The four basic components of marketing—product, place, price, and promotion—are also central to the planning, implementation, and evaluation of a social marketing program. In a social marketing approach, the *product* is the array of benefits associated with the desired behavior for a target audience; *price* represents the cost or sacrifice exchanged for the promised benefit that balances the perceived or actual benefits to a consumer; *place* refers to the distribution of products and the location of sales and services where the target audience either performs the behavior or accesses programs or services; and *promotion*—often the most visible component of marketing—refers to the means of communicating and reinforcing messages (Grier and Bryant, 2005; Wong et al., 2004).

Commercial marketers devote considerable resources to conduct marketing research, as do social marketers. Conducting formative research is essential for a social marketing program to gain an accurate understanding of a target audience's desires, behaviors, values, and lifestyles. Of special interest are the perceptions of the products, costs, benefits, and other factors relevant to changing behaviors and maintaining those changes. Additionally, a sustained commitment to the ongoing monitoring and evaluation of a social marketing program is essential at the beginning of the planning process to allow for modifications and refinements over the course of the program (Grier and Bryant, 2005). Part of the research includes assessment of the broader environment. In particular, attention to the policy context within which a social marketing program functions is a critical component that may influence the success of a social marketing program (Dorfman et al., 2005; Kraak and Pelletier, 1998).

Social Marketing Programs That Promote
Physical Activity and Nutrition

Several nationwide social marketing programs seek to promote physical activity and nutrition. One such effort, the *5 a Day for Better Health* program, was begun in the late 1980s by the NCI to promote the consumption of at least five servings of fruits and vegetables daily. This program was adopted as the *5 a Day for Better Health Campaign* in California and expanded nationally as a large-scale partnership between NCI and the Produce for Better Health Foundation (PBH). Partners have included the produce industry, trade organizations, supermarkets and foodservice outlets, voluntary and nonprofit organizations, all 50 state health departments and other government agencies including the USDA and CDC (PBH, 2005a). An evaluation of the various stages of the California *5 a Day* program found incremental increases in the reported number of daily services of fruits and vegetables, which could also be attributed to secular trends (Foerster et al., 1995), demographic shifts (Stables et al., 2002), or other factors (Keihner et al., 2005). On the other hand, program advocates emphasize that the resources invested in the national and state *5 a Day for Better Health Campaign* (e.g., approximately $9.55 million in 2004 on communications for both the national and California programs) are far smaller than needed to counter the marketing expenditures promoting high-calorie and low-nutrient foods and beverages (CPEHN and Consumers Union, 2005; Chapter 4).

As an active partner of the *5 a Day for Better Health* campaign, the PBH also has developed a broader national action plan that proposes an integrated framework built on the *5 a Day* concept to use marketing, public health, and communication strategies at national, state, and local levels, as well as public–private partnerships, to encourage children and adult consumers to access, prepare, and consume fruits and vegetables to support health (PBH, 2005b). Anticipated PBH public–private partnerships include vendors, produce suppliers, and food retailers that have developed educational materials and programs for children and youth; food service providers, full serve and quick serve restaurants; and children's television programming (PBH, 2005b).

Social marketing programs have also been used to encourage consumers to reduce dietary fat intake. In the late 1980s, the nationwide social marketing program, Project LEAN (Low-Fat Eating for American Now), was designed by the Henry J. Kaiser Family Foundation to encourage consumers to reduce their dietary fat consumption to 30 percent of total calories. The program used PSAs, publicity, and point-of-purchase programs in restaurants, supermarkets, and school and worksite cafeterias to increase the availability and accessibility of low-fat foods, promote the awareness of total fat and calorie intake, and foster collaboration between national organizations (Samuels, 1993). It was the first national nutrition social marketing effort undertaken by an organization outside the government, but was not able to marshal large-scale support or implement the advertising concepts developed for the campaign, and could not demonstrate sustained changes in dietary habits.

More recently, the CDC's youth media campaign, *VERB™—It's What*

You Do, was launched nationally in 2002 as a 5-year, multiethnic social marketing campaign to increase and maintain physical activity among 21 million U.S. tweens ages 9–13 years (CDC, 2005g; Wong et al., 2004). Parents and other intermediaries that influence tweens (e.g., teachers, youth program leaders) have been secondary target audiences of the *VERB*™ campaign. An initial literature review and formative research was conducted on the target group to inform the program design. The research showed that tweens would respond positively to messages that promoted moderate physical activity in a socially inclusive environment and that emphasized self-efficacy, self-esteem, and belonging to their peer group (Potter et al., 2004).

VERB™ is an example of behavioral branding (e.g., brands that encourage a behavior or lifestyle), similar to the American Legacy Foundation's truth® campaign (Evans et al., 2005b). The relationship between a brand and a consumer can be strong and long-lasting, with brands serving as symbolic instruments that allow groups of individuals to project a specific self-image (Evans et al., 2005b; Keller, 1998; Chapter 4). The developers of the *VERB*™ campaign partnered with advertising agencies experienced in youth marketing to create a recognizable brand awareness that encouraged children to associate *VERB*™ with physical activity. The primary goal during the first year of promoting the campaign was brand awareness, and all forms of media (e.g., print, broadcast and cable, electronic) were used to reach tweens of various racial/ethnic groups (Wong et al., 2004).

VERB™ expanded its promotional activities to enhance its reach. In 2005, through this campaign, the CDC launched a marketing strategy to connect tweens with places and events in their local areas where they can engage in various physical activities during the summer (CDC, 2005f). The campaign features television spots and celebrity promotions for the campaign website where tweens can participate in online games, monthly contests, and athlete trivia. The *VERB*™ campaign also uses the newer mobile marketing strategies (Chapter 4) to reach tweens ages 13 years and older to encourage them to sign-up to receive text messages about activity tours sponsored by the campaign near their cities.

Evaluation of the *VERB*™ campaign is still in progress, although preliminary tracking suggests positive results in protecting against declining activity levels. Those who saw the *VERB*™ campaign messages had a higher level of awareness and maintained the same levels of physical activity in 2003 that they had in 2002. Attitudes and behaviors toward physical activity changed modestly over the period of the first-year evaluation, with more positive attitude changes than behavioral improvement (Huhman et al., 2005).

Social Marketing Programs to Reduce
Youth Tobacco and Drug Use

Social marketing programs have also been used by the federal government and private groups over the past two decades to influence youth behaviors to reduce youth tobacco, underage alcohol consumption, and illicit drug use (IOM, 2005a). In the alcohol arena, youth are exposed to a variety of advertisements and other forms of marketing that promote alcohol consumption (NRC and IOM, 2003). Social marketing campaigns targeted to youth to reduce the rates of underage drinking have shown some positive results. For example, one study found that a social marketing campaign focused on correcting perceived social norms about drinking on a college campus among students reduced students' drinking rates (Mattern and Neighbors, 2004).

Better studied efforts may be found in those related to reducing youth drug use. The Partnership for a Drug-free America is a coalition of communication, health, medical, and educational professionals that has received donated media time valued at more than $3 billion to support antidrug advertisements that are positioned to air during large-audience viewing prime-time television (PDFA, 2005). Similarly, The National Youth Anti-Drug Media Campaign, sponsored by the Office of National Drug Control Policy, has sought to focus youth attention on active alternatives to using illicit drugs, alcohol, and tobacco (ONDCP, 2005). Evaluations of the $1 billion campaign (ONDCP, 2003) from 1999–2001 reported that while there was some effect on parental behavior, there was limited ability to attribute declines in youth drug use to the advertisements (NIDA, 2002). The most recent evaluation of the campaign in 2003 did not show a reduction in youth marijuana consumption (Hornik et al., 2003).

A particularly interesting example of the social marketing approach to youth behavior change can be found in the truth® campaign of the American Legacy Foundation, an effort to use branding to achieve a social good (similar to the *VERB*™ campaign). In 2000, the American Legacy Foundation launched truth®—a national, multimedia tobacco control social marketing campaign targeting youth, ages 12–17 years, to discourage tobacco use (Farrelly et al., 2005). The truth® brand represents an aspirational antismoking brand for teens that builds a positive image of youth as nonsmokers, cool and edgy, and rebellious against the tobacco industry. The truth® brand is a component of the social marketing campaign that encourages a set of behavioral objectives including encouraging youth to develop positive beliefs about not smoking by developing a brand that competes with cigarette brands; establishing high levels of brand awareness and brand recognition and value for the truth® brand; encouraging youth to adopt these positive beliefs and reduce the likelihood of smoking; and encouraging youth to adopt and pass on values of the truth® brand to their peers (Evans et al., 2005b).

The messages of the truth® campaign describe the tobacco industry's intentional attempts to market a harmful product to teens and its denial of the addictive and unhealthful effects of cigarettes, and were designed to empower youth to take action by joining the statewide youth antitobacco group (Niederdeppe et al., 2004). The campaign employed several activities, including a variety of television PSAs, billboards, print advertisements, and posters. An evaluation of the truth® brand has demonstrated that brand recognition and value may be a mediator for the relationship between the truth® campaign exposure and intermediate outcomes (e.g., antitobacco commitment) associated with reduced smoking (Evans et al., 2005b). Field marketing has been identified as a necessary component to enhance relevance of the truth® campaign to youth (Eisenberg et al., 2004). Two separate evaluations of the campaign suggest that it has contributed to a decline in youth tobacco use in Florida (Niederdeppe et al., 2004), and that it also has accounted for a significant portion of the recent national decline in youth smoking prevalence rates among students in grades 8, 10, and 12, which declined from 25.3 percent to 18 percent between 1999–2002 (Farrelly et al., 2005).

Challenges and Opportunities for Social Marketing Programs

Experience to date suggests that, in the near term, it is easier to create awareness in a social marketing campaign than it is to impact the attitudes and behaviors. Attitude changes may require sustained efforts over months and behavioral changes on a significant scale will take even longer. Maintaining those behavioral changes is an additional challenge, a lesson especially applicable to eating and physical activity, which are complex behaviors. An evaluation of populationwide communication initiatives on health matters has shown that in general, attitude and behavioral changes may occur more quickly if campaigns have the following characteristics: exposure to the campaign materials is high; messages are disseminated through multiple channels; campaign content is based on a valid change theory; the campaign conveys new information; the behavior is easy to perform; the target audience has opportunities to perform the behavior; services are available to support the new behavior; and family, friends, and social networks support the behavior (CDC, 2005d).

The complexity inherent in any effort that seeks at once to address the multiple factors that influence health, while striking a balance between efforts directed at the individual and the social-environmental context in which people live, requires very careful planning. Like commercial marketing, it is clear that social marketing efforts need to be based on insightful formative research. Many programs or campaigns have claimed to use social marketing principles, but have lacked formative research, planning, and evaluation to effectively launch and sustain a successful social marketing program. To facilitate the development of the *VERB*™ campaign, and to provide direction for its evaluation, the CDC used both consumer research and a logic model that linked expected program inputs and activities with anticipated program outcomes and benefits (Huhman et al., 2004). This research is necessary not only for the design of an effective media advocacy and communication component but for careful design of the other related change agents in the policy, legal, and regulatory environments (Andreasen, 2002; Dorfman et al., 2005; Wallack et al., 1993).

The character of social marketing efforts varies with the nature of the target change. The more complex are the changes sought, the broader the environmental scope that must be engaged. For example, a community-based campaign—the *1% or Less* campaign—was successful in using paid advertising and community education to encourage a shift from higher-fat to low-fat milk (Wootan et al., 2005), but efforts targeting the multiple behaviors and choices necessary to address this complex set of factors associated with childhood obesity must be layered with multiple strategies, engaging a broader environment.

Partnerships can be a key resource in these complicated circumstances, as reflected in the work of PBH (2005b), and national and state WIC program efforts (IOM, 2005c; Social Marketing Institute, 2005), which encouraged partners at the community level to provide the infrastructure necessary to manage complex community and regional activities. Accordingly, community involvement is key in program design for efforts whose success depends on change at the community level (Backer and Rogers, 1993). This is particularly true for the design of efforts to reach racial/ethnic minority audiences whose values, world views, orientations, and priorities must be identified and engaged throughout the planning process (Williams and Kumanyika, 2002).

A central challenge to large-scale social marketing efforts is discerning their impact. The reach and results of these campaigns are often diminished by ongoing secular trends (Hornick et al., 2003). Programs whose impact were likely important, but which were difficult to identify because of both the complexities of the interactions and the background of secular change, include some of the large-scale cardiovascular prevention trials of the 1970s and 1980s, and several large-scale multifactorial interventions for youth (Killen et al., 1988; Perry and Silvis, 1987). The challenge of crafting a reliable evaluation for these efforts may be even more difficult than designing the intervention itself.

Finding: Evidence for the effectiveness of social marketing programs to promote healthful behaviors is promising but mixed. Programs with the most positive results have had higher funding, been more sustained, been shaped by formative research, deployed an integrated marketing approach, and used ongoing monitoring and evaluation. These characteristics are the likely requirements for achievement of successful social marketing programs to improve the diets of children and youth.

LEGAL REGULATION OF ADVERTISING AND MARKETING

Implicit in the question of whether food and beverage marketing influences the health behaviors and outcomes of children and youth is the question of whether advertising should be legally regulated. Indeed, such proposals have been formally advanced here and abroad. Because of the prominence and complexity of this matter, the committee undertook a detailed analysis of the issues, precedents, and considerations. Typical to such analyses, the review is extensively documented in endnotes that can be found in Appendix G.

Public support for regulation of food and beverage advertising is mixed, but may be increasing. A Princeton Survey in 2004 found that 37 percent of parents favored restricting "junk food" advertisements during children's television shows, but 56 percent opposed such restrictions (Rideout, 2004). A national survey by RTI International in 2005 found that 57 percent of respondents believed that watching two or more hours of television daily contributed substantially to childhood obesity, with 91 percent believing that parents bore "a lot" of responsibility, followed by television advertisers at 45 percent (Evans et al., 2005a). A Wall Street Journal Online and Harris Interactive Internet Poll conducted in 2005 reported that 68 percent of those surveyed believed that government should be able to take companies to court if they mislead children and their parents about the nutritional value of the foods they sell, and 55 percent believed that the government should take a more active role in regulating the types of marketing and advertising practices that the food industry directs toward children (The Wall Street Journal Online and Harris Interactive, 2005).

From an historical perspective, legal regulation in the United States must be understood against the background of the common law, created by courts in the course of deciding litigated cases. Persons injured by consumer products could traditionally sue at common law for redress of injury or for compensation for the violation of contractual obligations. As a consequence of this history, litigation in the food domain has traditionally been used to protect those who have been harmed by food products. Common law standards that governed such lawsuits are now typically supplemented by explicit statutes. Litigation proceeds based upon the distinct standards of the 50 states, which are in a process of continuous evolution.

The private right of citizens to take legal action has played an instrumental role in protecting consumers from harmful practices and products in the United States. By compensating injured consumers, litigation not only raises public awareness about an issue or concern that may be detrimental to public health or society, it also creates incentives for an industry to engage in voluntary self-regulation and to limit or prevent harmful practices to consumers (Daynard et al., 2004).

The environment in which consumers' choices are shaped and informed is an important influence on their diet and health. But efforts to regulate the marketing of commercial products and services can be highly controversial. The constitutional policy of the First Amendment is that truthful and non-misleading advertising serves the public good by promoting informed decision making, and that truthful advertising also stimulates healthy competition that encourages industry innovation (Zywicki et al., 2004). Like all speech, advertising may nevertheless at times be regulated, especially if it is misleading or untruthful. Advertising to children raises special issues because they are too young to be regarded as fully autonomous decision-makers. There is cause for concern if advertising encourages children and youth to adopt eating behaviors that may have lifelong adverse effects on their health (Yach et al., 2005).

Legal Regulation of Food

Plaintiffs seeking redress for injuries caused by food products can allege that a defendant has negligently prepared or served food (*Clime* v. *Dewey Beach Enterprises, Inc.*, 1993); that a defendant has served food that is unreasonably dangerous, defective, or is otherwise in violation of an implied warranty of sale that food will be fit for the ordinary purposes for which it is served (*Cain* v. *Sheraton Perimeter Park South Hotel*, 1991); or that a defendant has engaged in deceptive or fraudulent advertising regarding food (*People* v. *Block & Kleaver, Inc.*, 1980). Because all such lawsuits tend to turn on the customary and reasonable expectations of consumers, they are awkward vehicles for legal efforts to regulate high-calorie and low-nutrient foods and beverages that contribute to obesity. A federal district court recently observed in rejecting claims brought by two obese adolescents that the contents of McDonald's Corporation products rendered them inherently dangerous:

> "It is well-known that fast food in general, and McDonald's products in particular, contain high levels of cholesterol, fat, salt, and sugar, and that such attributes are bad for one. . . . If a person knows or should know that eating copious orders of supersized McDonald's products is unhealthy

and may result in weight gain (and its concomitant problems) because of the high levels of cholesterol, fat, salt and sugar, it is not the place of the law to protect them from their own excesses" (*Pelman* v. *McDonald's Corporation*, 2003).[1]

Even the possibility that such litigation might develop, however, prompted tort reform legislation—the Personal Responsibility in Food Consumption Act (H.R. 339, 108th Congress, 1st Session, 2004)—still under consideration in Congress (H.R. 554, 109th Congress, 1st Session, 2005). The goal of the bill is "[t]o prevent legislative and regulatory functions from being usurped by civil liability actions brought or continued against food manufacturers, marketers, distributors, advertisers, sellers, and trade associations for claims of injury relating to a person's weight gain, obesity, or any health condition associated with weight gain or obesity." The bill sought "to prevent frivolous lawsuits against the manufacturers, distributors, or sellers of food or non-alcoholic beverage products that comply with applicable statutory and regulatory requirements." In effect, the bill seeks to exclude normal litigation as a means for legally regulating food to ameliorate harms associated with obesity. More than 19 states have considered or are considering similar tort reform bills for obesity-related claims (Daynard et al., 2004; TFAH, 2005). Louisiana, which has one of the highest adult overweight and obesity prevalence rates in the United States (CDC, 2002), is one state that has passed legislation to protect restaurants from obesity-related lawsuits (Daynard et al., 2004).

Legal Regulation of Advertising and Marketing

The legal regulation of food is frequently directed not merely at defects or dangers in the food itself, but also at the ways in which food is marketed. Common law and related statutory causes of actions have traditionally provided redress for harms caused by the fraudulent selling of food such as misbranded meat (*United States* v. *Jorgensen*, 1998), misleading or deceptive advertising related to food (*National Bakers Services, Inc.* v. *FTC*, 1964), and failure to warn with regard to dangerous food. The precise legal standards vary in the 50 states, and also change over time.

The regulation of consumer advertising is a central task of the Federal Trade Commission (FTC). The FTC is authorized to regulate "unfair or deceptive acts or practices in or affecting commerce" (15 U.S.C. § 45(a)(1), 2002),[2] and in particular, any "false advertisement . . . in or having an effect upon commerce, by any means, for the purpose of inducing, or which is likely to induce, directly or indirectly the purchase of food . . . ." (15 U.S.C. § 52(a)(1), 2002).[3] "[A]n advertisement is deceptive under the Act if it is likely to mislead consumers, acting reasonably under the circumstances, in a material respect. . . . In implementing this standard, the FTC examines the overall net impression of an advertisement and engages in a 3-part inquiry: (1) What claims are conveyed in an advertisement? (2) Are the claims false or misleading? (3) Are the claims material to prospective consumers" (*Kraft, Inc.* v. *FTC*, 1992)? The FTC regulates unfair and deceptive advertisements for food products (see, e.g., Nestlé Food Company, 1992; The Isaly Klondike Company, 1993).[4] Unlike courts, which are empowered only to resolve particular controversies, the FTC can promulgate general rules defining unfair, misleading, or false advertising (16 C.F.R. § 410.1, 2005; 16 C.F.R. § 239.1–5, 2005). In determining the acceptability of advertising to children, the law—in both its judicial and administrative manifestations—recognizes the special status and cognitive limitations of children. Advertisements that are acceptable if addressed to an adult, might be deceptive, unfair, or misleading when directed to a child (*Bunch* v. *Hoffinger Industries, Inc.*, 2004; *Swix* v. *Daisy Manufacturing Company*, 2004).[5] When an act or a practice is targeted to a specific audience such as children, the FTC will determine whether it is unfair or deceptive by reference to its effect on a reasonable member of that group (Federal Trade Commission Unfairness Policy Statement, appended to *International Harvester Company*, 104 F.T.C. 949, 1984). The FTC thus evaluates the legality of advertisements or sales practices directed to children in terms of how they are perceived by an ordinary child. The FTC has required those who sought to use television commercials containing characters such as Santa Clause or the Easter Bunny to promote 1-900 telephone numbers allowing children to speak with the fictional characters and to win prizes, to disclose a range of relevant information "in a manner understandable to children" (see *Audio Communications, Inc.*, 114 F.T.C. 414, 1991; *Phone Programs, Inc.*, 115 F.T.C. 977, 1992). Congress followed up on the FTC's efforts in this area by enacting the Telephone Disclosure and Dispute Resolution Act (P.L. 102–556, 106, 1992; codified at 15 U.S.C. § 5701 et seq., 2004), which, among other requirements, mandated that the FTC promulgate rules which prohibited marketers from directing advertisements for pay-per-call services at children under the age of 12 years, unless the service was for a *bona fide* educational service (15 U.S.C. § 5711(a)(1)(d), 2002).

In 1978 the FTC sought commentary on a proposed rule that would ban television advertisements addressed to children too young to understand the selling purpose of advertising and also ban television advertisements for food products posing the most serious dental health risks which are directed to, or seen by, audiences with a significant proportion of older children (Ratner et al., 1978). The proposed rulemaking, known as "kid-vid," proved intensely controversial (Beales, 2004), evoking criticism from

Congress (FTC Improvements Act of 1980, P.L. 96–252, 1980),[6] and resulted in a 1981 FTC staff recommendation that the FTC terminate the proposed rulemaking (Elliott et al., 1981).

There is an important legal distinction between regulations of food and regulations of advertising for food. The former poses few constitutional questions, whereas the latter directly raises issues of freedom of expression. Although the Supreme Court had held in 1942 that "the Constitution imposes no . . . restraint on government" regulation of "purely commercial advertising," (*Valentine* v. *Chrestensen*, 1942), it reversed course in 1976 (*Virginia State Board of Pharmacy* v. *Virginia Citizens Consumer Council, Inc.*, 1976) and created what is now known as "commercial speech doctrine," a complex web of rules restricting government regulations of private advertising. The precise nature of these rules remains contested and complex, but the doctrine which the Court uses most frequently to resolve constitutional issues of commercial speech is the *Central Hudson* test:

> In commercial speech cases, then, a four-part analysis has developed. At the outset, we must determine whether the expression is protected by the First Amendment. For commercial speech to come within that provision, it at least must concern lawful activity and not be misleading. Next, we ask whether the asserted governmental interest is substantial. If both inquiries yield positive answers, we must determine whether the regulation directly advances the governmental interest asserted, and whether it is not more extensive than is necessary to serve that interest (*Central Hudson Gas & Electric Corporation* v. *Public Service Commission*, 1980).[7]

Under the *Central Hudson* test, government can regulate advertisements which are misleading. There is some suggestion in the case law that advertisements that are merely potentially misleading, as distinct from inherently misleading, may not be prohibited altogether, but must instead be subject to milder correctives, such as mandatory disclosure requirements designed to ameliorate potential deception (*Peel* v. *Attorney Registration and Disciplinary Commission*, 1990).[8] Because "[t]he determination whether an advertisement is misleading requires consideration of the legal sophistication of its audience" (*Bates* v. *State Bar of Arizona*, 1977), it is likely that advertisements addressed to children may be deemed misleading even if they would not be if addressed to adults (*FTC* v. *R. F. Keppel & Brothers, Inc.*, 1934).[9]

The *Central Hudson* test imposes constitutional restraints on government efforts to restrict truthful, non-misleading advertisements in order to achieve desirable policy objectives like preventing smoking by children (*Lorillard Tobacco Company* v. *Reilly*, 2001) or promoting energy conservation (*Central Hudson Gas & Electric Corporation* v. *Public Service Commission*, 1980). Government regulations must directly advance a substantial state interest in a manner that is not more "extensive than is necessary." It is typically not difficult to demonstrate that well-designed regulation directly advances the interests it is designed to serve. Although the government "'must demonstrate that the harms it recites are real and that its restriction will in fact alleviate them to a material degree,'" (*Greater New Orleans Broadcasting Association* v. *United States*, 1999), the Supreme Court has generally proved receptive to the practical "theory that product advertising stimulates demand for products, while suppressed advertising may have the opposite effect" (*Lorillard Tobacco Company* v. *Reilley*, 2001).[10]

In recent years, however, the Supreme Court has tended to interpret the final prong of the *Central Hudson* test with increasing severity. It has used the "no more extensive than is necessary" requirement to strike down many government efforts to regulate truthful, non-misleading advertising (*Lorillard Tobacco Company* v. *Reilly*, 2001; *Thompson* v. *Western States Medical Center*, 2002). The Court has not been entirely consistent in its interpretation of this requirement. Although, on the one hand, the Court has "made it clear that 'the least restrictive means' is not the standard" and that case law instead requires merely "a reasonable 'fit between the legislature's ends and the means chosen to accomplish those ends'" (*Lorillard Tobacco Company* v. *Reilly*, 2001),[11] the Court has also, on the other hand, held "that if the Government could achieve its interests in a manner that does not restrict speech, or that restricts less speech, the Government must do so" (*Thompson* v. *Western States Medical Center*, 2002). What is clear is that a majority of the Court has grown decidedly unreceptive to the idea that the state can prohibit "the dissemination of truthful commercial information in order to prevent members of the public from making bad decisions with the information" (*Thompson* v. *Western States Medical Center*, 2002, at 374–375).

Because the focus of the Court's commercial speech doctrine has been to preserve the flow of accurate information to consumers (*First National Bank of Boston* v. *Bellotti*, 1978),[12] the Court has been somewhat more tolerant of regulations regarding the use of trademarks. It has regarded trademarks as "a form of commercial speech that has no intrinsic meaning" (*Friedman* v. *Rogers*, 1979), and hence it has concluded that the use of trademarks in advertising offers "significant possibility that trade names will be used to mislead the public." Efforts to restrict the use of trademarks must still survive scrutiny under *Central Hudson* (*Bad Frog Brewery, Inc.* v. *New York State Liquor Authority*, 1998; *Transportation Alternatives, Inc.* v. *City of New York*, 2002), but constitutional review will take account of the kind and quality of information conveyed by marks and images, as well as the high potential for marks and images to mislead.

The extent to which *Central Hudson* will govern restrictions on marketing as well as restrictions on advertising is not clear. In *Hoffman Estates*

v. *Flipside*, the Court considered a village ordinance that made it illegal for any person to "sell any items, effect, paraphernalia, accessory or thing which is designed or marketed for use with illegal cannabis or drugs" without first obtaining a license from the government (*Hoffman Estates* v. *Flipside, Hoffman Estates, Inc.*, 1982). Despite the fact that the restrictions of the ordinance were triggered because of "the presence of drug-related designs, logos, or slogans on paraphernalia," the Court ruled that "the village does not restrict speech as such, but simply regulates the commercial marketing of items that the labels reveal may be used for an illicit purpose." The Court added that "insofar as any *commercial* speech interest is implicated here, it is only the attenuated interest in displaying and marketing merchandise in the manner that the retailer desires. We doubt that the village's restriction on the manner of marketing appreciably limits Flipside's communication of information."

In *Lorillard Tobacco Company* v. *Reilly* (2001) the Court upheld against the First Amendment challenge a Massachusetts law that required retailers to place all tobacco products behind a counter and that prohibited retailers from permitting customers to handle tobacco products before they had contact with a salesperson. The Court held that even "[a]ssuming that petitioners have a cognizable speech interest in a particular means of displaying their products," the statute survived First Amendment scrutiny because it sought "to regulate the placement of tobacco products for reasons unrelated to the communication of ideas."

These decisions suggest that the line between regulating advertising and regulating the marketing of products is quite unclear. The Court has intimated that the latter may be subject to different and more lenient forms of constitutional scrutiny than the former, even if marketing regulations are triggered by communicative content. Yet lower courts have applied the *Central Hudson* test to restrictions on marketing that include telemarketing (*Mainstream Marketing Services, Inc.* v. *FTC*, 2004), "winback" marketing (*Southwestern Bell Telephone, L.P.* v. *Moline*, 2004), and the use of consumer information in marketing (*Trans Union, LLC* v. *FTC*, 2002).

The *Central Hudson* test governs regulations of advertising that apply to the general public. It is probable that the test will not pertain if government wishes to regulate advertising within specific and limited institutional contexts, like prisons or schools, in which the state exercises more comprehensive managerial control. The Court has held that in such environments state regulations of speech should be treated with special and considerable deference (*Burbridge* v. *Sampson*, 1999; *Hazelwood School District* v. *Kuhlmeier*, 1988; *Jones* v. *N.C. Prisoners' Labor Union, Inc.*, 1977; *Thornburgh* v. *Abbott*, 1988; *Turner* v. *Safley*, 1987; *Williams* v. *Spencer*, 1980).

Because "there is a compelling interest in protecting the physical and psychological well-being of minors" (*Sable Communications, Inc.* v. *FCC,* 1989) special constitutional rules may also apply to the regulation of advertising addressed to children. Although children retain First Amendment rights, it is also clear that in "at least . . . some precisely delineated areas, a child . . . is not possessed of that full capacity for individual choice which is the presupposition of First Amendment guarantees" (*Ginsberg* v. *New York,* 1968). For this reason "material which is protected for distribution to adults is not necessarily constitutionally protected from restriction upon its dissemination to children." Specific constitutional concerns may be raised if state regulations substantially interfere with the ability of parents to communicate information to their children (*Bolger* v. *Youngs Drug Products Corporation,* 1983), but even if "the supervision of children's reading may best be left to their parents, the knowledge that parental control or guidance cannot always be provided and society's transcendent interest in protecting the welfare of children justify reasonable regulation of the sale of material to them"(*Ginsberg* v. *New York,* 1968). Schools have broad discretion in restricting speech if that speech poses a material and substantial disruption (*Tinker* v. *Des Moines Independent School District,* 1969), bears the imprimatur of the school (*Hazelwood School District* v. *Kuhlmeier,* 1988),[13] or is inconsistent with its basic educational mission (*Bethel School District* v. *Fraser,* 1986).

The primary constitutional constraint which the Court has imposed on the regulation of children's advertising flows from the idea that "the governmental interest in protecting children from harmful materials . . . does not justify an unnecessarily broad suppression of speech addressed to adults" (*Reno* v. *American Civil Liberties Union,* 1997). Thus the Court ruled in a recent case that even if a state has an important interest in regulating the advertising of tobacco to children, it must nevertheless respect the fact that "tobacco manufacturers and retailers and their adult consumers still have a protected interest in communication"(*Lorillard Tobacco Company* v. *Reilly,* 2001). Regulation of children's advertising must not only satisfy the final prong of the *Central Hudson* test, but it must also respect the integrity of communications between an advertiser and adults. It may not "reduce the adult population . . . to reading only what is fit for children" (*Butler* v. *Michigan,* 1957). As the Court recently said in the context of striking down restrictions on commercial mail designed, in part, to limit children's access to certain information: "The level of discourse reaching a mailbox simply cannot be limited to that which would be suitable for a sandbox" (*Bolger* v. *Youngs Drug Products Corp.,* 1983; *Lorillard Tobacco Company* v. *Reilly,* 2001).

There are also distinct constitutional rules that apply to federal regulation of the broadcast media. Although "broadcasting is clearly a medium affected by a First Amendment interest" (*Red Lion Broadcasting Company*

v. FCC, 1969), it is accorded "special treatment" (*Action for Children's Television* v. *FCC*, 1995; *FCC* v. *Pacifica Foundation*, 1978). This is because broadcast frequencies are said to constitute "a scarce resource" that broadcasters hold in trust for the general public (*Columbia Broadcasting System, Inc.* v. *Democratic National Committee*, 1973; *Red Lion Broadcasting Company* v. *FCC*, 1969)[14] and because the broadcast media are said to constitute a "a uniquely pervasive presence in the lives of all Americans" that reach into "the privacy of the home," where they become "uniquely accessible to children, even those too young to read"(*FCC* v. *Pacifica Foundation*, 1978). The Court has concluded that "the government's interest in the 'well-being of its youth' and in supporting 'parents' claim to authority in their own household' . . . amply justifies special treatment of indecent broadcasting." In the special case of broadcast media, government regulation can infringe on adult communicative rights in order to ensure the protection of children.

Congress has largely entrusted the regulation of broadcast media to the Federal Communications Commission (FCC), which possesses a "broad" and "expansive" power "to assure that broadcasters operate in the public interest" (*McConnell* v. *FEC*, 2003; *Red Lion Broadcasting Company* v. *FCC*, 1969). The FCC has promulgated rules to protect the interests of children. Of particular pertinence are the FCC's rules enforcing the Children's Television Act, P.L. No. 101–437, 104 Stat. 996 (1990),[15] which sets advertising limits for children's programming. The Act requires television broadcasters to "limit the duration of advertising in children's television programming to not more than 10.5 minutes per hour on weekends and not more than 12 minutes per hour on weekdays" (47 U.S.C. § 303a(b), 2002).[16] The FCC interpreted children's programming to refer to "programs originally produced and broadcast primarily for an audience of children 12 years of age and under,"[17] and it crafted rules specifically designed to protect such children, who "constitute the audience primarily affected by overcommercialization because they are the persons who have the most difficulty distinguishing between commercial and programming material."[18] The FCC also regulates television stations' broadcast of "program-length commercials," which it defines as "a program associated with a product, in which commercials for that product are aired" (16 C.F.R. § 308.3(a)(6), 2005).[19] The FCC has applied these rules to prevent integrated cross-promotion. In one instance, it fined a television station which broadcast an advertisement for "Disney on Ice" during an episode of "Chip and Dale's Rescue Rangers." In holding the station responsible for violating the rule, the FCC noted that the policy was motivated by "a fundamental regulatory concern, that children who have difficulty enough distinguishing program content from unrelated commercial matter, not be all the more confused by a show that interweaves program content and commercial matter" (UTV of San Francisco [KBHK-TV], 10 FCC Record 10,986 [Oct. 4, 1995]). The FCC has held various other stations liable for violating this marketing restriction as well (North Carolina Broadcasting Partners [WCCB-TV], 16 FCC Record 5,627 [Mar. 7, 2001]; Gary M. Cocola [KXVO-TV], 15 FCC Record 9,192 [May 26, 2000]; Peak Media of Pennsylvania [WWCP-TV], 14 FCC Record 13,937 [Aug 27, 1999]).

Because of the special constitutional status of the broadcast media, there is little doubt that these FCC regulations meet First Amendment standards, even though they substantially interfere with the ability of advertisers to reach adults, who often view children's programs. The committee agreed that there was potential benefit from children's advertising closely aligned with healthful diets, and if an emphasis on the advertising of healthful foods and beverages could not be accomplished voluntarily, Congress should consider and, most felt, enact legislation mandating the shift on both broadcast and cable television. The customary deliberations of the legislative process would afford the opportunity for further assessment of the execution and implications of such a shift.

Government regulation of the Internet, by contrast, has been held subject to ordinary First Amendment principles (*Reno* v. *American Civil Liberties Union*, 1997). At the present time, the FTC is the lead federal agency in regulating commercial practices on the Internet. As of 2004, the FTC had pursued approximately 300 cases that challenged Internet practices involving substantial harms to consumers (North Carolina Broadcasting Partners [WCCB-TV], 16 FCC Record 5,627 [Mar. 7, 2001]; Gary M. Cocola [KXVO-TV], 15 FCC Record 9,192 [May 26, 2000]; Peak Media of Pennsylvania [WWCP-TV], 14 FCC Record 13,937 [Aug. 27, 1999]). Some of these cases involved deceptive or unfair marketing practices deployed in other media as well as the Internet, such as deceptive weight loss practices. Other cases have involved advertising or marketing practices that are unique to the Internet, such as the use of spyware (*FTC* v. *D Squared Solutions, LLC*, 2003). The FTC has also issued rules regulating websites' collection of personal information from children pursuant to its authority under the Children's Online Privacy Protection Act (COPPA) (15 U.S.C. §§ 6501–6506, 2002).[20] The regulations apply to operators of any websites or online services directed at children and to operators who knowingly collect or maintain personal information from a child.

The rules impose various requirements on operators, including that they post a clear and prominent link to a notice of their privacy policies with regard to children on the home pages of their websites or online service as well as in each additional area where personal information is collected from children. These notices must include information about the identity of the operator, the types of personal information that is being collected from children, how the operator uses that information, and whether that information is disclosed to third parties. In addition, the regulations require that the operators obtain parental permission before they collect, use, or disclose the personal information of children. Operators must provide parents with a reasonable means to review the personal information collected from their children and to stop its maintenance or continued collection if they desire. The regulations prohibit an operator from conditioning a child's "participation in a game, the offering of a prize, or another activity on the child's disclosing more personal information than is reasonably necessary to participate in such activity." Finally, the regulations require operators to establish and continue reasonable procedures to protect the confidentiality, security, and integrity of personal information collected from children (16 C.F.R. 312.8).[21]

It is likely that restrictions on Internet speech will be subject to the same kind of First Amendment scrutiny as would be deployed were the restrictions applicable to speech in movies or in newspapers. The nature of this scrutiny will depend upon whether the communication at issue is categorized as "public discourse" (*Hustler Magazine* v. *Falwell*, 1988), in which case constitutional review will be quite strict, or instead as "commercial speech," in which case it will be subject to the more lenient standard of the *Central Hudson* test. Regulation of the Internet poses unresolved constitutional issues because the constitutional status of much speech on the Internet is at this time highly uncertain.

Increasingly prominent are "advergames," which contain branded products built directly into a game through video games or Internet-based games with the intent to sell products (Chapter 4). Courts are just now beginning to rule that video games, if they are sufficiently artistic and complex, can be "analytically indistinguishable from other protected media, such as motion pictures or books, which convey information or evoke emotions by imagery, and are protected under the First Amendment" (*American Amusement Machine Association* v. *Kendrick*, 2001; *Interactive Digital Software Association* v. *St. Louis County*, 2003; *Video Software Dealers Association* v. *Maleng*, 2004; *Wilson* v. *Midway Games*, 2002). If advergames seem to have the primary purpose and effect of selling products, however, they might be categorized as advertisements rather than motion pictures or books, and hence subject to the standards of the *Central Hudson* test. There is also the question of how courts will categorize entire websites, such as Postopia.com®, hosted by Viacom International (compare *Ford Motor Company* v. *Texas Department of Transportation*, 2001 with *Fred Wehrenberg Circuit of Theatres, Inc.* v. *Moviefone, Inc.*, 1999). This website features Kraft Foods' food and beverage brands that contain both advergames and other types of commercial informational content (Viacom International, 2005).

Finding: Regulations for those who advertise and market food and beverage products to children will need to evolve as the food industry develops new techniques for promoting its products. How current law will be applied to rapidly changing areas like the Internet cannot currently be predicted with confidence. However, future regulatory interventions should certainly be taken on the basis of reliable data concerning the impacts on children of the marketing and advertising of food and beverage products. Currently, neither the Federal Trade Commission, nor any other responsible federal agency, collects or maintains such data.

OTHER POTENTIAL POLICY APPROACHES

The knowledge base supporting the importance of diet in promoting health and preventing disease has evolved during the last half century, which occurred after many U.S. agricultural policies had developed and been implemented. U.S. agricultural and economic policies have historically supported the production of a plentiful and affordable food supply, and health-promotion and disease-prevention objectives have not played a central role in these policies (Tillotson, 2004). Examining the historical context of the evolution of food and nutrition policies is important to understand the role they may have played in contributing to the rise in obesity rates and other chronic diseases. This section identifies potential actions that have been suggested in various quarters to create industry incentives or support agricultural subsidies to produce and market more healthful foods, as well as those to reduce the demand for less healthful foods.

Price Supports and Subsidies

An analysis of the agricultural production in the United States relative to recommended dietary guidelines showed that the food supply contains a substantial surplus of sugars and oils; approximately the expected amounts of meat, milk, and grains; and substantially less than what is needed for fruits and vegetables (Duxbury and Welch, 1999). Several agricultural policies and regulations that may affect the food sector and consumer food choices and dietary intake are federal farm assistance programs that include price- and income-support programs, producer-funded marketing orders, and research and promotion agreements (Ralston, 1999). Price and income support programs have historically affected the market supply of foods. From 1970 to 1985, poultry became a lower-priced alternative to red meat, and consumers switched from more expensive animal-based fats to lower-priced vegetable-based fats and oils (IOM, 1991).

Historically, price supports for milk were readily available based on the butterfat content of milk rather than the low-fat content of milk. In

1991, the Institute of Medicine (IOM) recommended that the dairy industry and companies that sell dairy products work toward changing the milk pricing system to encourage dairy producers to breed and manage their herds for the production of lower fat milk in accordance with changing consumer demand (IOM, 1991). Empirical research has shown that the dairy industry could receive economic benefits from the explicit promotion of low-fat milk, but the nutritional benefits of such promotion may be offset by dietary substitutions for fat from other types of foods (Pelletier et al., 1999).

Using price subsidies to encourage healthful food consumption, such as fruits and vegetables, in the United States has not been well explored but warrants further research. This type of research into subsidizing the growth, production, and consumption of healthier foods could improve knowledge about the feasibility of encouraging subsidies as a policy instrument to promote healthier food choices. An analysis of the U.S. produce production compared to the Dietary Guidelines for Americans showed sizable deficits in vegetable and fruit production in the United States. There are economic opportunities to increase the production of fruits and vegetables in different regions and to increase the U.S. government purchase of domestic surplus fruits, vegetables, and specialty crops that could be used for schools and other food service establishments (Branaman, 2003; Duxbury and Welch, 1999).

Tariff regulations cover a broad array of sectors other than agriculture, including trade policies, such as the North American Free Trade Agreement (NAFTA), restrictions on mergers, and environmental requirements. These regulations may affect the price or availability of specific food products. Other government regulations and programs may also affect food choices such as changes in welfare assistance regulations, which can increase or decrease household income and affect consumer food choices. How these regulations and polices impact individual dietary choices depends on how the regulations affect retail food prices and how responsive consumers are to the price changes (IOM, 1991). Ingredient costs are a small fraction of retail prices for many processed foods, but commodity prices are a larger proportion of food retail prices, especially for fresh meat, fish, poultry, eggs, milk, cheese, fruits, and vegetables. Consumers are not very responsive to price changes for poultry, eggs, fish, milk, and cheese, but they are more responsive to the prices of some fresh fruits and vegetables, as well as pork and beef (Ralston, 1999).

Tax Incentives

An imposition of taxes on certain foods and beverages, particularly ones that are salty, high-calorie, high-fat, high in added sugars, and low-nutrient has been suggested by certain public health advocates as a viable disincentive to discourage the consumption of less healthful foods and beverages (Brownell and Horgen, 2004; Kuchler et al., 2004, 2005; Swinburn and Egger, 2002). Empirical research is not readily available to assess the effectiveness of taxing certain foods and beverages in order to influence dietary choices, but some interesting work using economic models is beginning to emerge. For example, one assessment by the Food and Resource Economics Institute in Denmark used an econometric model to predict the effect of different tax (e.g., fat, saturated fat, sugar) or subsidy (e.g., fiber) approaches to changing diets. It found that each could have an impact on consumption, but with variable results by nutrient category and by socioeconomic and geographic status. The authors suggest that, for full effect, such economic incentives might require combination with other interventions, such as related public information campaigns (Smed et al., 2005).

Experience from tobacco policy in the United States has shown that taxing cigarettes, as a component of a comprehensive state-based program, is a cost-effective means of reducing tobacco use and achieving public health gains in adults (Warner, 2005) but does not necessarily discourage tobacco use in youth (DeCicca et al., 2002). The impact of implementing taxes on certain branded food items or high-calorie and low-nutrient food and beverage categories would depend on the size of the tax, how easily manufacturers could move their resources to produce and distribute untaxed products, and on how consumers would respond to the taxes (Kuchler et al., 2004).

In 2000, 18 states implemented a tax on specifically targeted food and beverages (e.g., candy, soft drinks, soft drink syrups, gum, ice cream, diluted juices, chocolate milk, and others) and 7 states had previously imposed taxes for certain foods, or categories of foods, but the legislation had been repealed (Brownell and Horgen, 2004; Jacobson and Brownell, 2000). The rationale for the repealed laws included lobbying by the soft drink and bottling industries, retailers, distributors, and industry employees; difficulties administering the taxes due to lack of clarity for a definition of which categories of foods and beverages to tax; and opposition to taxes linked to a general fund that could be used for purposes other than promoting public health objectives (Jacobson and Brownell, 2000).

Supporters of taxation have suggested several ways to implement such policies including taxing certain types of foods and beverages (e.g., high in salt, added sugars, fat, and total calories or low in nutrients) or taxing specific categories of foods and beverages (e.g., snack foods, candy, soft drinks, and fast foods) (Brownell and Horgen, 2004; Yach et al., 2003). The evidence does not exist at this time, however, to support a definite conclusion about whether imposing a sales tax on less healthful foods would have a significant effect on reducing sales. Consumers tend to favor taxes when the revenues will be used to fund health education programs (Jacobson and Brownell, 2000). Some have also advocated for simultaneous subsidization of fruits and vegetables to encourage more healthful diet (Brownell and Horgen, 2004; Kuchler et al., 2004). Opponents of taxation have suggested that taxation of certain categories of foods may produce unanticipated consequences for low-income consumers (Brownell and Horgen, 2004) and not produce the desirable effect of changing individuals' dietary patterns (Kuchler et al., 2004). One study determined that a small tax (1 cent per pound) as suggested in some research would not appreciably alter consumption, but would generate large tax revenues (Kuchler et al., 2004). The IOM (2005a) concluded that there is insufficient evidence to recommend either for or against taxing these foods, and that taxation or subsidies by themselves have not been substantial enough to create sustainable changes in people's eating behaviors. Research into a variety of factors is needed to determine the desirable combination of comprehensive policy instruments to encourage consumer behavior changes (Yach et al., 2003).

FOOD MARKETING POLICIES
OUTSIDE THE UNITED STATES

The rising concern about obesity in children and youth globally has led to public health responses in many countries and organizations. An estimated 85 percent of 73 countries surveyed by the World Health Organization (WHO) had some form of regulation for television advertising to children (Hawkes, 2004) (Appendix G, Table G-1). While television advertising may be the most efficient medium for food and beverage promotion, there are also statutory or voluntary regulations for other marketing approaches and channels used to reach children including in-school marketing, sponsorship, product placement, the Internet, and sales promotion (Appendix G, Table G-2). Options for advertising regulation in various countries include partial restrictions on advertising by type of food, target group, portion size, and the times of advertising exposure; establishing upper and lower limits of advertising exposure to children of certain ages; and a complete ban on advertising to children (Hawkes, 2004).

Where advertising legislation has been enacted, such as in Sweden and Norway, and in the Canadian province of Quebec, the regulations become less relevant when advertising through broadcast media (especially television and radio) is transmitted from outside national boundaries. Advertisements that are subject to the transmitting countries' guidelines and regulations, rather than those of the receiving countries' regulations, presents a dilemma for countries where the national border does not serve as an effective barrier to children's broadcast media and advertising.

Many countries use different definitions for children in developing regulations and some do not define an upper age limit. In regulations, children may be described as minors, juveniles, or young people, and the target ages may range from under 12 years to under 18 years (Hawkes, 2004). Similar marketing regulations can apply to various age groups in different countries and may create inconsistencies, especially when advertising messages transmitted externally from countries such as Sweden and Norway or the province of Quebec are subject to the transmitting countries' guidelines and regulations that may be more lenient or define children differently.

To enhance attention, action, and consistency across the international community, the WHO developed a *Global Strategy on Diet, Physical Activity and Health* that provides members states with a range of policy options to address less healthful dietary practices and physical inactivity, including provisions for marketing, advertising, sponsorship, and promotion. These provisions recommended that food and beverage advertisements should not exploit children's inexperience or credulity, should discourage messages that promote unhealthy dietary practices, and should encourage positive health messages. The Global Strategy was endorsed by the 57th World Health Assembly in 2004 (WHO, 2004).

International Chamber of Commerce

The International Chamber of Commerce (ICC) developed a series of self-regulatory codes of practice that set out ethical standards for different types of marketing, each of which includes a clause for children (Hawkes, 2004). The International Code of Advertising Practice covers television advertising. According to Article 14 of the Code, advertisements should not exploit the inexperience or credulity of children and young people (ICC, 1997). The International Code of Sales Promotion has a similar clause in Article 8 and adds that sales promotions should not harm children or young people mentally, morally, or physically, or strain their loyalty with parents or guardians (ICC, 2002). Article 7 of the International Code on Sponsorship presents an almost identical clause (ICC, 2003). The codes are frequently reflected in codes of professional associations in many countries.

Europe

The European Heart Network, concerned about the 20 percent of school-aged European children who are either obese or at risk for obesity, documented marketing trends for children in 20 European countries. The Network is developing an action plan to address childhood obesity throughout the European Union (EU) that includes protecting children from food marketing the network considers to be unhealthy (e.g., foods and beverages that are high in fat, sugar, salt, and low in nutrients) as one of many interventions to address childhood obesity (Matthews et al., 2005).

The EU Television Without Frontiers Directive is coordinated by the European Commission Directorate-General for Education and Culture that guides policy in Europe (TWFD, 2005). The Directive, most recently revised in 1997, upholds the basic freedom and legal right to advertise to children, provided a set of minimum criteria are observed. Article 16 of the EU Television Without Frontiers Directive states that "Television advertising shall not cause moral or physical detriment to minors." Many countries also implement regulations that restrict the timing and content of television advertising to children. As many as 25 European countries do not allow children's television programs of less than 30 minutes duration to be interrupted by advertising, which complies with Article 11 of the EU Television Without Frontiers Directive (Hawkes, 2004).

For EU Member States, the EU Television Without Frontiers Directive regulates sponsorship and product placement as well. Under Article 17, a sponsor may not influence the content of sponsored television, a sponsor must be clearly identified as such by its name at the beginning or end of the program, and the programs may not encourage the purchase of a sponsor's products. Article 10 prohibits hidden or surreptitious advertising. A total of 7 EU Member States and 6 other non-EU Member States appear to restrict some forms of product placement, and 4 EU Member States and Norway have explicitly banned product placement in television programs (Hawkes, 2004).

The Broadcasting Commission of Ireland introduced a new code in 2001 that bans the use of cartoon characters and celebrities to promote foods. The Children's Advertising Code defines certain categories of food, such as fast foods, that must carry a message stating that foods should be eaten in moderation and are part of a balanced diet. Confectionary products must have an auditory or visual message stating that sugar-sweetened products can damage teeth (BCI, 2001).

The self-regulatory body in the United Kingdom is the Advertising Standards Authority (ASA), an independent entity that investigates nonadherence to the Code of Advertising, Sales Promotions, and Direct Marketing that is developed by the Committee on Advertising Practice, an industry body with representatives from marketing and media that develop and enforce the advertising guidelines. Although the code states that child-directed advertising should contain nothing that is likely to result in the physical, mental, or moral harm of children, it contains no specific rules on food advertising (Hawkes, 2005).

In 2004, a United Kingdom (U.K.) Department of Trade and Industry bill established a new regulatory body, Ofcom (Office of Communication). As the new communications sector regulator, Ofcom inherited the duties of the five existing regulating bodies it replaced: the Broadcasting Standards Commission, the Independent Television Commission (ITC), Oftel, the Radio Authority, and the Radiocommunications Agency (Ofcom, 2004). Ofcom uses rules originally published by ITC on the amount and scheduling of advertising (Ofcom, 2005), stipulating that advertisements may not be inserted during programs designed to be broadcast in schools or during programs for children of less than half an hour scheduled duration. Ofcom recently conducted research to examine the effects of food advertising on childhood obesity and concluded that television advertising has a modest direct effect on children's food choices. Ofcom also concluded that changing the rules for the advertising of food products that are high in fat, salt, and sugar as a single approach to combat obesity would be highly unlikely to succeed (Ofcom, 2004).

Despite the Ofcom conclusions, the U.K. Food Standards Agency has embarked on a public consultation by a diverse expert committee to develop a nutrient profiling model that would use a simple scoring system to rate the overall balance of nutrients in foods. The model would support Ofcom's work to consider possible restrictions on advertising and other forms of marketing to children for foods that are high in fat, saturated fat, salt, or sugar (FSA, 2005). Additionally, the British Medical Association recommended, as a component of its childhood obesity prevention plan, a ban on advertising of foods that it considered to be unhealthful, including certain sponsorship programs targeted at school children and a ban on unhealthful food and beverage products from school vending machines (BMA, 2005).

The French government has recently passed legislation that mandatory health messages should accompany advertisements on television or radio for manufactured foods and sweetened beverages that are high in sugar, salt, or artificial colors. Advertisers can be exempted from including the obligatory health messages if they pay 1.5 percent of the expected profit to the French Health Education Institute to fund nutrition education programs (Carvajal, 2005). The French government's action is based on the findings of the Hastings et al. (2003) review, sponsored by the U.K. Food Standards Agency, which focused on the impact of promotion on the food choices of children. The key findings from the review were that food promotion affects children's preferences, purchase behaviors, and consumption, not just for different brands but also for different categories of foods (Hastings et al., 2003). The review provided evidence that fostered action to limit food and beverage promotion directed to children because of the impact on children's health.

In Sweden, all television and radio advertising aimed at children ages 12 and younger during children's programming was banned in 1991 (Bjurstrom, 1994; Hawkes, 2004). The ban was enacted based on the view that children younger than 12 years cannot clearly distinguish advertising messages from program content, and on the principle that children should have the right to grow up in a commercial-free environment, especially young children who are trusting and do not understand the difference between information and the persuasive intent of advertisements or commercials (Bjurstrom, 1994). The ban is enforced by the National Consumer Ombudsman in Sweden and applies only to the Swedish commercial channel but not the Swedish channels broadcast from the United Kingdom (Hawkes, 2004; National Food Administration and National Institute of Public Health, 2005). A comprehensive evaluation was not available to assess the effectiveness of the ban on reducing exposure to child-directed television advertising. What is clear is that Swedish children's exposure to advertising and other forms of marketing has not been eliminated, as satellite television channels originating from the United Kingdom and the United States to Sweden often provide exposure to commercial television with advertisements to children (Hawkes, 2004; MacCarthy, 2004; National Food Administration and National Institute of Public Health, 2005), which demonstrates the challenge of a global economy.

Norway enacted a ban on television advertisements to children ages 12 years and younger in 1992 (Hawkes, 2004; Norwegian Ministry of Children and Family Affairs, 2005). Although a comprehensive evaluation is not available to assess the effectiveness of the ban on reducing exposure to child-directed television advertising, the Norwegian government has developed *The Norwegian Action Plan to Reduce Commercial Pressure on Children and the Young People* (Norwegian Ministry of Children and Family Affairs, 2005).

Most of the countries that have regulations for in-school marketing are in Europe. Hungary is the only European country with self-regulatory guidelines that allows advertising only with the permission of the school principal (Hawkes, 2004). France, Greece, Luxembourg, and Portugal have statutory restrictions that prohibit in-school marketing. Finland and Germany permit advertising or marketing materials in schools as long as the school or the parents give consent. The governments of Denmark, Ireland, and the Netherlands issued guidelines that require advertisers and marketers to follow certain principles when targeting schools (Hawkes, 2004; Appendix G, Table G-2).

The Internet is a new medium for advertisers to market foods and beverages to consumers. In 2003, an estimated 13 percent of total spending on foods, carbonated soft drinks, and fast food advertising was done through the Internet in the United Kingdom (Matthews et al., 2005). The Internet is ranked as the second most important promotional medium that reaches children and youth after television. Given the high frequency of advertising and the novelty of this medium, countries worldwide are in the process of developing guidelines to regulate marketing to children via the Internet. In many European countries, it is presumed that national laws on advertising and consumer protection are also applicable to advertising using the Internet (Hawkes, 2004). The most stringent regulations have been developed by the Nordic Consumer Ombudsmen for Scandinavian countries, which has implemented guidelines on e-commerce and Internet marketing (Nordic Consumer Ombudsmen, 2002). These guidelines prohibit marketers from obtaining personal information from children and from urging children to make purchases over the Internet. Marketing is not to be designed or integrated as games or activity pages, and the guidelines specifically state that businesses should not send advertising directly to children (Nordic Consumer Ombudsmen, 2002).

Finland is the only country that has regulations in place with government oversight regarding broader sales promotion activities (Hawkes, 2004). Only three European countries have regulations specific to children—Finland, Ireland, and the United Kingdom. In Ireland, sales promotion codes of practice follow those of the ICC (ASAI, 2001). The British Code of Advertising, Sales Promotion, and Direct Marketing states that "promotions addressed to or targeted at children should not encourage excessive purchases in order to participate" (CAP, 2005).

Other Countries

Both government and self-regulatory mechanisms exist in Canada. The Broadcast Code for Advertising to Children is statutory and restricts the use of puppets and subliminal messages to encourage children to purchase products. Advertising Standards Canada (ASC), a self-regulating industry body, is responsible for ensuring adherence to the statutory code. The code states that advertising directed to children must not exploit their credulity or lack of experience and must not present information that may harm their physical, emotional, or moral well-being (ASC, 2004). The Canadian Broadcasting Corporation, the national public broadcaster, does not accept advertising of any kind in programs directed to children younger than 12 years of age (CBC, 2005).

In addition to television, Canada regulates in-school and Internet marketing. Specifically in the province of Quebec, the Law on State Education prohibits commercial solicitation in schools. Donations are allowed, however, and commercial funding cannot be used to persuade children to consume products. Voluntary guidelines developed by the Canadian Teachers Federation state that school-commercial relationships must share similar objectives and benefit both students and staff (Hawkes, 2004).

Also in Quebec, the Consumer Protection Act prohibits television advertising directed to children ages 13 and younger and has been in effect since 1980 (Hawkes, 2004; Quebec Government, 1980). The legislation only applies to commercial advertising, thus, educational advertising is allowed on television. In addition, the legislation cannot apply to signals originating from outside Quebec that are transmitted by cable television companies (Quebec Consumer Protection Act, 2005). Because of the television advertising ban, advertisers have changed commercials to make them less appealing to children. According to ASC, advertisements are more likely to be targeted to parents to urge them to purchase products for their children. Advertising dollars have also been diverted out of Quebec, thereby decreasing the amount of original French-language Quebec children's programming.

A study by Goldberg (1990) suggested that soon after its enactment in 1980, the Quebec ban served to reduce children's exposure to television commercials for sweetened breakfast cereals and consequently reduced children's consumption of these products. Even though children were still exposed to American commercials, only the English-speaking Canadian children could recognize and were more aware of products that were advertised, such as toys and sweetened breakfast cereals, and had more of these in their homes than did French-speaking Canadian children. The French-speaking children were also less likely to urge their parents to purchase these advertised products (Goldberg, 1990). On the other hand, a more recent study suggests that despite the advertising ban that has been in effect since 1980, television food commercials viewed by French-speaking Canadian children neither represent a balanced diet nor the foods recommended by the Canadian government (Lebel et al., 2005).

The Australian obesity prevention action plan supports stricter national regulations on food advertising directed to children, and is considering a ban on advertising during children's television viewing time (NSW Centre for Public Health Nutrition, 2005). Regulation of television in Australia is currently a combination of legislation and self-regulation with more emphasis on the statutory regulation. The Children's Television Standards (CTS) of the Australian Broadcasting Authority implements regulations limiting the amount of advertising to children according to program classification. Advertisements aired during programs directed at preschool children ('P' programs) are prohibited. Advertisements broadcast during programs directed at primary school-aged children ('C' programs) are limited to 5 minutes every 30 minutes (ABA, 2002). CTS also limits the repetition of advertisements and those featuring children's television personalities. Australia also has voluntary guidelines that were developed by the educational sector to regulate in-school marketing. Organizations are asked not to seek endorsement of products or services, as a condition of a sponsorship or participation in a promotion by the Australian Education Council (Hawkes, 2004).

A brief summary is provided for the regulatory and voluntary guidelines of selected countries in Africa, Asia, Latin America, and the Middle East (Appendix G, Table G-1).

Finding: Comprehensive evaluations are not available to assess the effect on children's diets of countrywide bans on child-directed television advertising. Limited evidence suggests that national borders may not serve as effective barriers to children's broadcast media and advertising where it is common to receive broadcasts from outside the receiving countries.

SUMMARY

Various public policies and programs implemented by government at all levels have the potential to influence the diets of children and youth. Dietary guidance, nutrition education and promotion, school nutrition policies and programs, food labeling, regulation of food marketing, and food production, distribution, and pricing policies, all have the potential to affect options and choices, and the milieu within which food and beverage marketing takes place. Several education and information programs and policies are sponsored by government at federal, state, and local levels and in many venues. The policy touchstones for federal education and information programs on nutrition are the Dietary Guidelines for Americans and its graphic representation, *MyPyramid*. Several federal partnerships promote nutrition and healthful diets as well, including the USDA and U.S. Department of Education *HealthierUS* School Challenge, the DHHS *Small Step* and *Small Step Kids!*, the DHHS *5 a Day for Better Health* program, and the DHHS/NIH *We Can!* childhood obesity prevention collaboration.

Nutrition labeling is one principal means of conveying nutrition information to the public. The importance of integrating and improving strategies for using the food label as an educational tool is emphasized by recent company initiatives to use proprietary logos or icons that communicate the nutritional qualities of their branded products. The DHHS Food and Drug Administration (FDA) is the primary agency responsible for overseeing the use of food and beverage labels to convey nutrition information and health claims, and is key to progress in ensuring the accuracy, consistency and effectiveness of industry and government initiatives using such graphics and standards to convey the nutritional qualities of foods and beverages in a form appealing and easily understood by children, youth, and their parents.

School-based interventions that reach the nation's children and youth include nutrition education, school food services, the Fruit and Vegetable Pilot Program, and the Department of Defense's Fresh Produce Program. Recent attention has been focused on competitive foods in schools. There are currently no comprehensive federal competitive food standards to guide the type of products that are available and marketed in America's schools and other venues. However, a variety of legislative initiatives pertaining to the availability, marketing, and sales of competitive foods and beverages in schools have been enacted or proposed at the state, district, and local levels.

Social marketing applies commercial marketing concepts and techniques to promote voluntary behavior change in specific groups or target audiences based on their socio-demographic, behavioral, and psychological characteristics. Evidence for the effectiveness of social marketing programs to promote healthful behaviors is promising but mixed. A central challenge to large-scale social marketing efforts is discerning their impact. Social marketing programs that have had positive results had higher funding, been sustained, been shaped by formative research, used an integrated marketing approach, and had ongoing monitoring and evaluation.

Like other dimensions of commerce, advertising and marketing is subject to regulation, including marketing that reaches children. Due to the prominence and complexity of this matter, the chapter presents a detailed analysis of the related issues, precedents, and considerations. The committee agreed that there was potential benefit from children's advertising closely aligned with healthful diets, and if an emphasis on the advertising of healthful foods and beverages could not be accomplished voluntarily, Congress should consider and, most felt*, enact legislation mandating the shift on both broadcast and cable television. The customary deliberations of the legislative process would afford the opportunity for further assessment of the execution and implications of such a shift. Other potential policy approaches that have been suggested are reviewed, including creating industry incentives and support for agricultural subsidies to produce and market more healthful foods, as well as to reduce the demand for less healthful foods.

The rising concern about obesity in children and youth globally has led to public health responses in many countries that have developed regulatory and voluntary advertising and marketing guidelines. Similarly, several international organizations, including the World Health Organization, have developed related policies.

---

*JHB excepted, based on his belief that the level of quantitative evidence on the salutary impact of more balanced television advertising on children's dietary patterns, in combination with a reported decline in the role of television advertising in the overall marketing of foods to children, would be insufficient for such a requirement to overcome the constitutional protection of freedom of speech.

REFERENCES

44 Liquormart, Inc. v. *Rhode Island,* 517 U.S. 484 (1996).

ABA (Australian Broadcasting Authority). 2002. *Children's Television Standards.* Australian Broadcasting Authority. [Online]. Available: http://www.aba.gov.au/contentreg/codes/television/documents/chstdvarn_03.pdf [accessed November 18, 2005].

Action for Children's Television v. *FCC,* 58 F.3d 654, 660 (D.C. Cir. 1995).

Ad Council. 2005. *What is Public Service Advertising?* [Online]. Available: http://www.adcouncil.org/np/tips_psa_definition/ [accessed June 23, 2005].

American Amusement Machine Association v. *Kendrick,* 244 F.3d 572, 574-78 (7th Cir. 2001).

Anderson PM, Butcher KF. 2005. *Reading, Writing and Raisinets: Are School Finances Contributing to Childhood Obesity?* Working Paper 11177. Cambridge, MA: National Bureau of Economic Research.

Andreasen AR. 1995. *Marketing Social Change. Changing Behavior to Promote Health, Social Development, and the Environment.* San Francisco, CA: Jossey-Bass.

Andreasen AR. 2002. Marketing social marketing in the social change marketplace. *Journal of Public Policy & Marketing* 21(1):3–13.

ASAI (Advertising Standards Authority of Ireland). 2001. *Code of Sales Promotion Practice, 3rd edition.* Dublin, Ireland: ASAI. [Online]. Available: http://www.asai.ie/ [accessed May 9, 2005].

ASC (Advertising Standards Canada). 2004. *Canadian Code of Advertising Standards.* Toronto, Canada: ASC.

Audio Communication, Inc. 114 F.T.C. 414 (1991).

Azuma A, Fisher A. 2001. *Healthy Farms, Healthy Kids: Evaluating the Barriers and Opportunities for Farm-to-School Programs.* Venice, CA: Community Food Service Coalition.

Backer TE, Rogers EM. 1993. *Organizational Aspects of Communication Campaigns: What Works?* Newbury Park, CA: Sage Publications, Inc.

Bad Frog Brewery, Inc. v. *New York State Liquor Authority,* 134 F.3d 87 (2d Cir. 1998).

Bates v. *State Bar of Arizona,* 433 U.S. 350, 383 (1977).

BCI (Broadcasting Commission of Ireland). 2001. *Children's Advertising Code.* Dublin, Ireland: BCI.

Beales JH. 2004. *Advertising to Kids and the FTC: A Regulatory Retrospective That Advises the Present.* [Online]. Available: http://www.ftc.gov/speeches/beales/040802adstokids.pdf [accessed April 8, 2005].

Bethel School District v. *Fraser,* 478 U.S. 675, 685–86 (1986).

Bjurstrom E. 1994. *Children and Television Advertising. A Critical Study of International Research Concerning the Effects of TV-Commercials on Children.* Report No. 1994/95:8. Stockholm, Sweden: Swedish Consumer Agency.

BMA (British Medical Association). 2005. *Preventing Childhood Obesity.* London, UK: BMA.

Bolger v. *Youngs Drug Products Corp.,* 463 U.S. 60, 74–75 (1983).

Boone LE, Kurtz DL. 1998. *Contemporary Marketing Wired.* 9th ed. Orlando, FL: The Dryden Press.

Branaman B. 2003. *Fruits and Vegetables: Issues for Congress.* Congressional Research Service. The Library of Congress.

Brown J. 2001. Media literacy and critical television viewing in education. In: Singer DG, Singer JL, eds. *Handbook of Children and the Media.* Thousand Oaks, CA: Sage Publications. Pp. 681–697.

Brownell KD, Horgen KB. 2004. *Food Fight: The Inside Story of the Food Industry, America's Obesity Crisis, and What We Can Do About It.* New York: The McGraw-Hill Companies.

Buckingham D. 2005. *The Media Literacy of Children and Young People: A Review of the Research Literature*. London, England: Centre for the Study of Children, Youth and Media Institute of Education, University of London, London Knowledge Lab. [Online]. Available: http://www.ofcom.org.uk/advice/media_literacy/medlitpub/?a=87101 [accessed April 12, 2005].

Bunch v. *Hoffinger Industries, Inc.*, 123 Cal. App. 4th 1278, 1298 (Cal. Ct. App. 2004).

Burbridge v. *Sampson*, 74 F. Supp. 2d 940 (C.D. Cal. 1999).

Butler v. *Michigan*, 352 U.S. 380, 383 (1957).

Buzby JC, Guthrie JF, Kantor LS. 2003. *Evaluation of the USDA Fruit and Vegetable Pilot Program: Report to Congress*. E-FAN-03-006. Washington, DC: USDA.

Cain v. *Sheraton Perimeter Park South Hotel*, 592 So. 2d 218, 220-22 (Ala. 1991).

CAP (Committee of Advertising Practice). 2005. *The British Code of Advertising, Sales Promotion, and Direct Marketing*. [Online]. Available: http://www.cap.org.uk/NR/rdonlyres/A44808F1-1573-482A-A0E5-D8045943DA57/0/The_CAP_Code_Ed11_1Oct2005.pdf [accessed May 9, 2005].

Carvajal D. 2005, October 2. Processed foods? Read this, France says. *International Herald Tribune Online* [Online]. Available: http://www.iht.com/articles/2005/10/02/business/food03.php [accessed October 24, 2005].

CBC (Canadian Broadcasting Corporation). 2005. *Summary of CBC Advertising Standards*. [Online]. Available: http://cbc.radio-canada.ca/docs/policies/advertising.shtml [accessed November 17, 2005].

CDC (Centers for Disease Control and Prevention). 2002. *Behavioral Risk Factor Surveillance System Survey Data. Prevalence Data: Risk Factors and Calculated Variables— 2002*. Atlanta, GA: U.S. Department of Health and Human Services, CDC. [Online]. Available: http://apps.nccd.cdc.gov/brfss/list.asp?cat=RF&yr=2002&qkey=4409&state=All/ [accessed April 10, 2005].

CDC. 2005a. *5 A Day. Home*. [Online]. Available: http://www.cdc.gov/nccdphp/dnpa/5aday/ [accessed October 14, 2005].

CDC. 2005b. *About CDC: CDC Organization*. [Online]. Available: http://www.cdc.gov/about/cio.htm [accessed October 15, 2005].

CDC. 2005c. Competitive foods and beverages available for purchase in secondary schools— Selected sites, United States, 2004. *MMWR* 54(37):917–921. [Online]. Available: http://www.cdc.gov/mmwr/preview/mmwrhtml/mm5437a1.htm [accessed October 10, 2005].

CDC. 2005d. *Guidance for Evaluating Mass Communication Health Initiatives: Summary of an Expert Panel Discussion*. Office of Communication, CDC. [Online]. Available: http://www.cdc.gov/communication/practice/epreport.pdf [accessed October 19, 2005].

CDC. 2005e. *Powerful Bones. Powerful Girls.*™ [Online]. Available: http://www.cdc.gov/powerfulbones/ [accessed October 14, 2005].

CDC. 2005f. *VERBNow.com*. [Online]. Available: http://www.verbnow.com [accessed November 11, 2005].

CDC. 2005g. *Youth Media Campaign. VERB*™. [Online]. Available: http://www.cdc.gov/youthcampaign/ [accessed July 30, 2005].

Central Hudson Gas & Electric Corporation v. *Public Service Commission*, 447 U.S. 557, 566 (1980).

Clime v. *Dewey Beach Enterprises, Inc.*, 831 F. Supp. 341, 344-46 (D. Del. 1993).

Columbia Broadcasting System, Inc. v. *Democratic National Committee*, 412 U.S. 94, 101-02 (1973).

Committee on Education and the Workforce. 2004. *Child Nutrition and WIC Reauthorization Act Bill Summary*. [Online]. Available: http://edworkforce.house.gov/issues/108th/education/childnutrition/billsummaryfinal.htm [accessed October 20, 2005].

Contento I, Balch G, Bronner YL, Lytle LA, Maloney SK, Olson CM, Sharaga SS. 1995. The effectiveness of nutrition education and implications for nutrition education policy, programs, and research: A review of research. *J Nutr Ed* 27(6):276–283.

Cooperative State Research, Education, and Extension Service. 2005. USDA Expanded Food and Nutrition Education Program. [Online]. Available: http://www.csrees.usda.gov/nea/food/efnep/about.html [accessed November 9, 2005].

CPEHN (California Pan-Ethnic Health Network) and Consumers Union. 2005. *Out of Balance: Marketing of Soda, Candy, Snacks and Fast Foods Drowns Out Healthful Messages.* Oakland and San Francisco, CA. [Online]. Available: http://www.consumersunion.org/pdf/OutofBalance.pdf [accessed September 15, 2005].

CSPI (Center for Science in the Public Interest). 2003. *School Foods Tool Kit. A Guide to Improving School Foods & Beverages. Part III: Case Studies. State Legislation to Improve School Foods and Beverages.* [Online]. Available: http://www.cspinet.org/schoolfoodkit/school_foods_kit_part3.pdf [accessed November 10, 2005].

CSPI. 2004. *Model School Foods Legislation.* [Online]. Available: http://www.cspinet.org/nutritionpolicy/school_food_legislation2.pdf [accessed June 15, 2005].

CSPI. 2005. *Schools and School Districts That Have Improved School Foods and Beverages and Not Lost Revenue.* [Online]. Available: http://www.cspinet.org/nutritionpolicy/improved_school_foods_without_losing_revenue2.pdf [accessed November 10, 2005].

Daynard RA, Howard PT, Wilking CL. 2004. Private enforcement: Litigation as a tool to prevent obesity. *J Public Health Policy* 25(3–4):408–417.

DeCicca P, Kenkel D, Mathios A. 2002. Putting out the fires: Will higher taxes reduce the onset of youth smoking? *J Political Economy* 110(1):144–169.

DHHS (U.S. Department of Health and Human Services). 2005a. *Head Start Bureau: Programs and Services.* [Online]. Available: http://www.acf.hhs.gov/programs/hsb/programs/index.htm [accessed October 14, 2005].

DHHS. 2005b. *Office of the Surgeon General.* [Online]. Available: http://www.surgeongeneral.gov/publichealthpriorities.html#schools [accessed October 5, 2005].

DHHS. 2005c. *Small Step.* [Online]. Available: http://www.smallstep.gov [accessed October 7, 2005].

DHHS. 2005d. *Small Step Kids!* [Online]. Available: http://www.smallstep.gov/kids/index.cfm [accessed November 1, 2005].

DHHS. 2005e. *Steps to a Healthier U.S. Initiative.* [Online]. Available: http://www.healthierus.gov/steps/ [accessed November 2, 2005].

DHHS, NIH (National Institutes of Health), NCI (National Cancer Institute). 2005. *Eat 5 to 9 Servings of Fruits and Vegetables a Day for Better Health.* [Online]. Available: http://www.5aday.gov [accessed October 21, 2005].

DHHS, USDA (U.S. Department of Agriculture). 2005. *Dietary Guidelines for Americans 2005.* [Online]. Available: http://www.healthierus.gov/dietaryguidelines [accessed March 28, 2005].

Dorfman L, Wilbur P, Lingas EO, Woodruff K, Wallack L. 2005. *Accelerating Policy on Nutrition: Lessons from Tobacco, Alcohol, Firearms, and Traffic Safety.* Berkeley Media Studies Group. [Online]. Available: http://home.mpowercom.net/~bmsg08/pdfs/BMSG_AccelerationReport.pdf [accessed July 30, 2005].

Duxbury JM, Welch RM. 1999. Agriculture and dietary guidelines. *Food Policy* 24(2–3):197–209.

Eisenberg M, Ringwalt C, Driscoll D, Vallee M, Gullette G. 2004. Learning from truth®: Youth participation in field marketing techniques to counter tobacco advertising. *J Health Commun* 9(3):223–231.

Elliott S, Wilkenfeld JP, Guarino ET, Kolish ED, Jennings CJ, Siegal D. 1981. *FTC Final Staff Report and Recommendation That the Commission Terminate Proceedings for the Promulgation of a Trade Regulation Rule on Children's Advertising.* TRR No. 215-60. Washington, DC: U.S. Federal Trade Commission.

ERS (Economic Research Service). 2002. *Farm Policy. Title IV Nutrition Programs.* [Online]. Available: http://www.ers.usda.gov/Features/farmbill/titles/titleIVnutritionprograms.htm [accessed August 22, 2005].

Evans WD, Finkelstein EA, Kamerow DB, Renaud JM. 2005a. Public perceptions of childhood obesity. *Am J Prev Med* 28(1):26–32.

Evans WD, Price S, Blahut S. 2005b. Evaluating the truth® brand. *J Health Commun* 10(2): 181–192.

Farrelly MC, Davis KC, Haviland ML, Messeri P, Healton CG. 2005. Evidence of a dose-response relationship between "truth" antismoking ads and youth smoking prevalence. *Am J Public Health* 95(3):425–431.

FCC v. Pacifica Foundation, 438 U.S. 726, 731 n.2 (1978).

FDA (U.S. Food and Drug Administration). 1993. Food labeling: Mandatory status of nutrition labeling and nutrient content revisions: Format of nutrition label. Final rule. *Federal Register* 58(3):2079–2205.

FDA. 2005a. Advanced notice of proposed rulemaking: Food labeling: Prominence of calories. *Federal Register* 70(63):17008–17010.

FDA. 2005b. Advanced notice of proposed rulemaking: Food labeling: Serving sizes of products that can reasonably be consumed at one eating occasion: updating of reference amounts customarily consumed: Approaches for recommending smaller portion sizes. *Federal Register* 70(63).

FDA. 2005c. *FDA's Plan to Tackle Obesity.* [Online]. Available: http://www.fda.gov/loseweight/obesity_plan.htm [accessed November 9, 2005].

First National Bank of Boston v. Bellotti, 435 U.S. 765, 783 (1978).

FMI (Food Marketing Institute). 1993. *Shopping for Health: A Report on Diet, Nutrition, and Ethnic Foods.* Washington, DC: FMI.

FMI. 2001. *Shopping for Health: Reaching Out to the Whole Health Consumer.* Washington, DC: FMI.

Foerster SB, Kizer KW, Disogra LK, Bal DG, Krieg BF, Bunch KL. 1995. California's "5 a Day for Better Health!" campaign: An innovative population-based effort to effect large-scale dietary change. *Am J Prev Med* 11(2):124–131.

Ford Motor Company v. Texas Department of Transportation, 264 F.3d 493 (5th Cir. 2001).

Fred Wehrenberg Circuit of Theatres, Inc. v. Moviefone, Inc., 73 F. Supp. 2d 1044 (E.D. Mo. 1999).

Friedman v. Rogers, 440 U.S. 1,12 (1979).

FSA (Food Standards Agency). 2005. *Food Promotions and Children's Diets—Consultation on Nutrient Profiling.* [Online]. Available: http://www.food.gov.uk/foodindustry/Consultations/completed_consultations/completeduk/notprofjuly05 [accessed July 30, 2005].

FTC v. D Squared Solutions, LLC, No. 03-CV-3108 (D. Md. 2003).

FTC v. R. F. Keppel & Brothers, Inc., 291 U.S. 304, 309, 313 (1934).

GAO (U.S. Government Accountability Office). 2003. *School Lunch Program: Efforts Needed to Improve Nutrition and Encourage Healthy Eating.* Report No. GAO-03-506. Washington, DC: U.S. Government Accountability Office.

GAO. 2004. *School Meal Programs: Competitive Foods Are Available in Many Schools; Actions Taken to Restrict Them Differ by State and Locality.* Washington, DC: GAO.

GAO. 2005. *School Meal Programs: Competitive Foods are Widely Available and Generate Substantial Revenues for Schools.* Report No. GAO-05-563. Washington, DC: GAO.

Ginsberg v. New York, 390 U.S. 629, 640, 649–50 (1968).

Gledhill L. 2005, September 16. Governor signs bill to trim obesity in schools. Toughest diet rules in nation for students. *The San Francisco Chronicle*. P. A1.

Goldberg ME. 1990. A quasi-experiment assessing the effectiveness of TV advertising directed to children. *J Marketing Res* 27(4):445–454.

Greater New Orleans Broadcasting Association v. *United States*, 527 U.S. 173, 188 (1999).

Grier S, Bryant CA. 2005. Social marketing in public health. *Annu Rev Public Health* 26: 319–339.

Hartwig M. 2004. *Harkin Enlists Institute of Medicine to Study Foods in Schools. U.S. Senator Tom Harkin of Iowa*, November 24. [Online]. Available: http://harkin.senate.gov/press/print-release.cfm?id=228717 [accessed June 25, 2005].

Hastings G, Stead M, McDermott L, Forsyth A, MacKintosh AM, Rayner M, Godfrey C, Caraher M, Angus K. 2003. *Review of Research on the Effects of Food Promotion to Children*. Glasgow, UK: Centre for Social Marketing.

Hawkes C. 2004. *Marketing Food to Children: The Global Regulatory Environment*. Geneva: World Health Organization.

Hawkes C. 2005. Self-regulation of food advertising: What it can, could and cannot do to discourage unhealthy eating habits among children. *Nutrition Bulletin* 30:374–382.

Hazelwood School District v. *Kuhlmeier*, 484 U.S. 260, 270 (1988).

Hobbs R, Frost R. 2003. Measuring the acquisition of media-literacy skills. *Reading Res Q* 38(3):330–356.

Hoffman Estates v. *Flipside, Hoffman Estates, Inc.*, 455 U.S. 489, 491-92 (1982).

Hornik R, Maklan D, Cadell D, Barmada CH, Jacobsohn L, Henderson VR, Romantan A, Niederdeppe J, Orwin R, Sridharan S, Chu A, Morin C, Taylor K, Steele D. 2003. *Evaluation of the National Youth Anti-Drug Media Campaign: 2003 Report of Findings*. Washington, DC: Westat.

Huhman M, Heitzer C, Wong F. 2004. The *VERB*™ campaign logic model: A tool for planning and evaluation. *Preventing Chronic Disease* 1(3):1–6.

Huhman M, Potter LD, Wong FL, Banspach SW, Duke JC, Heitzler CD. 2005. Effects of a mass media campaign to increase physical activity among children: Year-1 results of the VERB™ campaign. *Pediatrics* 116(2):e277–e284.

Hustler Magazine v. *Falwell*, 485 U.S. 46, 55 (1988).

ICC (International Chamber of Commerce). 1997. *ICC International Code of Advertising Practice*. Commission on Marketing, Advertising, and Distribution. [Online]. Available: http://www.iccwbo.org/home/statements_rules/rules/1997/advercod.asp [accessed May 9, 2005].

ICC. 2002. *ICC International Code of Sales Promotion*. Commission on Marketing and Advertising. [Online]. Available: http://www.iccwbo.org/home/statements_rules/statements/2002/code_of_sales_promotion.asp [accessed May 9, 2005].

ICC. 2003. *ICC International Code on Sponsorship*. Commission on Marketing and Advertising. [Online]. Available: http://www.iccwbo.org/home/statements_rules/rules/2003/International%20Code%20on%20Sponsorship.asp [accessed May 9, 2005].

Interactive Digital Software Association v. *St. Louis County*, 329 F.3d 954, 956–958 (8th Cir. 2003).

International Harvester Company, 104 F.T.C. 949, 1070 (1984).

IOM (Institute of Medicine). 1991. *Improving America's Diet and Health*. Washington, DC: National Academy Press.

IOM. 2003. *Dietary Reference Intakes: Guiding Principles for Nutrition Labeling and Fortification*. Washington, DC: The National Academies Press.

IOM. 2005a. *Preventing Childhood Obesity: Health in the Balance*. Washington, DC: The National Academies Press.

IOM. 2005b. *Nutrition Standards for Foods in Schools*. [Online]. Available: http://www.iom.edu/project.asp?id=30181 [accessed October 20, 2005].

IOM. 2005c. The *WIC Food Package: Time for a Change.* Washington, DC: The National Academies Press.

Jacobson MF, Brownell KD. 2000. Small taxes on soft drinks and snack foods to promote health. *Am J Public Health* 90(6):854–857.

Jones v. N.C. Prisoners' Labor Union, Inc., 433 U.S. 119, 125 (1977).

Keihner A. 2005, May 3. *Trends from the California Children's Healthy Eating and Exercise Practices Survey (1999–2003): Can Statewide Social Marketing Campaigns Impact Fruit and Vegetable Intake and Physical Activity Among 9- to 11-Year-Old Children?* Presented at the 2005 Lecture Series of the University of California Davis Center for Advanced Studies in Nutrition and Social Marketing, Davis, CA.

Keller KL. 1998. Branding perspectives on social marketing. *Advances in Consumer Research* 25:299–302.

KFF (Kaiser Family Foundation). 2003. *Key Facts: Media Literacy.* Menlo Park, CA: The Henry J. Kaiser Family Foundation. [Online]. Available: http://www.kff.org/entmedia/Media-Literacy.cfm [accessed April 12, 2005].

Killen JD, Telch MJ, Robinson TN, Maccoby N, Taylor CB, Farquhar JW. 1988. Cardiovascular disease risk reduction for tenth graders: A multiple-factor school-based approach. *J Am Med Assoc* 260(12):1728–1733.

Kraak V, Pelletier D. 1998. How marketers reach young consumers: Implications for nutrition education and health promotion campaigns. *Fam Econ Nutr Review* 11(4):31–41.

Kraft, Inc. v. FTC, 970 F.2d 311, 314 (7th Cir. 1992).

Kuchler F, Tegene A, Harris JM. 2004. Taxing snack foods: What to expect for diet and tax revenues. Agriculture Info Bull No. 747-08. Economic Research Service, U.S. Department of Agriculture. [Online]. Available: http://www.ers.usda.gov/publications/aib747/aib74708.pdf [accessed July 12, 2005].

Kuchler F, Golan E, Variyam JN, Crutchfield SR. 2005. Obesity policy and the law of unintended consequences. *Amber Waves* 3(3):26–33.

Lebel E, Hamelin AM, Lavallée M, Bedard A, Dubé A. 2005. Publicité télévisée sur les aliments visant les enfants: Valeurs nutritionnelles et culturelles. *Communication* 24(1): 65–84.

Lefebvre C. 1992. Social marketing and health promotion. In: Bunton R, MacDonald G, eds. *Healthy Promotion: Disciplines and Diversity.* London, UK: Routledge.

Lefebvre RC, Lurie D, Saunders Goodman L, Weinberg L, Loughrey K. 1995. Social marketing and nutrition education: Inappropriate or misunderstood? *J Nutr Ed* 27(3):146–150.

Lorillard Tobacco Company v. Reilly, 533 US 525, 121 (S. Ct. 2404, 2001).

MacCarthy C. 2004, June 8. Lean pickings for the anti-ad brigade Sweden is using these European elections to try to extend its kids advertising ban across the EU. But just how effective is it? *The Financial Times.* P.10.

Mainstream Marketing Services, Inc. v. FTC, 358 F.3d 1228 (10th Cir. 2004).

Mattern J, Neighbors C. 2004. Social norms campaigns: Examining the relationship between changes in perceived norms and changes in drinking levels. *J Stud Alcohol* 65(4): 489–493.

Matthews A, Cowburn G, Rayner M, Longfield J, Powell C. 2005. *The Marketing of Unhealthy Food to Children in Europe. A Report of Phase 1 of the Children, Obesity and Associated Avoidable Chronic Diseases Project.* Brussels: European Heart Network.

McConnell v. FEC, 540 U.S. 93, 237 (2003).

Morris J, Zidenberg-Cherr S. 2002. Garden-enhanced nutrition curriculum improves fourth-grade school children's knowledge of nutrition and preferences for some vegetables. *J Am Diet Assoc* 102(1):91–93.

National Bakers Services, Inc. v. FTC, 329 F.2d 365 (7th Cir. 1964).

National Food Administration and National Institute of Public Health. 2005. *Background Material to the Action Plan for Healthy Dietary Habits and Increased Physical Activity.* Stockholm, Sweden: National Food Administration.

NCES (National Center for Education Statistics). 1996. *Nutrition Education in Public Elementary and Secondary Schools.* Report No. NCES 96-852. Washington, DC: U.S. Department of Education, Office of Educational Research and Improvement.

NCSL (National Conference of State Legislatures). 2005, March 1. *Vending Machines in Schools.* [Online]. Available: http://www.ncsl.org/programs/health/vending.htm [accessed June 6, 2005].

Nestlé Food Company, 115 F.T.C. 67 (1992).

Ngo J. 1993. Social marketing and fat intake. *Eur J Clin Nutr* 47(suppl):S91–S95.

NIDA (National Institute on Drug Abuse). 2002. *Evaluation of the National Youth Anti-Drug Media Campaign.* Westat & the Annenberg School for Communication. [Online]. Available: http://www.nida.nih.gov/DESPR/Westat/exec_summ2.html [accessed June 28, 2005].

Niederdeppe J, Farrelly MC, Haviland ML. 2004. Confirming "truth": More evidence of a successful tobacco countermarketing campaign in Florida. *Am J Public Health* 94(2): 255–257.

NIH (National Institutes of Health). 2005a. *Milk Matters.* [Online]. Available: http://www.nichd.nih.gov/milk/ [accessed October 12, 2005].

NIH. 2005b. *We Can!* [Online]. Available: http://www.nhlbi.nih.gov/health/public/heart/obesity/wecan/ [accessed October 10, 2005].

Nordic Consumer Ombudsmen. 2002. *Position Statement of the Nordic Consumer Ombudsmen on E-commerce and Marketing on the Internet.* [Online]. Available: http://www.konsumentverket.se/Documents/in_english/nordic_statement_ecommerce_2002.pdf [accessed May 10, 2005].

Norwegian Ministry of Children and Family Affairs. 2005. *The Norwegian Action Plan to Reduce Commercial Pressure on Children and the Young People.* [Online]. Available: http://odin.dep.no/bfd/english/doc/handbooks/004061-990036/dok-bn.html [accessed May 30, 2005].

NRC (National Research Council) and IOM. 2003. *Reducing Underage Drinking: A Collective Responsibility.* Washington, DC: The National Academies Press.

NSW Centre for Public Health Nutrition. 2005. *Best Options for Promoting Healthy Weight and Preventing Weight Gain in NSW.* [Online]. Available: http://www.cphn.biochem.usyd.edu.au/resources/FinalHealthyWeightreport160305.pdf [accessed June 23, 2005].

Ofcom (Office of Communications). 2004. *Childhood Obesity—Food Advertising in Context. Children's Food Choices, Parents' Understanding and Influence, and the Role of Food Promotion.* London, UK: Ofcom.

Ofcom. 2005. *Rules on the Amount and Distribution of Advertising.* Ofcom. [Online]. Available: http://www.ofcom.org.uk/tv/ifi/codes/advertising/rules/rules.pdf [accessed May 10, 2005].

ONDCP (Office of National Drug Control Policy). 2003. *About the Campaign. Campaign Design.* [Online]. Available: http://www.mediacampaign.org/about/brochure/design.html [accessed November 14, 2005].

ONDCP. 2005. *National Youth Anti-Drug Media Campaign.* [Online]. Available: http://www.mediacampaign.org/ and http://www.freevibe.com/#/ [accessed June 28, 2005].

PBH (Produce for Better Health Foundation). 2005a. *5 a Day Mission & History.* [Online]. Available: http://www.5aday.com/html/background/mission.php [accessed November 11, 2005].

PBH. 2005b. *National Action Plan to Promote Health Through Increased Fruit and Vegetable Consumption.* Wilmington, DE: PBH.

PDFA (Partnership for a Drug-Free America). 2005. [Online]. Available: http://www. drugfree.org/Portal/About/AnnualReport/Download_the_2001-2002_Annual_Report/ [accessed November 14, 2005].

Peel v. Attorney Registration and Disciplinary Commission, 496 U.S. 91, 110 (1990).

Pelletier DL, Kendall A, Kettel Khan L, Mathios A. 1999. Nutrition and dairy industry benefits associated with promoting lowfat milk: Evidence from the 1989 CSFII. *Fam Econ Nutr Rev* 12(1):3–13.

Pelman v. McDonald's Corporation, 237 F. Supp. 2d 512, 532–533 (S.D.N.Y. 2003).

People v. Block & Kleaver, Inc., 427 N.Y.S.2d 133 (N.Y. Co. Ct. 1980).

Perry CL, Silvis GL. 1987. Smoking prevention: Behavioral prescriptions for the pediatrician. *Pediatrics* 79(5):790–799.

Phone Programs, Inc. 115 F.T.C. 977 (1992).

Posadas de Puerto Rico Associates v. Tourism Company, 478 U.S. 328 (1986).

Potter LD, Duke JC, Nolin MJ, Judkins D, Huhman M. 2004. *Evaluation of the CDC VERB Campaign: Findings from the Youth Media Campaign Longitudinal Survey, 2002–2003.* Rockville, MD: WESTAT.

Quebec Consumer Protection Act. 2005. *Consumer Protection Act. RSQ, Chapter P-40.* P-40.1 A. [Online]. Available: http://www2.publicationsduquebec.gouv.qc.ca/home.php# [accessed May 10, 2005].

Quebec Government. 1980. *Consumer Protection Act. RSQ, Chapter P-40.* P-40 A. [Online]. Available: http://www2.publicationsduquebec.gouv.qc.ca/home.php# [accessed June 6, 2005].

Ralston K. 1999. How government policies and regulations can affect dietary choices. In: Frazao E, ed. *America's Eating Habits: Changes and Consequences.* Agriculture Information Bulletin No. 750. Washington, DC: U.S. Department of Agriculture.

Ratner EM, Hellegers JF, Stern GP, Ogg RC, Adair S, Zacharias L. 1978. *FTC Staff Report on Television Advertising to Children.* Washington, DC: Federal Trade Commission.

Red Lion Broadcasting Company v. FCC, 395 U.S. 367, 386 (1969).

Reno v. American Civil Liberties Union, 521 U.S. 844, 875 (1997).

Rideout V. 2004. *Parents, Media and Public Policy: A Kaiser Family Foundation Survey.* Menlo Park, CA: Henry J. Kaiser Family Foundation.

Rubin v. Coors Brewing Company, 514 U.S. 476 (1995).

RWJF (The Robert Wood Johnson Foundation). 2003. *Active Living: Healthy Schools for Healthy Kids.* Princeton, NJ: RWJF.

Sable Communications, Inc. v. FCC, 492 U.S. 115, 126 (1989).

Samuels SE. 1993. Project LEAN—Lessons learned from a national social marketing campaign. *Public Health Reports* 108(1):45–53.

Smed S, Jensen JD, Denver S. 2005. *Differentiated Food Taxes as a Tool in Health and Nutrition Policy.* Frederiksberg, Denmark: Food and Resource Economics Institute.

Social Marketing Institute. 2005. *Success Stories. National WIC Breastfeeding Promotion Project.* [Online]. Available: http://www.social-marketing.org/success/cs-nationalwic.html [accessed June 23, 2005].

Southwestern Bell Telephone, L.P. v. Moline, 333 F. Supp. 2d 1073 (D. Kan. 2004).

Stables GJ, Subar AF, Patterson BH, Dodd K, Heimendinger J, Van Duyn MA, Nebeling L. 2002. Changes in vegetable and fruit consumption and awareness among US adults: Results of the 1991 and 1997 5 a Day for Better Health Program surveys. *J Am Diet Assoc* 102(6):809–817.

Swinburn B, Egger G. 2002. Preventive strategies against weight gain and obesity. *Obesity Rev* 3(4):289–301.

Swix v. Daisy Manufacturing Company, 373 F.3d 678, 685-87 (6th Cir. 2004).

TFAH (Trust for America's Health). 2005. *F as in Fat: How Obesity Policies Are Failing America*. [Online]. Available: http://healthyamericans.org/reports/obesity2005/ Obesity2005Report.pdf [accessed October 15, 2005].

The Isaly Klondike Company, 116 F.T.C. 74 (1993).

The Wall Street Journal Online and Harris Interactive. 2005. *Most of the American Public, Including a Majority of Parents, Believe That Childhood Obesity in the U.S. Is a Major Problem*. [Online]. Available: http://www.harrisinteractive.com/news/newsletters/ wsjhealthnews/WSJOnline_HI_Health-CarePoll2005vol4_iss03.pdf [accessed June 15, 2005].

Thompson v. Western States Medical Center, 535 U.S. 357, 367-68 (2002).

Thornburgh v. Abbott, 490 U.S. 401 (1988).

Tillotson JE. 2004. America's obesity: Conflicting public policies, industrial economic development, and unintended human consequences. *Annu Rev Nutr* 24:617–643.

Tinker v. Des Moines Independent School District, 393 U.S. 503 (1969).

Trans Union, LLC v. FTC, 295 F.3d 42 (D.C. Cir. 2002).

Transportation Alternatives, Inc. v. City of New York, 218 F. Supp. 2d 423 (S.D.N.Y. 2002).

Turner v. Safley, 482 U.S. 78 (1987).

TWFD (Television Without Frontiers Directive). 2005. *The European Commission Regulatory Framework*. [Online]. Available: http://europa.eu.int/comm/avpolicy/regul/regul_ en.htm#2 [accessed October 24, 2005].

United States v. Edge Broadcasting Company, 509 U.S. 418, 434 (1993).

United States v. Jorgensen, 144 F.3d 550 (8th Cir. 1998).

USDA (U.S. Department of Agriculture). 2000. *Changing the Scene—Improving the School Nutrition Environment*. Team Nutrition. [Online]. Available: http://www.fns.usda.gov/ tn/Resources/changing.html [accessed June 16, 2005].

USDA. 2002a. Amendments to the child nutrition infant meal patterns. Final rule. *Federal Register* 67(102):36779–36788.

USDA. 2002b. *School Lunch Salad Bars*. Nutrition Assistance Program Report Series. Food and Nutrition Service. CN-02-SB. Alexandria, VA: USDA.

USDA. 2002c. *School Meals: Foods of Minimal Nutritional Value*. Appendix B of 7 CFR Part 210. [Online]. Available: http://www.fns.usda.gov/cnd/menu/fmnv.htm [accessed June 15, 2005].

USDA. 2004a. *HealthierUS School Challenge*. [Online]. Available: http://www.fns.usda.gov/ tn/HealthierUS/index.html [accessed October 6, 2005].

USDA. 2004b. *Team Nutrition Demonstration Project 1999–2002*. Executive Summary. [Online]. Available: http://www.fns.usda.gov/oane/MENU/Published/Nutrition Education/Files/TNDP99-03.htm [accessed October 6, 2005].

USDA. 2004c. *Excerpt from P.L. 108-265 Child Nutrition and WIC Reauthorization Act of 2004*. [Online]. Available: http://schoolmeals.nal.usda.gov/Training/CO_Middle_School_ Marketing/1-2004_Middle_School_Marketing_Memos_and_Notices/WellnessPolicy Requirement.pdf [accessed June 15, 2005].

USDA. 2004d. *Local Wellness Policy*. Team Nutrition. [Online]. Available: http://www. fns.usda.gov/tn/Healthy/wellnesspolicy.html [accessed June 15, 2005].

USDA. 2005a. *Eat Smart, Play Hard™ Campaign. Campaign Overview*. [Online]. Available: http://www.fns.usda.gov/eatsmartplayhard/About/overview.html [accessed October 4, 2005].

USDA. 2005b. *Food and Nutrition Service, Nutrition Program Facts, National School Lunch Program*. [Online]. Available: http://www.fns.usda.gov/cnd/lunch/AboutLunch/ NSLPFactSheet.pdf [accessed March 24, 2005].

USDA. 2005c. *Food and Nutrition Service, Nutrition Program Facts, The School Breakfast Program*. [Online]. Available: http://www.fns.usda.gov/cnd/Breakfast/AboutBFast/ FactSheet.pdf [accessed November 9, 2005].

USDA. 2005d. *Food Stamp Program*. [Online]. Available: http://www.fns.usda.gov/fsp [accessed November 9, 2005].

USDA. 2005e. *MyPyramid: For Kids*. [Online]. Available: http://www.mypyramid.gov/kids/index.html [accessed July 6, 2005].

USDA. 2005f. *MyPyramid: Steps to a Healthier You*. [Online]. Available: http://www.mypyramid.gov [accessed April 25, 2005].

USDA. 2005g. *School Meals: Child Nutrition Labeling*. Washington, DC: USDA Food and Nutrition Service. [Online]. Available: http://www.fns.usda.gov/cnd/CNlabeling/default.htm [accessed July 13, 2005].

USDA. 2005h. Submission for OMB review: Comment request. Food and Nutrition Service. Child nutrition labeling program. *Federal Register* 70(82):22293.

USDA. 2005i. *The Food Assistance Landscape, March 2005*. Food Assistance and Nutrition Research Report No. 28-6. Washington, DC: USDA.

Valentine v. Chrestensen, 316 U.S. 52, 54 (1942).

Vallianatos M. 2005. *Healthy School Food Policies: A Checklist*. A working paper of the Center for Food and Justice, Urban and Environmental Policy Institute. Urban and Environmental Policy Institute. [Online]. Available: http://departments.oxy.edu/uepi/cfj/resources/healthy_school_food_policies_05.pdf [accessed June 14, 2005].

Viacom International. 2005. *Welcome to Postopia!* [Online]. Available: http://www.postopia.com [accessed July 9, 2005].

Video Software Dealers Association v. Maleng, 325 F. Supp. 2d 1180, 1184-85 (W.D. Wash. 2004).

Virginia State Board of Pharmacy v. Virginia Citizens Consumer Council, Inc., 425 U.S. 748 (1976).

Wallack L, Dorfman L, Jernigan D, Themba M. 1993. *Media Advocacy and Public Health: Power for Prevention*. Newbury Park, CA: Sage Publications.

Wansink B, Huckabee H. 2005. De-marketing obesity. *California Management Review* 47(4): 6–18.

Warner KE. 2005. Tobacco policy in the United States: Lessons learned for the obesity epidemic. In: Mechanic D, Rogut LB, Colby DC, Knickman JR, eds. *Policy Challenges in Modern Health Care*. New Brunswick, NJ: Rutgers University Press. Pp. 99–114.

WHO. 2004. *Global Strategy on Diet, Physical Activity, and Health*. WHA 57.17. Geneva: WHO. [Online]. Available: http://www.who.int/gb/ebwha/pdf_files/WHA57/A57_R17-en.pdf [accessed May 10, 2005].

Williams v. Spencer, 622 F.2d 1200, 1205 (4th Cir. 1980).

Williams JD, Kumanyika SK. 2002. Is social marketing an effective tool to reduce health disparities? *Social Market Q* 8(4):14–31.

Wilson v. Midway Games, 198 F. Supp. 2d 167, 181 (D. Conn. 2002).

Wong F, Huhman M, Heitzler C, Asbury L, Bretthauer-Mueller R, McCarthy S, Londe P. 2004. VERB™—A social marketing campaign to increase physical activity among youth. *Preventing Chronic Disease* 1(3):1–7.

Wootan MG, Reger-Nash B, Booth-Butterfield S, Cooper L. 2005. The cost-effectiveness of *1% or Less* media campaigns promoting low-fat milk consumption. *Preventing Chronic Disease* 2(4):1–10.

Yach D, Hawkes C, Epping-Jordan J, Galbraith S. 2003. The World Health Organization's Framework Convention on Tobacco Control: Implications for global epidemics of food-related deaths and disease. *J Public Health Policy* 24(3–4):274–290.

Yach D, McKee M, Lopez AD, Novotny T. 2005. Improving diet and physical activity: 12 lessons from controlling tobacco smoking. *Br Med J* 330(7496):898–900.

Zywicki TJ, Holt D, Ohlhausen M. 2004. *Obesity and Advertising Policy*. Law and Economics Working Paper Series. George Mason Law and Economics Research Paper No. 04-45.

7

Findings, Recommendations, Next Steps

Food and beverage marketing to children and youth has become ubiquitous on the American landscape. Although recent public announcements by some companies suggest an interest in change, the preponderance of the foods and beverages introduced and marketed to children and youth have been high in total calories, added sugars, salt, fat, and low in nutrients.

Multiple influences interact to shape the food preferences and choices, eating behaviors, total calorie intake, diet quality, and health outcomes of children and youth. There is evidence that commercial advertising and marketing of foods and beverages to children and youth through a growing variety of channels and media outlets—including the mass media, schools, child-care settings, grocery stores, shopping malls, theaters, sporting events, and even airports—are notable contributors to the environments in which the nutritional patterns of children and youth evolve.

This report has summarized the status and trends in the health, diet, and eating patterns of children and youth; reviewed the various factors that influence the food and beverage consumption habits of children and youth; described how food and beverages are developed and marketed to children and youth; systematically reviewed the evidence on the influence of food and beverage marketing on the diets and diet-related health of children and youth; and described the policy instruments that may be combined to enhance availability and access to healthful foods and to support healthful food and beverage choices and marketing practices affecting children and youth. This chapter summarizes the findings included throughout the report and offers recommendations on ways in which various sectors could help improve the diets and health of children and youth.

BOX 7-1
Broad Conclusions

- Along with many other intersecting factors, food and beverage marketing influences the diets and health prospects of children and youth.

- Food and beverage marketing practices geared to children and youth are out of balance with healthful diets, and contribute to an environment that puts their health at risk.

- Food and beverage companies, restaurants, and marketers have underutilized potential to devote creativity and resources to develop and promote food, beverages, and meals that support healthful diets for children and youth.

- Achieving healthful diets for children and youth will require sustained, multisectoral, and integrated efforts that include industry leadership and initiative.

- Public policy programs and incentives do not currently have the support or authority to address many of the current and emerging marketing practices that influence the diets of children and youth.

Overall, the committee identified five broad conclusions (Box 7-1), derived from the individual findings. These serve as the basis for the committee's recommendations.

HEALTH, DIET, AND EATING PATTERNS OF CHILDREN AND YOUTH

Health-related behaviors such as eating habits and physical activity patterns develop early in life and often extend into adulthood. A healthful and balanced diet provides recommended amounts of nutrients and other food components to promote normal growth and development, reduce chronic disease risk, and foster appropriate energy balance and a healthy weight. In order to develop eating habits that will have health-promoting benefits that carry them into adulthood, children and adolescents need to consume more fruits, vegetables, whole grains, and dairy products, and moderate their intakes of high-calorie and low-nutrient foods and beverages. The committee's review in Chapter 2 of the health, diet, and eating patterns of children and youth identified several issues and trends.

- More certain determinations of nutritional requirements for children and adolescents await the development of better techniques and data sets.

- More accurate methods are needed to assess the dietary intakes of children and youth, including calorie intakes and expenditures.
- Total calorie intake appears to have increased substantially over the past 25 years for preschool children and adolescent boys and girls, with more modest changes for children ages 6–11 years.
- Children and youth consume a large proportion of their total calories from foods and beverages that are of high-calorie and low-nutrient content.
- Carbohydrate intake has increased substantially among children and youth over approximately the past two decades.
- Total fat and saturated fat intakes among children and youth remain at levels that exceed dietary recommendations.
- Most preschool children consume added sugars well above suggested limits, and older children and adolescents consume about double the suggested limit of added sugars in their diet.
- Mean sodium intake of children and youth has increased over the past 35 years, and the majority of children and adolescents are consuming sodium in greater amounts than recommended levels.
- Over the past decade, most children and youth have not met the daily recommended servings for vegetables, fruits, or whole grains.
- Sweetened beverage consumption (e.g., carbonated soft drinks and fruit drinks) by children and adolescents has increased considerably over the past 35 years and is now a leading source of added sugars, especially in adolescents' diets. The consumption of milk, a major source of dietary calcium, has decreased among children and adolescents over the same period, and most have calcium intakes below the recommended adequate intake level.
- Breakfast consumption by children and adolescents has decreased considerably over the past 40 years and the occurrence of breakfast consumption declines with age. The frequency of breakfast consumption is predictive of lower body mass index (BMI) levels in children and adolescents.
- The prevalence of snacking and number of snacking occasions by children and youth have increased steadily over the past 25 years. There has been a steady increase in the proportion of calories that children and youth have received from away-from-home foods over the past 20 years. Approximately one-third or more of their calories are derived from foods purchased outside of the home, nearly one-half of which is obtained at restaurants and quick serve restaurants that contain higher fat content than food consumed at home.
- Calorie intake by infants and toddlers substantially exceeds their estimated requirements, although validation is needed on the reliability of food intake reporting by parents and caregivers, as well as on body weight estimates.

• Infants and toddlers are consuming diets disproportionately high in sweetened foods and beverages and fried potatoes, and disproportionately low in green leafy vegetables.

• Certain subgroups, such as low-income and minority children and adolescent girls, have inadequate dietary intakes of specific micronutrients (e.g., vitamins D and B_6, folate, iron, zinc, and magnesium).

FACTORS SHAPING FOOD AND BEVERAGE CONSUMPTION OF CHILDREN AND YOUTH

Children's dietary patterns and related health prospects are shaped by the interplay of many factors—genetics and biology, culture and values, economic status, physical and social environments, and commercial and media environments—all of which, apart from genetic predispositions, have undergone significant transformations over the past three decades. Interactions within and among these contexts affect behavior. The committee took an ecological perspective in assessing the processes and context of the influences shaping children's eating behaviors, identifying in Chapter 3 several broad issues relevant to child and adolescent eating behaviors and food and beverage choices.

• Food preferences develop as early as 2–3 years of age and are shaped by a child's early experiences, positive or negative conditioning, exposure to foods, and a biological predisposition to prefer sweet, high-fat, and salty foods.

• The availability and marketing of foods and beverages of larger portion sizes has increased steadily over the past three decades in many venues.

• Children are aware of food brands as young as 2–3 years of age and preschoolers demonstrate brand recognition when cued by spokescharacters and colored packages. The majority of children's food requests are for branded products. Brand loyalty is highest in teens for carbonated soft drinks and quick serve restaurants.

FOOD AND BEVERAGE MARKETING TO CHILDREN AND YOUTH

In multiple forms, media influences have assumed a central socializing role for children and youth. As media pervasiveness has grown in influence, so has its use for the marketing of branded food and beverage products. The substantial investment in commercial advertising and marketing of foods and beverages directed to children and youth over the past several decades has spawned a sizable and sophisticated marketing research enterprise to help companies translate desires and preferences into branded products and purchases for and by children and youth, making them a primary focus of food and beverage marketing initiatives. Last year an estimated more than $10 billion per year was spent for all types of food and beverage marketing to children and youth in America. The committee's review of food and beverage marketing to children and youth in Chapter 4 identified several key findings.

- Marketing research can provide important insights about how marketing techniques might help improve the diets of children and youth. Yet, much of the relevant marketing research on the profile and impact of food and beverage marketing to children and youth is currently unavailable to the public, including for use in designing and targeting efforts to improve the diets of children and youth.
- Children and youth ages 4–17 years have increasing discretionary income and purchasing capacity, are being targeted more directly by marketers, and frequently spend their discretionary income on high-calorie and low-nutrient foods and beverages.
- Child-targeted food and beverage products have steadily increased over the past decade, and are typically high in total calories, sugars, salt, fat, and low in nutrients.
- Television is the primary promotional medium for measured media marketing of food and beverage products to children and youth, but a notable shift is occurring toward unmeasured sales promotion (e.g., product placement, character licensing, in-school marketing, special event marketing).
- The use of child-oriented licensed cartoon and other fictional or real-life spokescharacters has been a prevalent practice used to promote low-nutrient and high-calorie food and beverage products. Use of such characters to promote more healthful foods, particularly for preschoolers, is relatively recent.
- Children are exposed to extensive advertising for high-calorie and low-nutrient foods and beverages and very limited advertising of healthful foods and beverages during their daily television viewing.
- The competitive multifaceted marketing of high-calorie and low-nutrient food and beverage products in school settings is widely prevalent and appears to have increased steadily over the past decade.
- Food and beverage marketing is increasingly delivered through integrated vehicles other than the traditional television advertising (e.g., Internet, event sponsorships, outdoor media, kid's clubs, video games, advergames, product placement, music, and schools) that are especially appealing to children and youth.

• Efforts by the Children's Advertising Review Unit (CARU)—*the children's arm of the advertising industry's self-regulation program for child-directed advertising and promotion in media*—have influenced certain elements of traditional advertising within its designated purview, but these standards do not address the impact of the volume of advertising, the appeal of its association with other elements of the popular culture for children and youth, or the influences of rapidly increasing marketing approaches. Furthermore, there is a need for a more formal evaluation of the effectiveness of CARU's impact and enforcement capacity.

• The consistency, accuracy, and effectiveness of the proprietary logos or icons introduced by several food companies as positive steps to communicate the nutritional qualities of some of their branded products to consumers have not been evaluated. Without an empirically validated industry-wide rating system and approach, efforts to use such graphic portrayals on food labels may fall short of their potential as guides to better food and beverage choices by children, youth, and their parents.

• Certain food and beverage companies and quick serve restaurants with products prominently consumed by children are actively exploring more balanced and health-promoting product development and marketing strategies. Prevailing industry practices, guidelines, and efforts remain limited.

• The food retail sector has taken some steps to promote healthful products to young consumers and their families, but there are abundant opportunities to do more to promote child-oriented foods and beverages that are healthful, visually accessible, and economically affordable.

INFLUENCE OF FOOD AND BEVERAGE MARKETING ON THE DIETS AND DIET-RELATED HEALTH OF CHILDREN AND YOUTH

The prevalence of obesity in children and youth has occurred in parallel with significant changes in the U.S. media and marketing environments. This relationship has prompted the committee's primary inquiry about the influence of food and beverage marketing on the diets and health of American children and youth. The committee's review of the published, peer-reviewed literature in Chapter 5 indicates that, among many factors, food and beverage marketing influences the preferences and purchase requests of children, influences consumption at least in the short term, is a likely contributor to less healthful diets, and may contribute to negative diet-related health outcomes and risks among children and youth. The literature indicates a relationship among marketing, dietary precursors, diets, diet-related health, and, in particular, adiposity (body fatness).

Specifically, the committee's systematic evidence review found that:

With respect to *dietary precursors*, food and beverage advertising on television has some influence on the preferences and purchase requests of children and youth:

• There is strong evidence that television advertising influences the food and beverage preferences of children ages 2–11 years. There is insufficient evidence about its influence on the preferences of teens ages 12–18 years.

• There is strong evidence that television advertising influences the food and beverage purchase requests of children ages 2–11 years. There is insufficient evidence about its influence on the purchase requests of teens ages 12–18 years.

• There is moderate evidence that television advertising influences the food and beverage beliefs of children ages 2–11 years. There is insufficient evidence about its influence on the beliefs of teens ages 12–18 years.

• Given the findings from the systematic evidence review of the influence of marketing on the precursors of diet, and given the evidence from content analyses that the preponderance of television food and beverage advertising relevant to children and youth promotes high-calorie and low-nutrient products, it can be concluded that television advertising influences children to prefer and request high-calorie and low-nutrient foods and beverages.

With respect to *diets*, food and beverage advertising on television has some influence on the dietary intake of children and youth:

• There is strong evidence that television advertising influences the short-term consumption of children ages 2–11 years. There is insufficient evidence about its influence on the short-term consumption of teens ages 12–18 years.

• There is moderate evidence that television advertising influences the usual dietary intake of younger children ages 2–5 years and weak evidence that it influences the usual dietary intake of older children ages 6–11 years. There is also weak evidence that it does *not* influence the usual dietary intake of teens ages 12–18 years.

With respect to *diet-related health*, food and beverage advertising on television is associated with the adiposity (body fatness) of children and youth:

• Statistically, there is strong evidence that exposure to television advertising is associated with adiposity in children ages 2–11 years and teens ages 12–18 years.

• The association between adiposity and exposure to television advertising remains after taking alternative explanations into account, but the research does not convincingly rule out other possible explanations for the association; therefore, the current evidence is not sufficient to arrive at any finding about a causal relationship from television advertising to adiposity. It is important to note that even a small influence, aggregated over the entire population of American children and youth, would be consequential in impact.

- Most children ages 8 years and under do not effectively comprehend the persuasive intent of marketing messages, and most children ages 4 years and under cannot consistently discriminate between television advertising and programming. The evidence is currently insufficient to determine whether or not this meaningfully alters the ways in which food and beverage marketing messages influence children.

- New research is needed on food and beverage marketing and its impact on diet and diet-related health and on improving measurement strategies for factors involved centrally in this research. Much of this research must be interdisciplinary and fairly large-scale in nature, although some highly-focused small-scale research is also desirable. Among the specific research needed are studies of newer promotion techniques, newer venues, and healthier products and portion sizes.

PUBLIC POLICY ISSUES IN FOOD AND BEVERAGE MARKETING TO CHILDREN AND YOUTH

Various public policies and actions at the federal, state, and local levels have been considered, implemented, or are in process to help improve the diets of children and youth. The committee reviewed efforts by government at the federal, state, and local levels to improve education and information to better inform the nutritional choices for children and youth; initiatives to enhance the influence that schools have on the nutritional status of students and their families; and the potential of social marketing as a means of improving dietary patterns and practices. It also surveyed the legal context for policies and regulations related to advertising and marketing. This review in Chapter 6 found a number of opportunities for improvement.

- A number of positive steps have been taken by the Food and Drug Administration to improve food and beverage labeling as a means of conveying helpful information to enable healthier choices, including exploration of ways to expand the provision of such information on menus and packaging in quick serve and full serve family restaurants. Still, the reach and effectiveness of such efforts—by the U.S. Food and Drug Administration (FDA), industry, and the two together—are far short of what they could or should be to provide children, youth, and their parents with the information they need, using consistent standards and graphics that are easily understood and engaging.

• National standards do not exist for the use or marketing of competitive foods and beverages in school settings or after-school venues such as in child-care settings. Cooperative initiative by the U.S. Department of Agriculture and the Department of Education has been limited in shaping policies and approaches related to healthier food and beverage promotion in schools.

• Evidence for the effectiveness of social marketing programs to promote healthful behaviors is promising but mixed. Programs with the most positive results have had higher funding, been more sustained, been shaped by formative research, deployed an integrated marketing approach, and used ongoing monitoring and evaluation. These characteristics are the likely requirements for achievement of successful social marketing programs to improve the diets of children and youth.

• Regulations for those who advertise and market food and beverage products to children will need to evolve as the food industry develops new techniques for promoting its products. How current law will be applied to rapidly changing areas like the Internet cannot currently be predicted with confidence. However, future regulatory interventions should certainly be taken on the basis of reliable data concerning the impacts on children of the marketing and advertising of food and beverage products. Currently, neither the Federal Trade Commission, nor any other responsible federal agency, collects or maintains such data.

• Comprehensive evaluations are not available to assess the effect on children's diets of countrywide bans on child-directed television advertising. Limited evidence suggests that national borders may not serve as effective barriers to children's broadcast media and advertising where it is common to receive broadcasts from outside the receiving countries.

RECOMMENDATIONS

Reflective of the responsibilities of multiple sectors, the committee's recommendations address actions related to food and beverage production, processing, packaging, and sales; marketing practice standards; media initiatives; parents, caregivers, and families; school environments; and public policy. Recommendations are also offered for research activities necessary to chart the path of future improvements, and the monitoring capacity to track improvements in marketing practices and their influence on children's and youths' diets and health. These recommendations reflect the current context and information in a rapidly changing environment, and should be implemented together as a package to support and complement one another.

Food and Beverage Production and Promotion

Central to making progress toward more healthful diets for children and youth will be carefully designed and sustained commitments by the food, beverage, and quick serve restaurant industries to promote the availability, accessibility, affordability, and appeal of nutritious foods and beverages.

Recommendation 1: *Food and beverage companies should use their creativity, resources, and full range of marketing practices to promote and support more healthful diets for children and youth.*

To implement this recommendation, companies should
- Shift their product portfolios in a direction that promotes new and reformulated child- and youth-oriented foods and beverages that are substantially lower in total calories, lower in fats, salt, and added sugars, and higher in nutrient content.
- Shift their advertising and marketing emphasis to child- and youth-oriented foods and beverages that are substantially lower in total calories, lower in fats, salt, and added sugars, and higher in nutrient content (see later recommendations on public policy and monitoring).
- Work with government, scientific, public health, and consumer groups to develop and implement labels and advertising for an empirically validated industrywide rating system and graphic representation that is appealing to children and youth to convey the nutritional quality of foods and beverages marketed to them and their families.
- Engage the full range of their marketing vehicles and venues to develop and promote healthier appealing and affordable foods and beverages for children and youth.

Recommendation 2: *Full serve restaurant chains, family restaurants, and quick serve restaurants should use their creativity, resources, and full range of marketing practices to promote healthful meals for children and youth.*

To implement this recommendation, restaurants should
- Expand and actively promote healthier food, beverage, and meal options for children and youth.
- Provide calorie content and other key nutrition information, as possible, on menus and packaging that is prominently visible at the point of choice and use.

Recommendation 3: *Food, beverage, restaurant, retail, and marketing industry trade associations should assume transforming leadership roles in harnessing industry creativity, resources, and marketing on behalf of healthful diets for children and youth.*

To implement this recommendation, trade associations should
- Encourage member initiatives and compliance to develop, apply, and enforce industrywide food and beverage marketing practice standards that support healthful diets for children and youth.
- Provide technical assistance, encouragement, and support for members' efforts to emphasize the development and marketing of healthier foods, beverages, and meals for children and youth.
- Exercise leadership in working with their members to improve the availability and selection of healthful foods and beverages accessible at eye level and reach for children, youth, and their parents in grocery stores and other food retail environments.
- Work to foster collaboration and support with public-sector initiatives promoting healthful diets for children and youth.

Marketing Practice Standards

A reliable barometer of the commitment of the members of the food, beverage, and restaurant industries to promote the nutritional health of children and youth will be the rigor of the standards they set and enforce for their own marketing practices.

Recommendation 4: *The food, beverage, restaurant, and marketing industries should work with government, scientific, public health, and consumer groups to establish and enforce the highest standards for the marketing of foods, beverages, and meals to children and youth.*

To implement this recommendation, the cooperative efforts should
- Work through the Children's Advertising Review Unit (CARU) to revise, expand, apply, enforce, and evaluate explicit industry self-regulatory guidelines beyond traditional advertising to include evolving vehicles and venues for marketing communication (e.g., the Internet, advergames, branded product placement across multiple media).
- Assure that licensed characters are used only for the promotion of foods and beverages that support healthful diets for children and youth.
- Foster cooperation between CARU and the Federal Trade Commission in evaluating and enforcing the effectiveness of the expanded self-regulatory guidelines.

Media and Entertainment Initiatives

Because no element of the lives of Americans has a broader reach than the media and entertainment industry, their opportunities and responsibilities are great to depict and promote healthful diets and eating habits among children and youth.

Recommendation 5: *The media and entertainment industry should direct its extensive power to promote healthful foods and beverages for children and youth.*

To implement this recommendation, media, and the entertainment industry should

- Incorporate into multiple media platforms (e.g., print, broadcast, cable, Internet, and wireless-based programming) foods, beverages, and storylines that promote healthful diets.
- Strengthen their capacity to serve as accurate interpreters and reporters to the public on findings, claims, and practices related to the diets of children and youth.

Parents, Caregivers, and Families

Parents and families remain the central influence on children's attitudes and behaviors, and social marketing efforts that aim to improve children's and youths' diets therefore must be tied directly to that influence.

Recommendation 6: *Government, in partnership with the private sector, should create a long-term, multifaceted, and financially sustained social marketing program supporting parents, caregivers, and families in promoting healthful diets for children and youth.*

To implement this recommendation

- Elements should include the full range of evolving and integrated marketing tools and widespread educational and community-based efforts, including use of children and youth as change agents.
- Special emphasis should be directed to parents of children ages birth to 4 years and other caregivers (e.g., child-care settings, schools, after-school programs) to build skills to wisely select and prepare healthful and affordable foods and beverages for children and youth.
- The social marketing program should have a reliable and sustained support stream, through public-appropriated funds and counterpart cooperative support from businesses marketing foods, beverages, and meals to children and youth.

School Environments

If schools and parents are to remain the strongest allies working to promote and advance the interests of American children and youth, the school environment must be fully devoted to preparing students for healthful lifelong dietary patterns.

Recommendation 7: *State and local educational authorities, with support from parents, health authorities, and other stakeholders, should educate about and promote healthful diets for children and youth in all aspects of the school environment (e.g., commercial sponsorships, meals and snacks, curriculum).*

To implement this recommendation, companies should
- Develop and implement nutrition standards for competitive foods and beverages sold or served in the school environment.
- Adopt policies and best practices that promote the availability and marketing of foods and beverages that support healthful diets.
- Provide visible leadership in this effort by public and civic leaders at all levels such as the National Governors Association, the state and local Boards of Education, and the National Parent Teacher Association, as well as trade associations representing private-sector businesses such as distributors, bottlers, and vending machine companies that directly interface with the school administration.

Public Policy

A first obligation of public policy is to protect the vulnerable and a second is to create the conditions for a desirable future. Both call for the careful use of policy initiatives to foster healthy prospects for children and youth.

Recommendation 8: *Government at all levels should marshal the full range of public policy levers to foster the development and promotion of healthful diets for children and youth.*

To implement this recommendation
- Government should consider incentives (e.g., recognition, performance awards, tax incentives) that encourage and reward food, beverage, and restaurant companies that develop, provide, and promote healthier foods and beverages for children and youth in settings where they typically consume them (e.g., restaurants, schools, amusement parks, sports venues, movie theaters, malls, and airports).

- Government should explore combining the full range of possible approaches (e.g., agricultural subsidies, taxes, legislation, regulation, federal nutrition programs) for making fruits and vegetables readily available and accessible to all children, youth, and families.
- The U.S. Department of Agriculture should develop and test new strategies for promoting healthier, appealing school meals provided through the School Breakfast Program and the National School Lunch Program as well as other federal programs designed for after-school settings (Special Milk Program) and child-care settings (Child and Adult Care Food Program).
- If voluntary efforts related to advertising during children's television programming are unsuccessful in shifting the emphasis away from high-calorie and low-nutrient foods and beverages to the advertising of healthful foods and beverages, Congress should enact legislation mandating the shift on both broadcast and cable television.*

Research

Knowledge is the bedrock of effective action and progress, yet current resources are scant to expand the knowledge base, from all sources, on the changing ways in which marketing influences the diets and health of children and youth.

Recommendation 9: *The nation's formidable research capacity should be substantially better directed to sustained, multidisciplinary work on how marketing influences the food and beverage choices of children and youth.*

To implement this recommendation
- The federal research capacity, in particular supported by the agencies of the U.S. Department of Health and Human Services (e.g., National Institutes of Health, Centers for Disease Control and Prevention, Food and Drug Administration), the U.S. Department of Agriculture, the National Science Foundation, and the Federal Trade Commission should be expanded to illuminate the ways in which marketing influences children's attitudes and behaviors. Of particular importance are studies related to newer promotion techniques and venues, healthier foods and beverages and portion sizes, product availability, the impact of television advertising on diet and diet-related health, diverse research methods that systematically control for alternative explana-

---

*See text at pages 349 and 262.

tions, stronger measurement, and methods with high relevance to every day life.

- A means should be developed for commercial marketing data to be made available, if possible as a publicly accessible resource, for better understanding the dynamics that shape the health and nutrition attitudes and behaviors of children and youth at different ages and in different circumstances, and for informing the multifaceted social marketing program targeting parents, caregivers, and families to promote healthful diets for children and youth.

Monitoring Progress

The saying goes that "what gets measured gets done." Yet no single public body exists with responsibility or authority to track the influences of marketing on the dietary practices and health status of children and youth in the United States.

Recommendation 10: *The Secretary of the U.S. Department of Health and Human Services (DHHS) should designate a responsible agency, with adequate and appropriate resources, to formally monitor and report regularly on the progress of the various entities and activities related to the recommendations included in this report.*

To implement this recommendation

- The Secretary should consult with other relevant cabinet officers and agency heads (e.g., U.S. Department of Agriculture, U.S. Department of Education, Federal Trade Commission, Federal Communications Commission) in developing and implementing the required monitoring and reporting.
- Within 2 years, the Secretary should report to Congress on the progress and on additional actions necessary to accelerate progress.

CLOSING THOUGHTS

The review and recommendations presented in this report are anchored in the presentation and interpretation of the evidence. This was the central charge to the committee, and the effort represents the most comprehensive and rigorous review of existing scientific literature done to date. It is important to point out that the committee was not charged with, nor did it engage in addressing some of the broader philosophical, social, and political issues related to food and beverage marketing to children and youth. Perspectives about basic responsibilities to shepherd the welfare of those most vulnerable or impressionable, conjecture about insights from studies not yet done or information not available on the strength of relationships between marketing and behavior of children and youth, and social urgency prompted by the rapidly increasing prevalence of childhood obesity, all are legitimate and important matters for public discussion. But they were not central features of the committee's charge or work. Neither was the related, but vital, matter of physical activity, which is so inextricably a part of the challenge of childhood obesity. What the committee can contribute to the ongoing and imperative public policy questions raised by this challenge is to conclude, based upon a thorough and impartial review of existing scientific data, that the dietary patterns of our children and youth put their health at risk, that the patterns have been reinforced if not encouraged by prevailing marketing practices, and that the turnaround required will depend upon aggressive and sustained leadership from all sectors, including the food and beverage industries. This is a public health priority of the highest order.

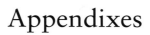

Appendixes

A

Acronyms

AAA	American Academy of Advertising
AAAA	American Association of Advertising Agencies
AAF	American Advertising Federation
AAP	American Academy of Pediatrics
ABA	Australian Broadcasting Authority
ACFN	American Council for Fitness and Nutrition
AI	Adequate Intake
AMA	American Medical Association; American Marketing Association
AMDR	Acceptable Macronutrient Distribution Range
ANA	Association of National Advertisers
ASA	Advertising Standards Authority
ASC	Advertising Standards Canada
BLS	U.S. Bureau of Labor Statistics
BMI	body mass index
CACFP	Child and Adult Care Food Program
CARU	Children's Advertising Review Unit
CBBB	Council of Better Business Bureaus
CDC	Centers for Disease Control and Prevention
CNLP	Child Nutrition Labeling Program
COPPA	Children's Online Privacy Protection Act
CSD	carbonated soft drink

CSFII	Continuing Survey of Food Intakes by Individuals
CSPI	Center for Science in the Public Interest
CTS	Children's Television Standards
DASH	Dietary Approaches to Stop Hypertension
DHHS	U.S. Department of Health and Human Services
DNPA	Division of Nutrition and Physical Activity
DRI	Dietary Reference Intake
DVD	digital video disc
EAR	Estimated Average Requirement
EER	estimated energy requirements
EFNEP	Expanded Food and Nutrition Education Program
FCC	Federal Communications Commission
FDA	U.S. Food and Drug Administration
FGP	Food Guide Pyramid
FITS	Feeding Infants and Toddlers Study
FMNV	foods of minimal nutritional value
FPA	Food Products Association
FSP	Food Stamp Program
FTC	Federal Trade Commission
GAO	U.S. Government Accountability Office
GMA	Grocery Manufacturers Association
HDL	high-density lipoprotein
HEI	Healthy Eating Index
ICC	International Chamber of Commerce
IOM	Institute of Medicine
ITC	International Trade Commission
IU	International Units
KFF	Kaiser Family Foundation
LDL	low-density lipoprotein
LND	low-nutrient dense
NAFTA	North American Free Trade Agreement
NARC	National Advertising Review Council
NASSP	National Association of Secondary School Principals
NCI	National Cancer Institute
NFCS	National Food Consumption Survey
NHANES	National Health and Nutrition Examination Surveys

NICHD	National Institute of Child Health and Human Development
NIH	National Institutes of Health
NLEA	Nutrition Labeling and Education Act
NRC	National Research Council
NSLP	National School Lunch Program
PBH	Produce for Better Health Foundation
PSA	public service announcement
QSR	quick serve restaurant
RDA	Recommended Dietary Allowance
REA	Recommended Energy Allowances
RTE	ready to eat
SBP	School Breakfast Program
SEMS	industry-sponsored educational materials
SES	Socioeconomic Status
SIP	National Family Opinion Research/Beverage Unit's Share of Intake Panel
UL	Tolerable Upper Intake Levels
USDA	U.S. Department of Agriculture
WHO	World Health Organization
WIC	Special Supplemental Nutrition Program for Women, Infants, and Children

B

Glossary

Acceptable Macronutrient Distribution Range Established for macronutrients and other dietary components as a percentage of total energy intake associated with reduced risk of chronic disease while providing recommended intakes of other essential nutrients.

Account Specific Marketing Retail promotional programs used to achieve incremental display activity and attain incremental sales volumes of select brands, including programs targeted at store personnel, managers, or consumers.

Added Sugars Sugars and syrups that are added to foods during processing or preparation. These do not include naturally occurring sugars such as lactose in milk or fructose in fruits.

Adequate Intake The recommended average daily intake level based on observed or experimentally determined approximations or estimates of nutrient intake by a group (or groups) of apparently healthy people that are assumed to be adequate, and is used when a Recommended Dietary Allowance cannot be determined.

Adiposity A term used to describe body fat.

Advergame A branded product that is built directly into a game through Internet-based materials, video games, or in print materials.

Advertising   A paid public presentation and promotion of ideas, goods, or services by a sponsor that is intended to bring a product to the attention of consumers through a variety of media channels such as broadcast and cable television, radio, print, billboards, the Internet, or personal contact.

Advertising Campaigns   A group of advertisements, commercials, and related promotional materials and activities that are designed to be used during the same period of time as part of a coordinated marketing plan to meet specified advertising objectives.

Advertising Intensity   The ratio of a food's share of advertising to its share of consumers' disposable income.

Audience Fragmentation   When a target group, such as a television viewing audience, watches a greater diversity of television programming and divides its attention and screen time across many media platforms.

Away-From-Home Foods   Foods categorized according to where they are obtained, such as restaurants and other places with wait service; quick serve restaurants and self-service or take-out eateries; schools, including childcare centers, after-school programs, and summer camp; and other outlets, including vending machines, community feeding programs, and eating at someone else's home.

Baby Boomer   The term is most often used to refer to people born during the post-World War II baby boom, 1946–1964, which was a period of increased birth rates relative to preceding or subsequent generations.

Balanced Diet   The overall dietary pattern of foods consumed that provide all the essential nutrients in the appropriate amounts to support life processes including growth and development in children without promoting excess body fat accumulation and excess weight gain.

Behavioral Branding   A strategy used by social marketing programs to create brands that individuals associate with a specific behavior or lifestyle. Examples include the *VERB*™ campaign, which encourages tweens to associate *VERB*™ with physical activity, and the truth® brand, which represents an aspirational antismoking brand for teens that builds a positive image of youth as nonsmokers, cool and edgy, and rebellious against the tobacco industry.

Body Mass Index   Body mass index (BMI) is an indirect measure of body fat calculated as the ratio of a person's body weight in kilograms to the square of a person's height in meters.

$$\text{BMI (kg/m}^2) = \text{weight (kilograms)} \div \text{height (meters)}^2$$
$$\text{BMI (lb/in}^2) = \text{weight (pounds)} \div \text{height (inches)}^2 \times 703$$

In children and youth, BMI is based on growth charts for age and gender and is referred to as BMI-for-age which is used to assess underweight, overweight, and risk for overweight. According to the Centers for Disease Control and Prevention (CDC), a child with a BMI-for-age that is equal to or greater than the 95th percentile is considered to be overweight. A child with a BMI-for-age that is equal to or between the 85th and 95th percentile is considered to be at risk of becoming overweight. In this report, the definition of obesity is equivalent to the CDC definition of overweight, and at risk of becoming obese is equivalent to the CDC definition of at risk for becoming overweight.

Brand Advantage   When marketers determine whether customers think a brand is improving or whether their interest in a specific brand is declining. Also called brand momentum.

Brand Awareness   Consumer's awareness about a brand and the competition for it. Also called brand image.

Brand Equity   When marketers build familiarity of a specific brand among consumers to enhance perceived quality, meet customers' expectations, or increase purchase intent of the brand. Also called brand relevance and brand performance.

Brand Loyalty   The degree to which consumers will consistently purchase the same brand within a product category. Also called brand bonding.

Brand Preference   A consumer preference for a particular brand that results in the continual purchase of it.

Branding   A marketing feature that provides a name or symbol that legally identifies a company, a single product, or a product line to differentiate it from other companies and products in the marketplace.

Buzz Marketing   Peer-to-peer marketing.

Buzz Spotters   A network of young people—from tweens to teens to young adults—who observe youth trends and provide this feedback to youth marketers.

Calorie   A kilocalorie is defined as the amount of heat required to change the temperature of one gram of water from 14.5 degrees Celsius to 15.5 degrees Celsius. In this report, calorie is used synonymously with kilocalorie as a unit of measure for energy obtained from foods and beverages.

Carbonated Soft Drinks A common marketing term used to refer to a category of cold, nonalcoholic, sweetened beverages that uses the process of carbonation to enhance its taste and texture.

Caregiver An individual, such as a parent, foster parent, or head of a household, who attends to the needs of a child or adolescent.

CARU The Children's Advertising Review Unit (CARU) was founded in 1974 to promote responsible children's advertising as a component of the strategic alliance with major advertising trade associations through the National Advertising Review Council. CARU is the children's arm of the advertising industry's self-regulation program and evaluates child-directed advertising and promotional material in all media to advance accuracy, truthfulness, and consistency of advertisements.

Causal Inference In this report, the evidence for a causal relationship between a marketing variable and an outcome precursor, diet, or diet-related health variable.

Causal Relationship A relationship between variables in which a change in one variable produces a change in another variable; changes in one variable affect another variable; and changes in one variable depend on changes in another variable.

Celebrity Endorsement Popular celebrities who allow their names to be associated with a specific product, brand, or company.

Channel One News A 12-minute current events program launched in 1990 that provides 2 minutes of commercials. It is viewed by more than 8 million adolescents daily in an estimated 12,000 U.S. public schools.

Character Merchandising The use of popular fictional characters to promote the sale of many types of products. The intellectual rights to the character frequently belong to another company. This form of consumer promotion is also known as out-licensing.

Co-branding A technique where two companies partner to create one product. It is used to reach new customers and to extend a company's name and trademark to new areas of the consumer market.

Commercialism   The means of communication that creates consumer awareness and induces the desire for products, thereby increasing consumer demand and commercial profit.

Community   A social entity that can either be spatial, based on where people live in local neighborhoods, residential districts, or municipalities; or relational, based on common ethnic, cultural, or other characteristics or similar interests.

Competitive Foods   Foods and beverages offered at schools other than meals and snacks served through the federally reimbursed National School Lunch Program (NSLP), School Breakfast Program (SBP), and the after-school snack programs. Competitive foods include food and beverage items sold through a la carte lines, snack bars, student stores, vending machines, and school fundraisers.

Consumer Promotion   A form of nonpersonal sales promotional efforts that are designed to have an immediate impact on sales. This form of promotion uses media and nonmedia marketing communications for a limited time to increase consumer demand, stimulate market demand, or increase product availability. Examples of consumer promotion include coupons, discounts and sales, contests, point of purchase displays, rebates, and gifts and incentive items. Also called sales promotion.

COPPA   Children's Online Privacy Protection Act of 1998 that requires online operators to seek parental permission before collecting personal information from children and to post links to their privacy policy on their homepage and every page where personal information is collected.

Correlate   To put or bring into causal, complementary, parallel, or reciprocal relation.

Cross-Promotion   A consumer sales promotion technique in which the manufacturer attempts to sell the consumer new or other products related to a product the consumer already uses or which the marketer has available.

Deception   According to Section 5 of the Federal Trade Commission statute, 15 U.S.C. § 45, a representation, omission, act, or practice that is likely to mislead consumers to act reasonably under given circumstances or affect consumers' conduct or decisions with respect to a product.

Dietary Guidelines Americans A federal summary of the latest dietary guidance for the American public based on current scientific evidence and medical knowledge. The Guidelines are issued jointly by the U.S. Department of Health and Human Services and U.S. Department of Agriculture and revised every 5 years.

Dietary Reference Intakes A set of four distinct nutrient-based reference values that replaced the former Recommended Dietary Allowances in the United States. They include Estimated Average Requirements (EARs), Recommended Dietary Allowances (RDAs), Adequate Intakes (AIs), and Tolerable Upper Intake Level (UL).

Digital Divide The socioeconomic gap between groups or communities that have access to computers and the Internet and those who do not have access. It also refers to a gap that exists between groups regarding their ability to use information and communications technology effectively due to differing levels of literacy and technical skills.

Direct Marketing Sending a promotional message directly to consumers through direct mail or telemarketing rather than through a mass medium such as television or the Internet.

Disclaimer A repudiation or denial of responsibility or connection.

Disclosure The act or process of revealing or making something evident.

Discretionary Fat The ability of a person to selectively add dietary fat (e.g., salad dressing, butter, oil) at one's own discretion, according to dietary preferences, and which contributes to total calorie intake. This is distinct from obligatory fat that has been added to foods prior to consumption and cannot be removed. It may also represent the amount of fat in a person's "energy allowance" or discretionary calories after consuming sufficient amounts of high-calorie and low-nutrient foods to meet one's daily calorie and nutrient needs while promoting weight maintenance.

Ecological Validity The extent to which an investigation's research setting, stimuli, and response demands are similar to those of naturally occurring settings, stimuli, and response characteristics of the behavioral system being studied.

Energy Balance A state where calorie intake is equivalent to energy expenditure, resulting in no net weight gain or weight loss. In this report, energy balance in children is used to indicate equality between energy intake and energy expenditure that supports normal growth and development without promoting excess weight gain.

Energy Density   The amount of calories stored in a given food per unit volume or mass. Fat stores 9 kilocalories/gram (g), alcohol stores 7 kilocalories/g, carbohydrate and protein each store 4 kilocalories/g, fiber stores 1.5 to 2.5 kilocalories/g, and water has no calories. Foods that are almost entirely composed of fat with minimal water (e.g., butter) are more calorie dense than foods that consist largely of water, fiber, and carbohydrates (e.g., fruits and vegetables).

Energy Expenditure   Calories used to support the body's basal metabolic needs plus those used for thermogenesis, growth, and physical activity.

Energy Intake   Calories ingested as foods and beverages.

Environment   The aggregate of social and cultural conditions that influence the life of an individual or community.

Estimated Average Requirement   The average daily nutrient intake level estimated to meet the requirement of half the healthy individuals in a particular life stage and gender group.

Estimated Energy Requirements   The calorie needs calculated for different groups based on age, gender, and physical activity level, published by the Institute of Medicine in 2002, which replaced the Recommended Energy Allowance (REA).

Exclusive Contracting   When a school district enters into an exclusive contract with a soft drink company to sell only a particular beverage product on the school premises. Also called pouring rights.

Explicit Learning   The ability to acquire knowledge through a fully conscious and hypothesis-driven mode, such as learning a concept or learning how to solve a problem.

Fast Food   Foods and meals designed for ready availability, use, or consumption and sold at eating establishments for quick availability or take-out.

Flavor   The sensory impression of a food or other substance that is determined by the chemical senses of taste and smell. A substance added to food to give it a particular taste.

Focus Group A research method whereby a moderator convenes a group of participants who often have common characteristics (e.g., age, gender, ethnicity) to discuss the attributes of a specific concept or product. It is often used in the marketing development phase to generate ideas and provide insights into consumer reactions and perceptions.

Food Guide Pyramid An educational tool designed for the public that translates and graphically illustrates recommendations from the Dietary Guidelines for Americans and nutrient standards such as the Dietary Reference Intakes into food group-based advice that promotes a healthful diet for the U.S. population. In 2005, it was replaced by an interactive food guidance system, *MyPyramid*.

Gatekeeper Refers to the person who controls decisions, such as a parent for a child or teen, by controlling the purchasing or decision-making process. It also refers to the person who controls the flow of information from the mass media to a group or other individuals.

Generation X A term used in marketing, the social sciences, and popular culture to describe people born in the 1960s and 1970s.

Generation Y People born between 1981 and 1995 in the United States, also know as Echo Boomers and the Millennium Generation.

Global Brand Value Represents the total monetary worth of a company's collective brands.

Global Revenues Represent a company's total sales and earnings worldwide.

Health Represents a state of complete physical, mental and social well-being and not merely the absence of disease or infirmity.

Health Promotion The process of enabling people to increase control over and to improve their health through networks and initiatives that create healthy environments. To reach a state of complete physical, mental, and social well-being, an individual or group must be able to identify and to realize aspirations, to satisfy needs, and to change or cope with the environment. Health is a resource for everyday life, not the objective of living, and is a positive concept emphasizing social and personal resources, as well as physical capacities.

Healthful Diet For children and adolescents, a healthful diet provides recommended amounts of nutrients and other food components within estimated energy requirements (EER) to promote normal growth and development, a healthy weight trajectory, and energy balance. A healthful diet also reduces the long-term risk for obesity and related chronic diseases associated with aging, including type 2 diabetes and metabolic syndrome.

Healthy Weight In children and youth, a level of body fat that supports normal growth and development and where there are no observed co-morbidities. In adults, a BMI between 18.5 and 24.9 kg/m^2.

Host Selling Refers to the same character appearing in a television program as well as an advertisement placed next to a television show in which the character appears.

Implicit Learning The ability to learn under passive, automatic, and unconscious acquisition of abstract knowledge. This type of learning remains robust over time.

Incentive Programs Sponsors that agree to give discounts or free products if students collect a certain number of coupons or shop at certain stores.

Integrated Marketing A planning process designed to assure that all promotional activities, including media advertising, direct mail, sales promotion, and public relations, produce a unified, customer-focused promotion message that is relevant to a customer and consistent over time.

Interactive Product Placement A technique that merges television and the Internet through channels such as digital television and Web television.

Internet Marketing A promotional activity that occurs on the Internet, which connects consumers to companies' brands and products for the purpose of stimulating sales.

Licensing Agreement A contractual agreement that allows copyright holders to loan their intellectual property to another company in exchange for payment. In the children's media industries, companies can license the characters and images of their media products to food and beverage companies for a fee.

Lifestyle Marketing A promotional activity created around the interests, attitudes, opinions, and ways of life of consumers to connect with how they want to live.

Marketing   An organizational function and a set of processes for creating, communicating, and delivering value to customers and for managing customer relationships in ways that benefit an organization and its stakeholders. Marketing encompasses a wide range of activities including market research, analyzing the competition, positioning a new product, pricing products and services, and promoting them through advertising, consumer promotion, trade promotions, public relations, and sales.

Marketing Mix   Combining the four strategy elements of market decision making—product, placement, price, and promotion—to reach consumers.

Marketing Research   Activities that link the consumer, customer, and public to the marketer through information that is used to identify and define marketing opportunities and problems; generate, refine, and evaluate marketing actions; monitor marketing performance; and improve understanding of marketing as a process. Marketing research specifies the information required to address these issues, designs the method for collecting information, manages and implements the data collection process, analyzes the results, and communicates the findings and their implications.

Marketplace   The set of commercial activities where goods and services are bought and sold.

Market Segmentation   The division of a market into different groups of consumers that have common characteristics.

Measured Media   The categories tracked by media research companies including television (e.g., network, spot, cable, syndicated, Spanish-language network), radio (e.g., network, national spot, local), magazines (e.g., local, Sunday magazine), business publications, newspapers (e.g., local, national), outdoor, direct mail, the Yellow Pages, and the Internet.

Media Advocacy   The strategic use of the mass media to advance a social or public policy initiative.

Media Literacy   The ability to access, analyze, evaluate, and produce communication in a variety of forms. A media-literate person can understand and think critically about the nature, technique, and impact of the mass media, including print and broadcast media, the Internet, and newly emerging technologies. Also called media education.

Mediator   The mechanism by which one variable affects another variable.

Millennial   A person born between 1981 and 1995 in the United States, also know as an Echo Boomer or Generation Y.

Moderator   A variable that changes the impact of one variable on another.

Naming Rights   An owner of an object sells the rights for someone else to name the object.

National School Lunch Program   The National School Lunch Program (NSLP) is a federally funded meal program established in 1946 that operates in public and nonprofit private schools and residential child-care institutions. The NSLP provides nutritionally balanced, reduced-cost, or free lunches to children every school day.

Nutrient Density   The amount of nutrients that a food contains per unit volume or mass. Nutrient density is independent of energy density although, in practice, the nutrient density of a food is often described in relationship to the food's energy density. Fruits and vegetables are nutrient dense, but not energy dense. Compared to foods of high fat content, carbonated soft drinks are not particularly energy dense because these are made up primarily of water and carbohydrate, but because they are otherwise low in nutrients, their energy density is high for the nutrient content.

Nutrition Facts Panel   Standardized detailed nutritional information on the contents and serving sizes of nearly all packaged foods sold in the marketplace. The panel was designed to provide nutrition information to consumers and was mandated by the Nutrition Labeling and Education Act of 1990.

Obesity   An excess amount of subcutaneous body fat in proportion to lean body mass. In adults, a BMI of 30 or greater is considered obese. In this report, obesity in children and youth refers to the age- and gender-specific BMI that is equal to or greater than the 95th percentile of the CDC BMI charts. At-risk for obesity in children and youth is defined as a BMI-for-age and gender that is between the 85th and 95th percentiles of the CDC BMI curves. In most children, these values are known to indicate elevated body fat and to reflect the co-morbidities associated with excessive body fatness.

Obesogenic   Environmental factors that may promote obesity and encourage the expression of a genetic predisposition to gain weight.

Older Children   In this report, refers to children ages 6–11 years.

Overweight Defined by the CDC as a BMI-for-age and gender that is greater than or equal to the 95th percentile of the 2000 CDC BMI curves developed for U.S. children and adolescents ages 2 to 20 years. At-risk for overweight is defined by the CDC as a BMI-for-age and gender that is between the 85th and 95th percentiles of the 2000 CDC BMI curves.

Persuasive Intent Refers to the cognitive awareness and demonstrated ability of children and youth to recognize and comprehend the inherent bias, exaggeration, and self-interest of commercial messages. They understand that a commercial message has other interests and perspectives than the receiver of the message; that the purveyor of the persuasive message is guided by commercial self-interest; that persuasive messages are biased; and that biased messages demand different interpretive strategies than unbiased messages.

Pester Power The ability children have to badger their parents into purchasing items they would otherwise not buy or performing actions they would otherwise not do.

Physical Activity Body movement produced by the contraction of skeletal muscles that result in energy expenditure above the basal level. Physical activity consists of athletic, recreational, housework, transport or occupational activities that require physical skills and utilize strength, power, endurance, speed, flexibility, range of motion, or agility.

Portion Size Represents the amount of food an individual is served at home or away from home and chooses to consume for a meal or snack. Portions can be larger or smaller than serving sizes listed on the food label or the Food Guide Pyramid.

Pouring Rights When a school district enters into an exclusive contract with a soft drink company to sell only a particular beverage product on the school premises. Also called exclusive contracting.

Precision Refers to the sensitivity or coarseness of a measure.

Prevention With regard to obesity, primary prevention represents avoiding the occurrence of obesity in a population; secondary prevention represents early detection of disease through screening with the purpose of limiting its occurrence; and tertiary prevention involves preventing the sequelae of obesity in childhood and adulthood.

Product Placement A marketing technique that uses a message, brand logo, or product in a visual or graphic medium in a variety of forms of media entertainment, including television programs, films, music, videos/DVDs, video games, and advergames.

Promotion The means by which a business or company communicates with its target audience or customers to inform, persuade, or influence customers' purchase decisions.

Proprietary Privately owned and operated; something that is held under patent, trademark, or copyright by a private person or company.

Public Relations A company's communications and relationships with various groups including customers, employees, suppliers, stockholders, government, general public, and society.

Public Service Announcement An advertisement or commercial that is carried by an advertising vehicle at no cost as a public service to its readers, viewers, or listeners. A promotional message for a nonprofit organization or for a social cause printed or broadcast at no charge by the media.

Purchase Influence The array of behaviors related to a child's or an adolescent's influence on family purchases.

Quick Serve Restaurant A category of restaurants characterized by food that is supplied quickly after ordering and with minimal service. Foods and beverages purchased may be consumed at the restaurant or served as take-out.

Recommended Dietary Allowance The average daily dietary nutrient intake level sufficient to meet the nutrient requirement of nearly all (97 to 98 percent) healthy individuals in a particular life stage and gender group.

Recommended Energy Allowance The average energy needs of individuals as presented in the 10th edition of the Recommended Dietary Allowances which were updated by the IOM in 2002 and replaced with the estimated energy requirements (EER).

Relationship Marketing A marketing approach that acquires information about a customer during the history of that customer's relationship with a company. This information is used to market to the customer to promote trust and loyalty. Five components of relationship marketing are awareness, recognition, preferences, commitment, and endorsement.

Reliability   Assesses the extent to which the same measurement technique, applied repeatedly, is likely to yield the same results.

Safety   The condition of being protected from or unlikely to cause danger, risk, or injury that either may be perceived or objectively defined.

Sales Promotion   Marketing activities other than advertising, personal selling, and publicity that stimulate consumer purchases at the point-of-sale such as a display, product demonstration, trade show, contest, coupon, premium, prize, toy, or price discount. Also called consumer promotion.

School Breakfast Program   A federally administered program that provides cash assistance to states to operate nonprofit breakfast programs in U.S. public schools and residential child-care institutions.

School Meal Initiative For Healthy Children   A program launched by the U.S. Department of Agriculture in 1995 to improve the nutritional quality of school lunches and breakfasts.

Screen Time   The number of hours a child or adolescent spends watching various types of electronic media (e.g., broadcast and cable television, video and/or digital video disc, movie, computer) per day, week, month, or year.

Secular Trend   A long-term trend in numbers (up or down).

Sedentary   A way of living or lifestyle that requires minimal physical activity and that encourages inactivity through limited choices, disincentives, and/or structural or financial barriers.

Serving   A standardized unit of measure used to describe the total amount of foods recommended daily from each of the food groups from the Food Guide Pyramid or a specific amount of food that contains the quality of nutrients listed on the Nutrition Facts panel. This may differ from a portion which represents the amount of food an individual is served at home or away from home and chooses to consume for a meal or snack.

Social Marketing   The application of commercial marketing principles to the analysis, planning, implementation, and evaluation of programs designed to influence voluntary behavior changes in target audiences in order to improve their personal welfare and for the benefit of society.

Spam   Unwanted, unsolicited e-mail messages that are typically of a commercial nature.

Sponsored Educational Materials   Materials in which the sponsor assumes responsibility for the production and usually the content of the materials as well as the advertising that appears within it.

Stealth Marketing   A marketing strategy used to present products or services that consumers do not identify as an attempt to influence their purchase behaviors. Viral marketing is a form of stealth marketing.

Subsidy   A monetary grant given by government in support of an activity regarded as being in the public interest. A payment that a government makes to a producer to supplement the market price of a commodity. A subsidy can keep consumer prices low while maintaining a higher income for domestic producers.

Target Market   A group of individuals to whom a company markets its products or ideas that are designed to satisfy their specific needs and preferences. Target markets may be segmented by demographic characteristics (e.g., age, gender, income, race or ethnicity), psychographic characteristics (i.e., values, attitudes, beliefs, lifestyles), behavioral patterns (e.g., brand loyalty, product usage rates, price), and geographic characteristics (e.g., region, population density).

Taste   The sense that distinguishes the sweet, sour, salty, and bitter qualities of dissolved substances in contact with the taste buds on the tongue.

Teen   In this report, refers to young people ages 12–18 years.

Tolerable Upper Intake Level   The highest average daily nutrient intake level that is likely to pose no risk of adverse health effects to almost all individuals in the general population. As intake increases above the Tolerable Upper Intake Level (UL), the potential risk of adverse effects may increase.

Trade Promotion   Promotion activities directed to marketing intermediaries, such as grocery stores, convenience stores, and other food retail outlets, and uses strategies that include in-store displays, shelf space and positioning, free merchandise, buy-back allowances, merchandise allowances, and sales contests to encourage wholesalers or retailers to sell more of a company's specific product or lines.

Tween   In this report, refers to young people ages 9–13 years. Marketers distinguish the tween market segment from children and teens, defining it as young people who have attitudes and behaviors that are "in between" the ages of 8–12 years or 9–14 years.

Unmeasured Media   The difference between a company's reported or estimated advertising costs and its measured media spending. Unmeasured media spending includes activities such as sales promotions, coupons, direct mail, catalogs, and special events, and it is not systematically tracked.

Validity   Refers to the extent to which an instrument directly and accurately measures what it is intended to measure.

Variable   Anything that is not constant but that can and does change in different circumstances.

Viral Marketing   A strategy used to build brand awareness and promote purchases by encouraging people to pass a marketing message to a target audience, often through electronic or digital platforms. Customers act as agents to promote and endorse a company's products, and incentives are often provided to customers to distribute the promotional messages and offers.

Virtual Advertisements   Digital advertisements that are inserted into programs, into films, or onto stadium walls at sporting events.

Well-being   A view of health that takes into account a child's physical, social, and emotional health.

Younger Children   In this report, refers to children ages 2–5 years.

C

Literature Review

To conduct a thorough review of the scientific literature, the Institute of Medicine (IOM) committee and staff conducted online bibliographic searches of relevant databases, including the following: ABI/INFORM, Academic Search Premier, AGRICOLA, Communication and Mass Media Complete, EconLit, EMBASE, ERIC, LexisNexis, MEDLINE, NTIS, PsycINFO, Science Direct, Sociological Abstracts, Web of Science, and WorldCat/FirstSearch (Box C-1).

To begin the process of identifying the primary literature in this field, the IOM staff at the beginning of the study conducted general bibliographic searches on topics related to marketing aimed toward children and youth. These references were categorized and annotated by the staff, and reference lists of key citations were provided to the committee. After examining the initial search in each of the databases, a comprehensive search strategy was designed in consultation with librarians at the George E. Brown Jr. Library of the National Academies. Search terms incorporated relevant MeSH (Medical Subject Headings) terms as well as terms from the EMBASE thesaurus. To maximize retrieval, the search strategy incorporated synonymous terms on the topics of dietary patterns and factors that shape them; food and/or beverage marketing (e.g., sources, venues, scope, trends, market segmentations, investment); effects of marketing on diets and health; and public policy issues (e.g., self-regulation, monitoring efforts, legal, social, and economical). The searches were limited to English language and targeted to retrieve citations related to infants, children, or youth (less than 18 years of age). The searches were not limited by date of publication.

BOX C-1
Online Databases

ABI/INFORM contains information on more than 60,000 companies as well as executive profiles, reports on market conditions, and in-depth case studies of global business trends. The database contains content from thousands of journals that help researchers track business conditions, trends, management techniques, corporate strategies, and industry-specific topics worldwide.

Academic Search Premier is a large academic multidisciplinary database. It provides full text for nearly 4,700 publications, including full text for more than 3,600 peer-reviewed journals. Coverage spans virtually every area of academic study and offers information dating as far back as 1975. This database is updated on a daily basis via EBSCO*host.*

AGRICOLA is a bibliographic database of citations to the agricultural literature. Production of these records in electronic form began in 1970, but the database covers materials in all formats, including printed works from the 15th century. The records describe publications and resources encompassing aspects of agriculture and allied disciplines, such as agricultural economics; animal and veterinary sciences; earth and environmental sciences; entomology; extension and education; farming and farming systems; fisheries and aquaculture; food and human nutrition; forestry; and plant sciences. AGRICOLA indexes more than 2,000 serials as well as books, pamphlets, conference proceedings, and other resources. This database is updated and maintained by the National Agricultural Library.

Communication and Mass Media Complete provides research solutions in areas related to communication and mass media. This database originated with the acquisition and subsequent merging of two popular databases in the fields of communication and mass media studies—*CommSearch* (formerly produced by the National Communication Association) and *Mass Media Articles Index* (formerly produced by Pennsylvania State University).

EconLit is the American Economic Association's bibliographic database of economics literature published in the United States and other countries from 1969 to the present. EconLit contains citations and abstracts from more than 500 economics journals. Some full-text articles are available. The database also indexes books, book chapters, book reviews, dissertations, essays, and working papers. The database covers subjects including accounting, consumer economics, monetary policy, labor, marketing, demographics, modeling, economic theory, and planning. EconLit contains more than 350,000 records and is updated monthly.

EMBASE (Excerpta Medica) database is a major biomedical and pharmaceutical resource containing more than 9 million records from 1974 to the present from over 4,000 journals; approximately 450,000 records are added annually. Over 80 percent of recent records contain full author abstracts. This bibliographic database indexes international journals in the following fields: drug research, pharmacology, pharmaceutics, toxicology, clinical and experimental human medicine, health policy and management, public health, occupational health, environmental

continues

BOX C-1 Continued

health, drug dependence and abuse, psychiatry, forensic medicine, and biomedical engineering/instrumentation. EMBASE is produced by Elsevier Science.

ERIC (Educational Resources Information Center) is a national education database containing nearly 100,000 citations and abstracts published from 1993 to the present. ERIC contains more than 1 million citations of research documents, journal articles, technical reports, program descriptions and evaluations, and curricular materials in the field of education. ERIC is sponsored by the U.S. Department of Education, Office of Educational Research and Improvement.

LexisNexis provides access to full-text information from more than 5,600 sources, including national and regional newspapers, wire services, broadcast transcripts, international news, and non-English-language sources; U.S. federal and state case law, codes, regulations, legal news, law reviews, and international legal information; and business news journals, company financial information, Securities and Exchange Commission filings and reports, and industry and market news. It is produced by Reed Elsevier, Inc.

MEDLINE is the National Library of Medicine's bibliographic database containing citations from the mid-1960s to the present. It covers the fields of medicine, nursing, dentistry, veterinary medicine, the health care system, and the preclinical sciences. PubMed provides online access to more than 12 million MEDLINE citations and additional life science journals. MEDLINE contains bibliographic citations and author abstracts from more than 4,600 biomedical journals published in the United States and 70 other countries. PubMed includes links to many sites providing full-text articles and related resources. This database can be accessed at http://www.ncbi.nlm.nih.gov/PubMed.

NTIS serves the United States as a central resource for government-funded scientific, technical, engineering, and business-related information available. NTIS offers information on more than 600,000 information products covering over 350 subject areas from 200-plus federal agencies.

PsycINFO is a bibliographic database of psychological literature with journal coverage from the 1800s to the present and book coverage from 1987 to the present. It contains more than 1.9 million records including citations and summaries of journal articles, book chapters, books, and technical reports, as well as citations to dissertations, all in the field of psychology and psychological aspects of related disciplines. Journal coverage includes full-text article links to 42 American Psychological Association journals including peer-reviewed international journals. PsycINFO is produced by APA.

Science Direct is a large electronic collection of science, technology, and medicine full-text and bibliographic information.

Sociological Abstracts indexes the international literature in sociology and related disciplines in the social and behavioral sciences from 1963 to the present. This bibliographic database contains citations (from 1963) and abstracts (only after 1974) of journal articles, dissertations, conference reports, books, book chapters, and reviews of books, films, and software. Approximately 1,700 journals and 900 other serials published in the United States and other countries in more than 30

BOX C-1 Continued

languages are screened yearly and added to the database bimonthly. The Sociological Abstracts database contained approximately 600,000 records in 2003. A limited number of full-text references are available. Sociological Abstracts is prepared by Cambridge Scientific Abstracts.

Web of Science provides access to current and retrospective multidisciplinary information from approximately 8,700 high-impact research journals. *Web of Science* also provides a unique search method, cited reference searching.

WorldCat/FirstSearch is an online service that gives library professionals and end users access to a wide collection of reference databases. With FirstSearch, materials in a library's collection are highlighted in results from searches in dozens of databases. Underlying FirstSearch is the WorldCat database, a comprehensive and up-to-date bibliographic resource.

As the study progressed, additional focused searches were conducted. Topics of these searches included emerging technologies, integrated advertising, stealth advertising, and food preference and intake. Additional references were identified by reviewing the reference lists found in major review articles, key reports, prominent websites (e.g., marketing research and surveys), and relevant books. Committee members, workshop presenters, consultants, and IOM staff also supplied references. Requests for literature suggestions were made to experts in relevant fields. An e-mail request was sent to nearly 50 researchers, academicians, industry professionals, advocates, and policy analysts, seeking their advice on important literature that should be considered for the committee's review. Requests were also made to individuals who attended a public workshop and forum on marketing foods and beverages to children and youth (Appendix H). Furthermore, public comment on the committee's task was requested through the National Academies' website.

The committee maintained the reference list in a database that could be searched by keywords, staff annotations, or other criteria. Additionally, an Internet-based website was developed from the search of some of the key resources. Bibliographies were updated throughout the study and as committee members requested the full text of journal articles and other resources as needed for their information and analysis. The literature was categorized into a taxonomy of peer-reviewed articles and marketing firm research or commercial reports, as described in Box C-2.

A number of reviews of literature have been published on topics relevant to the committee's work. Studies included in these literature reviews were considered for inclusion in the committee's review.

BOX C-2
Research Taxonomy

Descriptive studies

- Prevalence of disease, risk, and condition
- Dietary intakes and trends, including portion sizes
- Dietary intake influences
- Other behavioral influences
- Product profiles and trends
- Purchaser profiles and trends
- Television viewing patterns
- Commercial marketing activities (all forms)
    Television: placement analyses of advertising
    Television: content analyses of advertising
    Print advertising
    Toys and characters
    Internet
    Video games
- Social marketing activities
- Economic factors in food availability and choice
- Industry profiles and practices
- Ethics, guidelines and adherence
- Regulatory agencies and actions
    United States
    International

Surveys

- Children's and adolescents' views
    Of advertising
    Of food and nutrition
- Parents' views
    Of advertising
    Of food and nutrition
- Marketing surveys

Observational studies

- Children's and adolescents' development and understanding
- Relation of diet to disease risk
- Children's food and beverage consumption behaviors
    Influence of advertising
    Influence of television content
    Influence of television viewing time
    Influence of product design and packaging
    Influence of price
    Influence of school meals/vending
    Family variables/parent—child interactions
    Peer influences
- Other behaviors among children and youths
- Methodologic studies
    Dietary intake estimates
    Assessing advertising effects

Intervention studies

- On awareness and food preference
- On food and beverage choices
    School curriculum
    Television viewing
- On other youth behaviors
- Media literacy

Reviews/literature syntheses/recommendations

- Factors in childhood and youth development
- Diet and health/children's health/adolescents' health
- Influence of food marketing on children's and adolescents' diets
- Lessons from studies on behaviors other than diet
- Social marketing
- Research recommendations

D

Chapter 2 Appendix

TABLE D-1 Estimated Energy Requirements for Proposed Food Intake Patterns of U.S. Children and Adolescents, Ages 2–18 Years

Boys

Age	Sedentary EER	Target Pattern	Low Active EER	Suggested Patterns	Active EER	Suggested Patterns
2	1,050	1,000	1,050	1,000–1,400	1,050	1,000–1,400
3	1,162		1,324		1,485	
4	1,215	1,400	1,390	1,400–1,600	1,566	1,600–2,000
5	1,275		1,466		1,658	
6	1,328		1,535		1,742	
7	1,394		1,617		1,840	
8	1,453		1,692		1,931	
9	1,530	1,800	1,787	1,800–2,200	2,043	2,000–2,600
10	1,601		1,875		2,149	
11	1,691		1,985		2,279	
12	1,798	2,200	2,113	2,400–2,800	2,428	2,800–3,200
13	1,935		2,276		2,618	
14	2,090		2,459		2,829	
15	2,223		2,618		3,013	
16	2,320		2,736		3,152	
17	2,366		2,796		3,226	
18	2,383		2,823		3,263	

Girls

Age	Sedentary EER	Target Pattern	Low Active EER	Suggested Patterns	Active EER	Suggested Patterns
2	997	1,000	997	1,100–1,200	997	1,000–1,400
3	1,080		1,243		1,395	
4	1,133	1,200	1,310	1,400–1,600	1,475	1,400–1,800
5	1,189		1,379		1,557	
6	1,247		1,451		1,642	
7	1,298		1,515		1,719	
8	1,360		1,593		1,810	
9	1,415	1,600	1,660	1,600–2,000	1,890	1,800–2,000
10	1,470		1,729		1,972	
11	1,538		1,813		2,071	
12	1,617	1,800	1,909	2,000	2,183	2,400
13	1,684		1,992		2,281	
14	1,718		2,036		2,334	
15	1,731		2,057		2,362	
16	1,729		2,059		2,368	
17	1,710		2,042		2,353	
18	1,690		2,024		2,336	

NOTE: This table shows target and suggested energy intake levels for each age and gender group for proposed Food Guide Pyramid (FGP) intake patterns. These target and suggested levels are based on Estimated Energy Requirements (EER) calculated by gender, age, and activity level for

continues

TABLE D-1 Continued

reference-sized individuals (IOM, 2002). *Sedentary* is defined as a lifestyle that includes only the physical activity of independent living. *Low active* is defined as a lifestyle that includes a physical activity equivalent to walking about 1.5 to 3 miles per day at 3 to 4 miles per hour, in addition to the activities of independent living. *Active* is defined as a lifestyle that includes a physical activity equivalent to walking more than 3 miles daily at 3 to 4 miles per hour, in addition to the activities of independent living. Target patterns are the energy levels assigned to each age and gender group that are used to determine the nutrient adequacy of the food guidance system daily food intake patterns for each group. One target pattern is set for each age and gender group, and is appropriate for most sedentary individuals in the group, based on the calculated EER. For children ages 9 to 13, energy levels for the target patterns were selected at the higher end of the age range to allow for growth spurts during this period. Suggested patterns are the food guidance system daily food intake patterns that are generally appropriate for low active or active individuals for each age and gender group, based on their EER. These suggested patterns are not used to determine nutritional adequacy of the pattern but to suggest appropriate food selections for those requiring more calories than the target patterns provide.

SOURCES: IOM (2002–2005); USDA (2003).

TABLE D-2 Dietary Reference Intake Recommendations of Macronutrients for Children and Adolescents, Ages 1–18 Years

Age	Carbohydrate	Protein	Fat	Saturated Fat	Trans Fat	Cholesterol	Added Sugars	Fiber[a]	Total Daily Water AI[b]
1–3				As low as possible while consuming a nutritionally adequate diet	As low as possible while consuming a nutritionally adequate diet	As low as possible while consuming a nutritionally adequate diet	Limit to no more than 25% of total calorie intake		
(% Energy AMDR)	45–65	5–20	30–40						
(g/d)	130	13						19	1.3 L/d (~44 oz)
4–8									
(% Energy AMDR)	45–65	10–30	25–35						
(g/d)	130	19						25	1.7 L/d (~60 oz)
9–13									
Boys									
(% Energy AMDR)	45–65	10–30	25–35						
(g/d)	130	34						31	2.4 L/d (~84 oz)
Girls									
(% Energy AMDR)	45–65	10–30	25–35						
(g/d)	130	34						26	2.1 L/d (~72 oz)
14–18									
Boys									
(% Energy AMDR)	45–65	10–30	25–35						
(g/d)	130	52						38	3.3 L/d (~112 oz)
Girls									
(% Energy AMDR)	45–65	10–30	25–35						
(g/d)	130	46						26	2.3 L/d (~92 oz)

NOTE: AMDR = Acceptable Macronutrient Distribution Range. AI = Adequate Intake.

[a]Extrapolated from the adult value. This level represents the best estimate based on limited or uncertain available evidence when it was determined.

[b]The AI for "total daily water" includes fluids from all foods and beverages consumed, including drinking water. Conversion factors: 3 L = 33.8 fluid oz; 1 L = 1.06 qt; 1 cup = 8 fluid oz.

SOURCES: IOM (2002–2005, 2005).

TABLE D-3 Dietary Reference Intake Recommendations of Micronutrients for U.S. Children and Adolescents, Ages 1–18 Years

Age	Vitamin A (µg/d)	Vitamin C (mg/d)	Vitamin E (mg/d)	Vitamin B$_6$^{a} (mg/d)	Folate (µg/d)	Ca^{a,b} (mg/d)	Iron (mg/d)	Na^a (mg/d)	K^a (mg/d)	Mg (mg/d)
1–3	300	15	6	0.5	150	500	7	1,000	3,000	80
4–8	400	25	7	0.6	200	800	10	1,200	3,800	130
9–13										
Boys	600	45	11	1.0	300	1,300	8	1,500	4,500	240
Girls	600	45	11	1.0	300	1,300	8	1,500	4,500	240
14–18										
Boys	900	75	15	1.3	400	1,300	11	1,500	4,700	410
Girls	700	65	15	1.2	400	1,300	15	1,500	4,700	360

NOTE: Both the Recommended Dietary Allowances (RDAs) and Adequate Intakes (AIs) may be used as goals for individual intake. RDAs are established to meet the needs of nearly all individuals (97–98 percent) in a group. The AI for life stages and gender groups other than breastfed infants is believed to cover the needs of all individuals in a group. However, lack of data or uncertainty in the data preclude being able to specify with confidence the percentage of individuals covered by this intake.

^{a}Indicates an AI since an RDA value could not be determined.

^{b}Extrapolated from the adult value. This level represents the best estimate based on limited or uncertain available evidence when it was determined.

SOURCES: IOM (1997, 1998, 2000, 2001, 2005).

TABLE D-4 Survey of National Dietary Data for U.S. Individuals, 1971–2000

Survey	Dates	Population	Sample Size	Dietary Intake Methodology
NHANES I	1971–1974	Ages 1–74 years; oversampling of women of childbearing age, ages 5 and younger, adults ages 60–74, and persons with income below poverty	20,749[a]	Single 24-hour dietary recall, no weekend intakes
NHANES II	1976–1980	Ages 6 months–74 years; oversampling of children ages 5 years and younger, adults ages 60–74 years, and persons with income below poverty	20,322[a]	Single 24-hour dietary recall, no weekend intakes
NFCS	1977–1978	All ages; oversampling of low income[b] and elderly; 48 states	30,467[c]	Three consecutive days (single 24-hour dietary recall and 2-day food record)
NHANES III	1988–1994	Ages 2 months and older; oversampling of Mexican Americans, African Americans, ages 2 months–5 years, and ages 60 years and older	31,311[a]	Single 24-hour dietary recall and 3-month food frequency questionnaire; second 24-hour recall on a subsample (~5%)
CSFII	1989–1991	All ages; oversampling of low income[b]; 48 states	15,192[c]	Two nonconsecutive 24-hour dietary recalls
CSFII	1994–1996, 1998[d]	All ages; oversampling of low income; ages 0–9 years; 50 states	15,968[c]; 5,559[c]	Two nonconsecutive 24-hour dietary recalls
NHANES	1999–2000[e]	All ages; oversampling of Mexican Americans, African Americans, ages 12–19 years, ages 60 years and older, pregnant women, and low income[b]	8,604[c]	Single 24-hour dietary recall, and second recall on a subsample (~10%)

NOTE: NHANES = National Health and Nutrition Examination Survey. NFCS = National Food Consumption Survey. CSFII = Continuing Survey of Food Intakes by Individuals. IU = International Units.

[a]Examined persons.

[b]Low income is defined as household income at or below 130 percent of the poverty line, the income cut-off level for eligibility for the Food Stamp Program.

[c]Persons with 1-day intakes.

[d]Supplemental sample of children ages 0–9 years added to the CSFII 1994–1996.

[e]NHANES started a continuous data collection beginning in 1999. The most recent data were available for 1999–2000. CSFII is now incorporated into NHANES.

SOURCE: Adapted from Briefel and Johnson (2004). Reprinted with permission.

TABLE D-5 Mean Intakes and Changes[a] or Trends[b] in Intakes of Selected Nutrients of Girls and Boys, Ages 6–11 Years and 12–19 Years, as Reported in CSFII 1994–1996, 1998 and Compared to NFCS 1977–1978 and CSFII 1989–1991

Nutrient	Girls 6–11 yrs	Girls 12–19 yrs	Boys 6–11 yrs	Boys 12–19 yrs
Energy (kcal)	1,825	1,910	2,050	2,766 ↑
Protein (% kcal)	13.9 ↓	14.0 ↓	14.0 ↓*	14.4 ↓
Fat (% kcal)	32.6 ↓*	32.2 ↓*	32.6 ↓**	33.1 ↓**
Saturated fat (% kcal)[c]	12	11	12	12
Carbohydrate (% kcal)	54.9 ↑**	55.0 ↑**	54.8 ↑**	53.2 ↑**
Fiber (g)[c]	12	13	14	17
Vitamin A (IU)	4,475	4,817	5,242	6,361
Vitamin C (mg)	95	95	103 ↑	119
Thiamin (mg)	1.48 ↑	1.44 ↑	1.77 ↑*	2.13 ↑
Riboflavin (mg)	1.91	1.75	2.28 ↑	2.58
Niacin (mg)	18.1	19.0 ↑	21.5 ↑	27.8 ↑*
Vitamin B_6 (mg)	1.52	1.53 ↑	1.84 ↑	2.21 ↑
Vitamin B_{12} (µg)	3.87 ↓*	3.80 ↓	4.53 ↓	5.85 ↓
Calcium	865	771	984	1,145
Phosphorous (mg)	1,138	1,108	1,292	1,633
Magnesium (mg)	219	223	249	311
Iron (mg)	13.8 ↑	13.8 ↑**	16.6 ↑**	19.8 ↑*

NOTE: CSFII = Continuing Survey of Food Intakes by Individuals. NFCS = National Food Consumption Survey. IU = International Units.

[a]Significant increase (↑) or decrease (↓) in mean intakes (or percentages) between 1977–1978 and 1994–1996, 1998 (p < 0.001).

[b]Significant, progressive rise or fall in mean intakes (or percentages) from 1977–1978 through 1989–1991 to 1994–1996, 1998; *p < 0.05, **p < 0.01.

[c]Data from 1977–1978 and 1989–1991 are not provided.

SOURCES: Adapted from Enns et al. (2002, 2003).

TABLE D-6 Food Sources of Energy Among U.S. Children and Adolescents, Ages 2–18 Years (CSFII 1989–1991)

Rank	Food Group	Girls and Boys 2–18 Years	Girls and Boys 2–5 Years	Girls and Boys 6–11 Years	Boys 12–18 Years	Girls 12–18 Years
		% Energy				
1	Milk	11.7	15.4	12.4	9.5	8.8
2	Yeast bread	9.3	8.7	9.1	9.8	9.7
3	Cakes/cookies/quick breads/donuts	6.2	5.8	6.4	6.3	6.0
4	Beef	5.7	4.3	5.4	7.0	6.4
5	Ready-to-eat cereal	4.5	5.3	4.8	4.1	3.3
6	Carbonated soft drinks	4.3	2.5	3.2	6.1	6.3
7	Cheese	3.7	3.3	3.4	3.8	4.4
8	Potato chips/corn chips/popcorn	3.1	2.0	2.9	3.3	4.6
9	Sugars/syrups/jams	3.0	2.6	3.3	3.0	2.9
10	Poultry	2.6	2.8	2.4	2.5	3.2
		% Carbohydrate				
1	Yeast bread	13.0	12.1	12.7	14.0	13.7
2	Carbonated soft drinks	8.5	4.9	6.1	12.3	12.3
3	Milk	7.9	10.2	8.2	6.6	6.1
4	Ready-to-eat cereal	7.4	8.6	7.9	6.9	5.5
5	Cakes/cookies/quick breads/donuts	7.2	6.6	7.4	7.4	7.1
6	Sugars/syrups/jams	6.0	5.1	6.5	6.1	5.8
7	Fruit drinks	4.3	5.4	4.4	3.5	3.9
8	Pasta	3.9	4.4	4.0	3.2	4.1
9	White potatoes	3.7	3.0	3.8	4.0	4.0
10	Orange/grapefruit juice	2.9	3.0	2.5	3.1	3.5
		% Fat				
1	Milk	13.8	19.0	15.0	10.7	10.3
2	Beef	9.7	7.3	9.1	11.7	10.6
3	Cheese	7.4	7.1	7.0	7.4	8.8
4	Margarine	6.8	7.5	6.7	7.0	6.0
5	Cakes/cookies/quick breads/donuts	6.6	6.4	6.8	6.7	6.2
6	Potato chips/corn chips/popcorn	4.9	3.4	4.5	5.1	7.3
7	Salad dressings/mayonnaise	4.3	2.6	3.7	5.3	6.1
8	Oils	4.2	3.7	4.3	4.2	4.3
9	Yeast bread	3.8	3.6	3.8	3.9	3.9
10	Other fats	3.5	2.8	3.5	3.6	4.1

SOURCE: Subar et al. (1998). Reproduced by permission of *Pediatrics* 102(4 Pt 1):913–923, ©1989–1991.

TABLE D-7 Top 10 Foods and Beverages Contributing to Energy Intake in the U.S. Population, NHANES 1999–2000 and NHANES III[a]

Rank	Food	% Total Energy	Cumulative % Total Energy
NHANES 1999–2000			
1	Regular soft drinks	7.1	7.1
2	Cake, sweet rolls, doughnuts, pastries	3.6	10.6
3	Hamburgers, cheeseburgers, meat loaf	3.1	13.8
4	Pizza	3.1	16.8
5	Potato chips, corn chips, popcorn	2.9	19.7
6	Rice	2.7	22.4
7	Rolls, buns, English muffins, bagels	2.7	25.0
8	Cheese or cheese spread	2.6	27.6
9	Beer	2.6	30.2
10	French fries, fried potatoes	2.2	32.4
NHANES III 1988–1994			
1	Regular soft drinks	6.0	6.0
2	Cake, sweet rolls, donuts, pastries	3.9	9.9
3	Pizza	3.3	13.2
4	White bread including Italian or French	3.3	16.5
5	Hamburgers, cheeseburgers, meatloaf	3.1	19.6
6	Beer	2.7	22.3
7	Rolls, buns, English muffins, bagels	2.6	24.9
8	Potato chips, corn chips, popcorn	2.6	27.5
9	Rice	2.3	29.8
10	French fries, fried potatoes	2.3	32.1

[a]Includes both adults and children of both sexes.
SOURCE: Adapted from Block (2004). Reprinted from Journal of Food Composition and Analysis, Vol 17, Block G, Foods contributing to energy intake in the US: Data from NHANES II and NHANES 1999–2000, Pages 439–447, 2004, with permission from Elsevier.

TABLE D-8 Mean Sodium Intake (mg) for U.S. Children and Adolescents, 1971–2000[a]

Age/Sex Years	NHANES I 1971–1974	NHANES II 1976–1980	NHANES III 1988–1994	NHANES 1999–2000
Both Sexes				
1–2	1,631	1,828	1,983	2,148
3–5	1,925	2,173	2,594	2,527
6–11	2,393	2,716	3,164	3,255
Boys				
12–15	2,923	3,405	4,240	3,858
16–19	3,219	4,030	4,904	4,415
Girls				
12–15	2,094	2,567	3,200	3,034
16–19	1,812	2,336	3,160	3,048

[a]Includes food sources and sodium used in food preparation but not salt added to food at the table.
SOURCE: Reprinted, with permission, adapted from Briefel and Johnson (2004).

TABLE D-9 Trends in Sweetened Beverage and Milk Consumption by Children and Adolescents, Ages 2–18 Years

Measurement	Years	Sweetened Beverages[a]	Milk
Percentage of total daily calorie intake[b]	1977–1978	4.8	13.2
	1989–1991	6.1	11.2
	1994–1996	8.5	8.8
	1999–2001	10.3	8.3
Percentage of consumers	1977–1978	74.5	94.3
	1989–1991	74.2	90.3
	1994–1996	84.7	84.6
Servings[c]	1977–1978	2.02	3.46
	1989–1991	2.2	2.89
	1994–1996	2.55	2.75
Portions[d] (fluid ounces)	1977–1978	13.1	15.4
	1989–1991	15.8	14.1
	1994–1996	18.9	13.6

[a]Includes soft drinks and fruit drinks.
[b]Based on mean per capita intake.
[c]Servings are the number of discrete times an individual consumes an item.
[d]Portions are the amount consumed by an individual at one eating occasion.
SOURCE: Adapted from Nielsen and Popkin (2004). Reprinted from *American Journal of Preventive Medicine*, Vol 27, Nielsen SJ, Popkin BM, Changes in beverage intake between 1997 and 2001, Pages 205–210, 2004, with permission from *American Journal of Preventive Medicine*.

REFERENCES

Block G. 2004. Foods contributing to energy intake in the US: Data from NHANES III and NHANES 1999–2000. *J Food Comp Analysis* 17(3-4):439–447.

Briefel RR, Johnson CL. 2004. Secular trends in dietary intake in the United States. *Annu Rev Nutr* 24:401–431.

Enns CW, Mickle SJ, Goldman JD. 2002. Trends in food and nutrient intakes by children in the United States. *Fam Econ Nutr Rev* 14(2):56–68.

Enns CW, Mickle SJ, Goldman JD. 2003. Trends in food and nutrient intakes by adolescents in the United States. *Fam Econ Nutr Rev* 15(2):15–27.

IOM (Institute of Medicine). 1997. *Dietary Reference Intakes for Calcium, Phosphorus, Magnesium, Vitamin D, and Fluoride.* Washington, DC: National Academy Press.

IOM. 1998. *Dietary Reference Intakes for Thiamin, Riboflavin, Niacin, Vitamin B_6, Folate, Vitamin B_{12}, Pantothenic Acid, Biotin, and Choline.* Washington, DC: National Academy Press.

IOM. 2000. *Dietary Reference Intakes for Vitamin C, Vitamin E, Selenium and Catotenoids.* Washington, DC: National Academy Press.

IOM. 2001. *Dietary Reference Intakes for Vitamin A, Vitamin K, Arsenic, Boron, Chromium, Copper, Iodine, Iron, Manganese, Molybdenum, Nickel, Silicon, Vanadium, and Zinc.* Washington, DC: National Academy Press.

IOM. 2002–2005. *Dietary Reference Intakes for Energy, Carbohydrate, Fiber, Fat, Fatty Acids, Cholesterol, Protein, and Amino Acids.* Washington, DC: The National Academies Press.

IOM. 2005. *Dietary Reference Intakes for Water, Potassium, Sodium, Chloride, and Sulfate.* Washington, DC: The National Academies Press.

Nielsen SJ, Popkin BM. 2004. Changes in beverage intake between 1997 and 2001. *Am J Prev Med* 27(3):205–210.

Subar AF, Krebs-Smith SM, Cook A, Kahle LL. 1998. Dietary sources of nutrients among US children, 1989–1991. *Pediatrics* 102(4 Pt 1):913–923.

USDA. 2003. *Federal Register Notice on Technical Revisions to the Food Guide Pyramid.* Table 2: Energy Levels for Proposed Food Intake Patterns. Center for Nutrition Policy and Promotion. [Online]. Available: http://www.cnpp.usda.gov/pyramid-update/FGP%20docs/TABLE%202.pdf [accessed March 28, 2005].

E

Chapter 4 Appendix

This table represents examples of selected marketing research firms and marketing reports that the committee considered through its data-gathering process.

TABLE E-1 Marketing Research Conducted on U.S. Children and Youth

Sources	Report	Description
Children's Marketing Services (2004a)	TeenTrends™, 2004	Examined the interests and behavior of tweens and teens ages 12–18 years. A personal interview was conducted for 300 teens.
Children's Marketing Services (2004b)	KidTrends2004™, 2004	Examined the interests and behavior of older children ages 6–11 years. A personal interview was conducted for 300 older children.
Harris Interactive (2004)	Youth Pulse, 2004	Examined the interests and behavior of older children and teens ages 8–21 years through a large-scale study of youth lifestyles and attitudes via an online questionnaire.

continues

TABLE E-1 Continued

Sources	Report	Description
Just Kid Inc., Nickelodeon, and Research International (Friend and Stapylton-Smith, 1999)	The Global Kids Study, 1996 and 1998	Surveyed 400 children ages 7–12 years and their mothers in 12 countries: the United States, United Kingdom, France, Germany, Japan, China, Australia, India, Italy, Argentina, Brazil, and Mexico. An interview and questionnaire were used that provided a detailed picture of the attitudes, beliefs, and consumer dynamics of children and tweens.
Just Kid Inc. (2001)	Kid ID Study, 2001	Surveyed 4,000 children ages 8–14 years in schools to examine the emotional, psychological, and social forces that drive their behaviors.
Kidsay (2005)	Trend Tracker, conducted bimonthly	Examines the interests and behaviors of tweens and young teens ages 8–15 years.
KidShop/KidzEyes (2003)	Kid Food Findings. Brand New Research	Examined the product brand, food category, and restaurant preferences of 629 tweens ages 8–12 years.
Mediamark Research (2005)	Teen Study (Teenmark), conducted annually	Collects data about media exposure by more than 4,000 teens ages 12–19 years through a mailed questionnaire.
Mintel International Group Ltd. (2004)	Kids' and Teens' Eating Habits U.S., 2004	Examined eating habits of children ages 6–11 and 12–17 years based on the Simmons Kids and Teens surveys.
Mintel International Group Ltd. (2003a)	Kids' Snacking U.S., 2003	Examined snacking trends of children ages 6–8 and 9–11 years based on a variety of surveys, including the Simmons Kids Study.
Mintel International Group Ltd. (2003b)	Kids' Lifestyles U.S., 2003	Examined the lifestyle trends and attitudes of children ages 6–11 years.
Porter Novelli (2004)	Combined YouthStyles Survey and HealthStyles Survey	Provided parent–child dyads of information to develop understanding about the contexts in which youth act and live. The YouthStyles Survey examined children's values, goals, and motivations combined with behavioral data through a mail survey of an estimated 8,000 children and youth ages 10–19 years. Provided a combination of behavioral, motivational, and communication data.

TABLE E-1 Continued

Sources	Report	Description
Roper Youth Report (2003)	Roper Youth Report	Examined the purchasing power of young consumers ages 8–17 years. The report is based on 500 in-depth, personal interviews of a nationally representative sample of the U.S. tween and teen population.
Simmons (2005a)	Simmons Kids Study, conducted twice annually	Examines the media, consumer, and personal behaviors that drive the purchasing decisions of children ages 6–11 years.
Simmons (2005b)	Simmons Teens Study, conducted twice annually	Examines the media, consumer, and personal behaviors that drive the purchasing decisions of 5,000 teens ages 12–17 years based on in-home interviews and mail surveys.
Simmons (2005c)	Simmons Tweenz Study, conducted twice annually	Examines the media, consumer, and personal behaviors that drive the purchasing decisions of 5,000 tweens ages 8–14 years based on in-home interviews and mail surveys.
Simmons (2005d)	Simmons Youth Study, conducted twice annually	Examines the information of media, consumer, and personal behaviors that drive the purchasing decisions of children and youth ages 6–17 years.
Strottman International (2005)	Nutrition from a Kid's Perspective	Conducted brand-specific marketing research for clients from the food, beverage, and restaurant industries.
Teenage Research Unlimited (2004)	TRU Teenage Marketing and Lifestyle Study, 2004	Examined the spending power of 2,000 teens ages 12–19 years based on mail questionnaire.
The Geppetto Group (2005)	Case studies of market research conducted for food and beverage companies	A child and teen advertising agency and marketing consulting company that conducts research for clients about the motivations of childhood, kid archetypes, psyche of mothers as the family gatekeeper, understanding tweens' and teens' perspectives and lifestyles.
The Intelligence Group/Youth Intelligence (2005)	Nickelodeon/ Youth Intelligence Tween Report, 2004	Examined the lifestyles of tweens and teens ages 9–14 years including snacking and lifestyle habits.

continues

TABLE E-1 Continued

Sources	Report	Description
The NPD Group (2004)	Snacking in America Report, 2004	Examined the snacking behaviors of 10,000–12,000 children, teens, and adults from 1997–2003.
Yankelovich (2003)	Youth Monitor™, conducted annually	Examines the trends and information on media, brands, goals, technology, family, and self-image of 1,200 children ages 6–17 years through in-home personal interviews.
Yankelovich (2005)	Preschool Study	Surveyed a nationally representative sample of 650 parents and guardians of children ages 2–5 years to provide insights into the attitudes, concerns, and expectations of parents of preschoolers; healthy eating patterns; shopping habits; children's preferences; children's daily activities; developmental issues; and television viewing.
Zandl Group (2005)	Hot Sheet	Examined the attitudes, interests, entertainment, and product preferences of 3,000 children, youth, and young adults ages 8–24 years based on open-ended questionnaires.

TABLE E-2 New Food and Beverage Products Targeted to Children and Adolescents by Company, Manufacturer, or Distributor, 1994–2004

Company / Manufacturer / Distributor	Number of New Food Products
General Mills	166
Philip Morris	138
Kellogg Company	132
Nestlé S.A.	105
Wrigley	73
Unilever	65
Hasbro	60
Mars	56
ConAgra	53
Altria Group	52
Campbell Soup Company	44
Quaker Oats	42
Topps	40
OddzOn	38
Foreign Candy Company	36
Hershey Foods	36
Imaginings 3	34
PepsiCo	29
Felfoldi Potpourri Ltd.	27
RJR Nabisco	27
Philadelphia Chewing Gum Corp.	26

Company / Manufacturer / Distributor	Number of New Beverage Products
The Coca-Cola Company	37
Philip Morris	30
Nestlé S.A.	24
In Zone Brands	18
Cadbury Schweppes	15
Altria Group	12
PepsiCo	12
Danone	9
In Zone Brands	8
J. M. Smucker	8

SOURCE: Williams (2005b).

TABLE E-3 Selected Leading Companies Ranked by Total U.S. Revenues and Total Advertising Spending, 2004 and 2003

Company	Headquarters	Total U.S. Revenues ($ millions) 2004	Total U.S. Revenues ($ millions) 2003	Total Advertising Spending ($ millions) 2004	Total Advertising Spending ($ millions) 2003
Entertainment/Media					
Time Warner	New York, NY	33,572	32,123	3,283	3,073
Walt Disney	Burbank, CA	24,012	22,124	2,241	2,036
Viacom	New York, NY	18,812	17,488	1,207	1,151
Food and Beverage					
Altria Group[a]					
Kraft Foods	New York, NY	39,966	38,370	1,399	1,386
	Glenview, IL				
PepsiCo	Purchase, NY	18,329	17,377	1,262	1,211
General Mills	Minneapolis, MN	9,441	9,144	913	954
Kellogg Company	Battle Creek, MI	5,968	5,608	647	577
The Coca-Cola Company	Atlanta, GA	6,643	6,344	541	447
Campbell Soup Company	Camden, NJ	4,581	4,549	425	430
ConAgra	Omaha, NE	13,222	15,439	364	561
Food Retail					
Kroger Company	Cincinnati, OH	56,434[b]	53,791[b]	686	655
Safeway	Pleasanton, CA	31,463	31,679	606	536

Fast Food/Quick Serve Restaurant					
McDonald's Corporation	Oak Brook, IL	6,525[c]	6,039[c]	1,389	1,370
Yum! Brands	Louisville, KY	5,763	5,655	779	753
Burger King Corporation	Miami, FL	7,710	7,900	542	526
Wendy's International	Dublin, OH	2,475	2,197	436	387

NOTE: The majority of media and spending categories are monitored by TNS Media Intelligence, formerly TNS Media/Competitive Media Reporting (TNS Media Intelligence, 2005), and certain measured media categories, such as television and Internet advertising spending and impressions, are tracked by Nielsen Media Research and Nielsen//Net Ratings. Unmeasured media expenditures are not shown in the table.

[a]The Altria Group is the parent company for Kraft Foods and is separated into two sales divisions—food and tobacco. In 2004, total combined North America sales and earnings were $39.9 billion. Total division sales worldwide were $89.6 billion representing approximately $32.2 billion in food sales and $57 billion in tobacco sales. The company's brands represent five consumer sectors: snacks, beverages, cheese and dairy, grocery, and convenience meals (Brown et al., 2004, 2005; Kraft Foods, 2004).

[b]U.S. sales not available. This figure represents total worldwide sales.

[c]McDonald's Corporation worldwide sales in 2004 totaled $24.4 billion (BrandWeek, 2005).

SOURCES: Adapted from Brown et al. (2004, 2005). Reprinted with permission from the June 27, 2005 issue of *Advertising Age*. © Crain Communications, Inc., 2005.

REFERENCES

BrandWeek. 2005. *A Special Report: Superbrands. Plus: America's Top 2000 Brands.* [Online]. Available: http://www.brandweek.com [accessed August 8, 2005].

Brown K, Endicott RC, Macdonald S, Schumann M, Macarthur G, Sierra J, Matheny L, Green A, Ryan M. 2004. 100 leading national advertisers. *Advertising Age* June 28. Pp.1–83.

Brown K, Endicott RC, Macdonald S, Schumann M, Macarthur G, Sierra J, Matheny L, Green A, Ryan M. 2005. 50th annual 100 leading national advertisers. *Advertising Age* June 27. Pp.1–84. [Online]. Available: http://www.adage.com/images/random/lna2005. pdf [accessed September 16, 2005].

Children's Marketing Services. 2004a. *TeenTrends™*. [Online]. Available: http://www. kidtrends.com/new/reports.html [accessed May 3, 2005].

Children's Marketing Services. 2004b. *KidTrends™*. [Online]. Available: http://www. kidtrends.com/new/reports.html [accessed May 3, 2005].

Friend B, Stapylton-Smith M. 1999. *Through the Eyes of Children.* Presentation at the ESOMAR Marketing in Latin America Conference. Santiago, Chile. April 1999.

Harris Interactive. 2004. *Youth Pulse.* [Online]. Available: http://www.harrisinteractive.com/ expertise/youthpulse.asp [accessed May 3, 2005].

Just Kid Inc. 2001. *Kid ID Study.* [Online]. Available: http://www.justkidinc.com/ whatwedo.html [accessed May 13, 2005].

Kidsay. 2005. *Trend Tracker: Lifestyles of the Young and Influential.* [Online]. Available: http://www.kidsay.com/html/tracker/get_tracker_body.html [accessed September 17, 2005].

KidShop/KidzEyes. 2003. *Kid Food Findings. Brand New Research.* [Online]. Available: http://www.kidshopbiz.com/ [accessed October 3, 2005].

Kraft Foods. 2004. *Form 10-K Annual Report for the Fiscal Year Ended December 31, 2004.* [Online]. Available: http://kraft.com/pdfs/KraftAR04_10K.pdf [accessed June 6, 2005].

Mediamark Research. 2005. *Teen Study (Teenmark).* [Online]. Available: http://www. mediamark.com/mri/techguide/fall2004/tg_tm04.htm [accessed May 3, 2005].

Mintel International Group Ltd. 2003a. *Kids' Snacking US, 2003.* [Online]. Available: http:// reports.mintel.com/sinatra/mintel/searchexec/type=reports&variants=true&fulltext =kids+snacking/report/repcode=0093&anchor=noaccess0093/ [accessed May 3, 2005].

Mintel International Group Ltd. 2003b. *Kids' Lifestyles US, 2003.* [Online]. Available: http: //reports.mintel.com/sinatra/mintel/searchexec/type=reports&variants=true&fulltext =kids+lifestyles/report/repcode=2915&anchor=noaccess2915/ [accessed May 3, 2005].

Mintel International Group Ltd. 2004. *Kids' and Teens' Eating Habits US, 2004.* [Online]. Available: http://reports.mintel.com/sinatra/mintel/searchexec/type=reports&variants= true&fulltext=kids+and+teens+eating+habits/report/repcode=0240&anchor= noaccess0240/ [accessed May 3, 2005].

Porter Novelli. 2004. *YouthStyles and HealthStyles.* [Online]. Available: http://pn2. porternovelli.com/services/research/styles/ [accessed September 17, 2005].

Roper Youth Report. 2003. *Roper Youth Report. American Youth Wielding More Household Buying Power.* [Online]. Available: http://www.nopworld.com/news.asp?go= news_item&key=59/ [accessed April 11, 2005].

Simmons. 2005a. *Simmons Kids Study.* [Online]. Available: http://www.smrb.com/products_ kids.html [accessed May 3, 2005].

Simmons. 2005b. *Simmons Teens Study.* [Online]. Available: http://www.smrb.com/products _teens.html [accessed May 3, 2005].

Simmons. 2005c. *Simmons Tweenz Study.* [Online]. Available: http://www.smrb.com/products _tweenz.html [accessed May 3, 2005].

Simmons. 2005d. *Simmons Youth Study*. [Online]. Available: http://www.smrb.com/products _youth.html [accessed May 3, 2005].

Strottman International. 2005. *Nutrition from a Kid's Perspective. Findings, Implications, and Applications*. Presentation to the IOM Committee on Food Marketing and the Diets of Children and Youth. March 22.

Teenage Research Unlimited. 2004. *The TRU Study*. [Online]. Available: http://www. teenresearch.com/PRview.cfm?edit_id=168 [accessed May 3, 2005].

The Geppetto Group. 2005. [Online]. Available: http://www.geppettogroup.com/TheGeppetto Group5b.swf [accessed September 17, 2005].

The Intelligence Group/Youth Intelligence. 2005. *Nickelodeon/Youth Intelligence Tween Report 2004*. [Online]. Available: http://www.youthintelligence.com/cassandra/cassarticle. asp?cassArticleId=3 [accessed September 16, 2005].

The NPD Group. 2004. *Snacking in America Report*. Press release. January 28. [Online]. Available: http://www.npd.com/press/releases/press_040128a.htm [accessed September 15, 2005].

TNS Media Intelligence. 2005. *Delivering Information at Its Best*. [Online]. Available: http:// www.tns-mi.com [accessed April 30, 2005].

Yankelovich. 2003. *Youth Monitor™. Youth Today: Shaping Tomorrow*. Chapel Hill, NC: Yankelovich Partners, Inc.

Yankelovich. 2005. *Youth Monitor™*. [Online]. Available: http://www.yankelovich.com/prod-ucts/youth2005_ps.pdf [accessed May 3, 2005].

Williams J. 2005b. *Product Proliferation Analysis for New Food and Beverage Products Targeted to Children 1994–2004*. University of Texas at Austin Working Paper.

Zandl Group. 2005. *Hot Sheet*. [Online]. Available: http://www.zandlgroup.com/hot_sheet. shtml [accessed May 3, 2005].

F-1

Evidence Table Codebook

Each research study included in the systematic evidence review was coded on several descriptive and evaluative dimensions. Text description and commentary was also provided. This Codebook was used by each coder to ensure consistency in the information and judgments entered into the Evidence Table. Anything in bold should be entered exactly as described so that information on that variable can be sorted later.

Reference: Author Name(s)

Enter the **last name(s)** of the author(s) in order. If two authors, enter both last names separated by a comma. If more than two authors, use "**et al.**" after the last name of the first author.

Reference: Year

Enter the publication **year**; use all four digits for the year.

Link Number (#)

Enter the **number** of the link (relationship) that is being studied: 1 if the relationship is between marketing and a precursor (mediator) to diet, 3 if the relationship is between marketing and diet, and 5 if the relationship is between marketing and diet-related health. If the study has information or sub-studies about more than one link, make each link a separate line in the Evidence Table.

For studies in which television viewing was measured and interpreted as an indicator of exposure to televised advertising, add **TV** after the link number.

Link? Y/N

Enter **Y** (yes) if the link is significant at p equal to or less than .05; enter **N** (no) otherwise. For studies with statistical tests of more than one measure of the cause and/or effect or with statistical tests of various subgroups (e.g., boys and girls)—all for the same link—enter **Y** if any of the tests were significant and describe them all in the abstract. If none are significant, enter **N**.

Research Method

Enter one of the following six abbreviations (in parentheses). See the definitions that follow the terms.

- *Natural experiment* (**Exp-N**)
- *Randomized trial* (**Exp**)
- *Panel* (**L-Pnl**)
- *Cohort* (**L-Coh**)
- *Trend* (**L-Trnd**)
- *Cross-sectional* (**CS**)

Experimental Studies

- *Natural experiment (Exp-N):* Treatment assigned serendipitously but randomly. For example, in the early 1990s in the Milwaukee School Voucher program, there were more students who applied for school vouchers than vouchers available. All applicants were entered in a lottery, with only the winners getting vouchers.
- *Randomized trial (Exp):* Treatment assigned deliberately and randomly.

Nonexperimental (Observational) Studies

Longitudinal Studies:

- *Panel (L-Pnl):* Measures the *same* sample of individuals at different points in time.
- *Cohort (L-Coh):* Similar subjects (age, demographics, etc.) are followed over time and compared on outcome or descriptive measures (e.g., health). Cohort studies typically involve a sample in which some individuals have a property and some do not (e.g., smokers versus nonsmokers).
- *Trend (L-Trnd):* Samples *different* groups of people at different points in time from the *same* population, using the same measures.

Cross-Sectional Studies:

- *Cross-sectional (CS):* Nonexperimental study at a single point in time.

Cause Variable

Briefly describe the marketing variable considered the causal (initiating, independent) variable in the research. To describe it, use short, simple terms such as "vending machines in school," "exposure to food ads," and "television viewing." If there are multiple cause variables, all for the same link number, describe them all. Do not create separate lines for each variable. If some are significant and some are not (again all testing the same link in the model), enter **Y** in the link-significant column and describe all of the p-values for all the cause variables (testing the same link) in the mini-abstract. Do not describe the specifics of how the variable was measured.

In this column, to the extent possible, use a very short, general descriptor, closely tied to (if not the same as) one of the terms in the initiating variable box for the link in the Conceptual Framework that is being studied.

Cause Variable Measure

Describe the way(s) in which the independent variable was measured (for a nonexperimental study) or implemented in treatment conditions (for experimental study). Do so only for the link identified in this line of the Evidence Table. As examples, measurement techniques could be "self-report questionnaire," "parent interview," "sound-activated videotaping in rooms with television sets," or "ads taken from cable stations and inserted into cartoons taken from similar cable stations."

Cause Variable Category

Based on a description of the cause variable and how it was measured, determine which of the following possible categories best describes it. If more than one cause variable (with the same link) or more than one measure of the same cause were used, choose the best description for each.

- TV ads: Experiment
- TV ads: Viewing only
- TV ads: Observed in natural setting
- TV ads: Viewing + other media
- TV ads: Campaign
- Product placement in film
- Print ads
- Radio ads
- Multimedia campaign
- Price and promotion
- Other

Effect Variable

Briefly describe the variable considered the effect (consequent, dependent) variable in the research. It will be a precursor, diet, or diet-related health variable. To describe it, use simple terms such as "food preferences," "belief food is good for you," "increased drinking of Pepsi." If there are multiple effect variables, all for the same link number, describe them all. Do not create separate lines for each variable. If some are significant and some are not (again all testing the same link in the model), enter Y in the link significant column and describe all of the p-values for all the effect variables (testing the same link) in the mini-abstract. In this column, don't describe the specifics of how the variable was measured.

In this column, to the extent possible, use a very short, general descriptor, closely tied to (if not the same as) one of the terms in the box for the link in the Conceptual Framework that is being studied.

Effect Variable Measure

Describe the way(s) in which the dependent variable was measured. Describe all measures for every variable treated as a dependent variable for the link identified in this line of the evidence table. As examples, measurement techniques could be "self-report questionnaire," "parent interview," "observations at school cafeteria," "total sales," or "body mass index (BMI) calculated from weight and height measured by health professional."

Effect Variable Category

Based on a description of the effect variable and how it was measured, determine which of the following possible categories best describes it. If more than one effect variable (with the same link) or more than one measure of the same effect were used, choose the best description for each. In parentheses is the link number for which each effect variable term can be used.

- **Preferences** (Link 1)
- **Requests** (Link 1)
- **Beliefs** (Link 1)
- **Short-term consumption** (Link 3)
- **Usual diet** (Link 3)
- **Adiposity** (Link 5)
- **Other** (Links 1, 3, 5)

Sample Size

Enter the sample size as a **number**. If the number is 1,000 or greater, use a comma. Choose the number that is included in the analyses not the number the researcher started with, if these numbers are different. If there is significant participant loss, note that in the "Other Comments" column. If more than one sample was studied, make each sample a separate line.

In the mini-abstract, if useful, include more information about the sample; for example, include text description and numbers for different sectors of the sample (e.g., 100 children/teens and 100 parents, one parent for each child/teen). You might also decide to mention participant loss/attrition here.

Sample Age

Enter **IT, YC, OC,** or **T** if the sample is respectively all infants and toddlers (under 2 years of age), younger children (2–5 years), older children (6–11 years), or teens (12–18 years). If the sample is largely just one of these groups, enter that age group only or enter where the mean of the group falls (e.g., "mean 5.7," "preschool and some kindergarten," and "age 4 plus/minus 2 years" are all entered as YC). If the sample is described as more than one of these groups, enter the relevant letters, following the IT, YC, OC, T order (e.g., "OCT" not "TOC" for a sample of teenagers and older children). Do not use commas to separate the letters. If the sample was tested more than once, enter the age group for the sample when first tested. If at the later testing(s), the sample has grown into an older age group, add that. If still in the same age group, add nothing. If the article has no information about the age of the participants, enter **No Info.**

Indicate in the mini-abstract if the sample age clusters in one part of the indicated age range (e.g., if the sample of "older children" is only 6- and 7-year-olds, indicate this in the mini-abstract).

Note that it is not uncommon to see a child's age described as "3-11" or "6-1" to denote that the child was 3 years, 11 months, or 6 years, 1 month, respectively. When read in context, the reviewer should be able to figure out whether "3-11" means 3 years, 11 months, or 3 to 11 years.

Measure Quality

Enter **H, M,** or **L** to indicate high, medium, or low, following the guidance below. In the "Other Comments" column, include a brief description of the rationale for your rating choice. In general, the quality of the measure of the independent/cause variable is more important than the quality of the measure of the dependent/effect variable in determining this rating. Measurement of the control variables in a non-experimental study is also important. Finally, if any self-report measure is used, the best rating possible is **M** for overall measurement quality.

There are three primary criteria for evaluating the quality of measures in a study: *validity, reliability,* and *precision,* each of which is explained in more detail below.

- *Validity* refers to the extent to which an instrument directly and accurately measures what it is intended to measure.
- *Reliability* assesses the extent to which the same measurement technique, applied repeatedly, is likely to yield the same results.
- *Precision* refers to the fineness or coarseness of a measure.

Validity

Validity refers to the extent to which an operationalized measure directly and accurately measures the concept it is intended to measure. In measuring a child's food preferences in response to an ad, for example, a measure in which a child's actual food consumption was recorded is more valid than a measure in which a child's self-report of his/her future intentions was recorded. The total amount of TV watched is often used as a measure of the total exposure to advertising, but such a measure is lower in validity than is a direct measure of advertising exposure. For example, some people might channel surf or do chores during ads or they might watch programs with ads that are unlikely to be relevant to children.

Bias affects validity, but certain kinds of bias are much worse than others. A highly reliable bathroom scale that is set 7 pounds light is biased, but its bias is constant, the scale measures what it is supposed to, and thus the scale still has high validity, especially when measuring change in weight over time. Self-reports of socially undesirable behaviors are usually biased, and the amount of bias usually varies with the amount of social undesirability (e.g., heavy candy eaters are likely to underreport more severely than are those who eat less candy).

Reliability

Reliability assesses the extent to which the same measurement technique, applied repeatedly, is likely to yield the same results when it is believed that the variable measured has not changed. Measuring a child's weight with a good bathroom scale is highly reliable, but measuring the child's cumulative exposure to environmental lead since birth by measuring the concentration of lead in drawn blood is not reliable (it varies greatly from day to day). Almost no one can remember every bit of food he or she consumed last week, so measures that depend on recall are typically low in reliability (and also typically low on validity).

Reliability is often important in studies involving subjective coding of observed behavior. One, we want the same coder to score the same behavior in the same way across times (intracoder reliability), and two, we want different coders to score the same behavior in the same way (intercoder reliability).

Precision

Precision refers to the fineness or coarseness of a measure. For example, recording family income as low, medium, or high is less precise than recording the number of dollars in family income, such as $18,500.

Overall Scoring for Measure Quality

Studies that rank high on all three factors—high on validity AND on reliability AND on precision—would be considered to have **H**, *high measure quality*.

Studies that rank high on one or two of the three factors and low on none would be considered to have **M**, *medium measure quality*.

Studies that do not rank high on any of the three factors or that rank low on at least one would be considered to have **L**, *low measurement quality*.

Causality Evidence

Enter **H**, **M**, or **L** to indicate high, medium, or low, following the guidance below. In the "Other Comments" column, include a brief description of the rationale for your rating choice.

The rating of causality evidence is entirely separate from that for ecological validity. The idea is to rate the quality of the case that can be made for interpreting a statistically significant association as causal and not just an association. We separate experimental studies from observational studies in explaining how to do the rating.

Experimental Studies

1. *Treatment Bias*

The essential feature of an experimental study that allows causal inference is that assignment of treatment be independent of any potential confounder, that is, any property that might also have an influence on the outcome. When treatment is assigned randomly, treatment bias is (at least in theory) eliminated. In natural experiments, or experiments without randomized assignment of treatment, treatment bias is a real concern.

For example, an experiment comparing an online course on computer programming to a human-taught course on the same topic in which participants were allowed to choose the condition would obviously suffer from treatment bias, as those with high computing aptitude and/or experience are more likely to choose the online condition.

The antidote to treatment bias is analogous to what is required in observational studies: we must measure and statistically control for the confounding property, perhaps with a pretest. For example, if the online/human study measured computer aptitude prior to the course and then controlled for it, treatment bias would not be a large concern.

2. *Dropout/Attrition Bias*

Experiments in which dropout during the trial is associated with a potential confounder are suspect for causal inference. For example, in the Milwaukee School Voucher evaluation "natural experiment," in which all participants wanted vouchers but only those who won a lottery received them, both groups experienced fairly high dropout rates between the enrollment period and the post-test. Researchers were concerned that, among the students who did not win the lottery, those who dropped out were the ones with aggressive concerned parents, leaving behind those likely to learn less.

3. *Measurement*

Studies in which the measures have low validity are suspect for causal inference. For example, an experiment in which the cause of interest was advertising exposure—but only overall TV watching was experimentally manipulated—suffers from this problem because overall TV exposure is a weak measure of advertising exposure.

4. *Experimental Studies—Summary*

Experimental studies with no treatment bias, no dropout bias, and reasonable validity in measurement should be given **H**, High Causality Evidence. Studies with serious treatment bias should be given **L**, Low Causality Evidence.

Observational Studies

In an observational study, an association between a putative cause X and an effect Y might be due to any combination of (1) X is a cause of Y, (2) some third factor is a common cause of both, or (3) Y is a cause of X. The overall assessment of causal validity rides on how convincingly the study eliminates possibilities 2 and 3.

1. *Time*

One common strategy is to use time order to eliminate possibility 3. The fact that X is measured prior to Y, however, does nothing to eliminate possibility 2, that there is a confounder that occurs prior to both X and Y that is responsible for both X and Y and accounts for the apparent association between X and Y.

2. *Confounders/Controls/Omitted Variables/Covariates*
2a. *Inclusion*

The most common obstacle to causal inference in observational studies is the possibility that the statistical association between the putative cause and effect might be spurious, that is, due to an omitted variable that is a cause of both. Such factors are commonly referred to as confounders, covariates, third variables, omitted variables, etc.

To be rated **H**, High on causal inference validity, an observational study must include—that is, measure and statistically control for—all confounders that are significantly associated with both the cause and effect. A study that controls for most significant but not all possible confounders can still be rated **M**, Medium on causal inference validity.

2b. *Measures*

Measurement is crucial to causal inference in observational studies, but not in a simple way. If any of the measures lacks validity, then the case for causality is weakened.

Although a lack of precision or reliability in the dependent variable will affect the statistical inference (the standard errors and p-values), it will not bias the coefficient estimate and is of little or no consequence to the causal inference validity.

When the cause, or independent, variable is measured with low reliability, then the estimate of its effect is biased toward zero, making it *harder* to find a significant p-value, and thus in some sense strengthening the case for causation.

When a covariate, that is, a variable being "controlled for" in the analysis, is measured with low reliability or precision, however, the estimate of the association between cause and effect will be biased.[1] In some cases the bias will be toward zero, and in others away from zero. The direction of the bias is the same as the case in which the variable is entirely left out of the analysis.

3. *Observational Studies—Summary*

An observational study should score **H**, High on Causality Evidence when (a) the possibility that the response variable is a cause of the independent variable can be eliminated (perhaps by time), (b) the cause and effect are measured with high validity, and (3) all significant confounders have been included and measured with high validity, reliability, and precision.

Ecological Validity

Enter **H**, **M**, or **L** to indicate high, medium, or low, following guidance below. In the "Other Comments" column, include a brief description of the rationale for your rating choice.

Ecological validity refers to the extent to which an investigation's research setting, stimuli, and response demands are similar to those of the naturally occurring settings, stimuli, and responses characteristic of the behavioral system being studied.

H, *high ecological validity*, occurs when the research setting and stimuli/cause and effect/response are similar to those of the system under investigation.

---

[1]The sign of the bias is the same as the bias that would result if the variable was omitted from the analysis entirely, and the size of the bias is proportional to the size of the measurement problem. A covariate with a highly imprecise measure will result in more bias than one with a mildly imprecise measure.

An example would be an experiment that manipulated the signage on the vending machines in schools with the measured responses being the purchases made from the vending machines. Another example would be a survey in which parents and children reported on the children's home television viewing and daily diet.

M, *medium ecological validity*, occurs when the research setting or the stimuli or the responses are similar to those of the system under investigation.

An example would be an experiment in which children are brought to a university laboratory, shown a children's TV program with embedded food commercials, and then allowed to choose food from a selection of food items. The foods chosen and the amounts eaten are the responses. In this case, the setting is not a natural setting for the child, but the stimuli (children's TV program and commercials) and the responses are at least moderately similar to natural stimuli and responses.

L, *low ecological validity*, occurs when neither the research setting nor the stimuli nor the responses are similar to those of the system under investigation. An example would be an experiment in which a child is brought to a university laboratory, hears a description of a television commercial, explains the intent underlying the broadcast of the commercial, and chooses a food from several pictures of food. In this case neither the setting, nor the stimuli, nor the response demands would be characteristic of the behavioral system under investigation.

Mini-Abstract
Provide a brief description of the main elements of the study. If the research was conducted outside the United States, indicate where it was conducted.

Lead Reviewer
Enter the last name of the person designated as lead reviewer.

Other Comments: Lead Reviewer
The lead reviewer adds any comments about unusual results or features of the research, questions he or she had in reviewing the research or filling in the Evidence Table, opinions about the overall quality of the work, arguments for why the apparently positive causal relationship should be discounted, and other information that seems pertinent. Also be sure to include the rationales for the Measure Quality, Causality Evidence, and Ecological Validity ratings.

Second Reviewer
Enter the last name of the person designated as the second reviewer.

Other Comments: Second Reviewer

The second reviewer adds any comments about unusual results or features of the research, questions he or she had in reviewing the research or filling in the Evidence Table, opinions about the overall quality of the work, arguments for why the apparently positive causal relationship should be discounted, and other information that seems pertinent. Also be sure to include the rationales for the Measure Quality, Causality Evidence, and Ecological Validity ratings.

F-2

Summary Evidence Table

Relationship	Precursors	Relationship between marketing and precursors to diet
	Diet	Relationship between marketing and diet
	Health	Relationship between marketing and diet-related health
	(TV)	Exposure to advertising on television measured by television viewing
Significance	Y	Study reported one or more statistically significant relationships between marketing and an outcome variable at p less than or equal to 0.05
	N	Study reported no statistically significant relationship between marketing and an outcome variable
Research Method	CS	Cross-sectional
	Exp	Randomized trial
	Exp-N	Natural experiment
	L-Pnl	Longitudinal—Panel
	L-Trnd	Longitudinal—Trend
Cause Variable Category		The general category that the independent variable was measuring, e.g., "TV ads—Experiment," "TV ads—Viewing only," and "Multimedia campaign"
Effect Variable Category		The general category that the dependent variable was measuring, e.g., "Preferences," "Short-term consumption," and "Adiposity"
Sample Age	IT	Infants and toddlers under 2 years of age
	YC	Younger children ages 2–5 years
	OC	Older children ages 6–11 years
	T	Teens ages 12–18 years
Measure Quality/ Causality Evidence/ Ecological Validity	H	High
	M	Medium
	L	Low

447

Reference				
Author(s)	Year	Relationship	Significance	Research Method
Andersen et al.	1998	Health (TV)	Y	CS
Anderson et al.	2001	Health (TV)	N	L-Pnl
Anderson et al.	2001	Health (TV)	Y	CS
Armstrong et al.	1998	Health (TV)	Y	CS
Auty, Lewis	2004	Diet	Y	Exp
Bao, Shao	2002	Precursors	Y	Exp
Bao, Shao	2002	Precursors	Y	L-Trnd
Barry, Gunst	1982	Precursors	N	Exp
Berkey et al.	2000	Health (TV)	Y	L-Pnl
Berkey et al.	2003	Health (TV)	Y	CS
Bogaert et al.	2003	Health (TV)	N	L-Pnl
Bolton	1983	Diet (TV)	Y	CS
Borzekowski, Poussaint	1998	Precursors (TV)	Y	CS
Borzekowski, Poussaint	1998	Diet (TV)	Y	CS
Borzekowski, Robinson	2001	Precursors	Y	Exp
Boynton-Jarrett et al.	2003	Diet (TV)	Y	L-Pnl
Brody et al.	1981	Precursors	Y	Exp
Burke et al.	2005	Health (TV)	Y	L-Pnl
Cantor	1981	Diet	Y	Exp
Carruth et al.	1991	Diet (TV)	N	CS
Christenson	1982	Precursors	Y	Exp
Clancy-Hepburn et al.	1974	Precursors (TV)	N	CS

Cause Variable Category	Effect Variable Category	Sample Size	Sample Age	Measure Quality	Causality Evidence	Ecological Validity
TV ads—Viewing only	Adiposity	4,063	OCT	L	L	H
TV ads—Viewing only	Adiposity	570	YCT	M	M	H
TV ads—Viewing only	Adiposity	570	T	L	L	H
TV ads—Viewing + other media	Adiposity	588	OC	L	L	H
Product placement in film	Short-term consumption	105	OC	H	H	M
Radio ads	Preferences	180	T	L	M	L
Multimedia campaign	Preferences	2,276	T	L	L	H
TV ads—Experiment	Preferences	172	YCOC	L	M	L
TV ads—Viewing + other media	Adiposity	10,769	OCT	L	M	H
TV ads—Viewing + other media	Adiposity	10,896	OCT	L	L	H
TV ads—Viewing only	Adiposity	41	OC	L	L	H
TV ads—Viewing only	Usual Diet	262	YCOC	M	M	H
TV ads—Viewing only	Requests	128	YC	L	L	M
TV ads—Viewing only	Usual Diet	128	YC	L	L	M
TV ads—Experiment	Preferences	39	YC	H	H	M
TV ads—Viewing only	Usual Diet	548	OC	L	M	H
TV ads—Experiment	Requests	57	YC	M	H	M
TV ads—Viewing only	Adiposity	1,430	OC	L	M	H
TV ads—Experiment	Short-term consumption	37	YCOC	H	H	M
TV ads—Viewing only	Usual diet	887	T	M	L	H
TV ads—Experiment	Preferences and other	90	OC	M	H	M
TV ads—Viewing only	Preferences	105	OC	L	L	H

continues

Reference				Research
Author(s)	Year	Relationship	Significance	Method
Clarke	1984	Precursors	N	Exp
Coon et al.	2001	Diet (TV)	Y	CS
Crespo et al.	2001	Diet (TV)	Y	CS
Crespo et al.	2001	Health (TV)	Y	CS
Crooks	2000	Health (TV)	N	CS
Dawson et al.	1988	Precursors	N	Exp
Deheeger et al.	1997	Health (TV)	Y	CS
Dennison et al.	2002	Health (TV)	Y	CS
Dennison et al.	2002	Health (TV)	Y	CS
Dietz, Gortmaker	1985	Health (TV)	Y	CS
Dietz, Gortmaker	1985	Health (TV)	Y	L-Pnl
Donkin et al.	1993	Precursors (TV)	Y	CS
Donkin et al.	1993	Diet (TV)	Y	CS
Donohue	1975	Precursors (TV)	Y	CS
Dowda et al.	2001	Health (TV)	Y	CS
duRant et al.	1994	Health (TV)	N	CS
duRant et al.	1996	Health (TV)	N	CS
Dwyer et al.	1998	Health (TV)	N	CS
Eisenmann et al.	2002	Health (TV)	Y	CS
Faber et al.	1984	Precursors	Y	Exp
Fontvieille et al.	1993	Health (TV)	Y	CS

Cause Variable Category	Effect Variable Category	Sample Size	Age	Measure Quality	Causality Evidence	Ecological Validity
TV ads— Experiment	Preferences	80	YC	M	M	M
TV ads— Viewing only	Usual Diet	91	OC	M	L	H
TV ads— Viewing only	Usual Diet	4,069	OCT	L	L	H
TV ads— Viewing only	Adiposity	4,069	OCT	L	L	H
TV ads— Viewing + other media	Adiposity	54	OC	L	L	H
TV ads— Experiment	Preferences	80	OC	M	H	L
TV ads— Viewing only	Adiposity	86	OC	L	L	H
TV ads— Viewing only	Adiposity	2,761	YC	M	L	M
TV ads— Viewing only	Adiposity	1,182	YC	M	L	M
TV ads— Viewing only	Adiposity	13,636	OCT	M	L	M
TV ads— Viewing only	Adiposity	2,153	OCT	M	M	M
TV ads— Viewing only	Requests	254	OC	L	L	H
TV ads— Viewing only	Usual diet	254	OC	L	L	H
TV ads— Viewing only	Requests	162	YC	L	L	M
TV ads— Viewing only	Adiposity	2,791	OCT	L	L	H
TV ads— Observed in natural setting	Adiposity	110	YC	M	L	H
TV ads— Observed in natural setting	Adiposity	138	YCOC	M	L	H
TV ads— Viewing + other media	Adiposity	3,214	OC	M	L	M
TV ads— Viewing only	Adiposity	15,143	T	L	L	H
TV ads— Experiment	Beliefs and preferences	162	YCOCT	M	M	L
TV ads— Viewing + other media	Adiposity	85	OC	L	L	L

continues

| Reference | | | | |
Author(s)	Year	Relationship	Significance	Research Method
Francis et al.	2003	Diet (TV)	Y	L-Pnl
Francis et al.	2003	Health (TV)	Y	L-Pnl
French et al.	2001a	Diet	Y	Exp-N
French et al.	2001b	Diet (TV)	Y	CS
Galst	1980	Diet	Y	Exp
Galst, White	1976	Precursors	Y	CS
Giammattei et al.	2003	Health (TV)	Y	CS
Goldberg	1990	Diet (TV)	Y	Exp-N
Goldberg et al.	1978	Precursors	Y	Exp
Gordon-Larsen et al.	2002	Health (TV)	Y	L-Pnl
Gorn, Florsheim	1985	Precursors	N	Exp
Gorn, Florsheim	1985	Precursors	Y	Exp
Gorn, Goldberg	1980	Diet	N	Exp
Gorn, Goldberg	1980	Precursors	Y	Exp
Gorn, Goldberg	1982	Diet	Y	Exp
Gortmaker et al.	1996	Health (TV)	Y	L-Pnl
Gracey et al.	1996	Health (TV)	N	CS
Graf et al.	2004	Health (TV)	Y	CS
Gray, Smith	2003	Health (TV)	Y	CS
Greenberg, Brand	1993	Precursors	Y	Exp-N
Greenberg, Brand	1993	Diet	N	Exp-N
Grund et al.	2000	Health (TV)	Y	CS

Cause Variable Category	Effect Variable Category	Sample Size	Age	Measure Quality	Causality Evidence	Ecological Validity
TV ads—Viewing only	Usual diet	173	YCOC	M	M	H
TV ads—Viewing only	Adiposity	173	YCOC	M	M	H
Price and promotion	Usual diet	55	T	H	H	H
TV ads—Viewing only	Usual diet	4,344	T	L	L	H
TV ads—Experiment	Short-term consumption	65	YC	H	H	L
TV ads—Viewing only	Requests	41	YC	H	L	M
TV ads—Viewing only	Adiposity	319	OC	M	L	H
TV ads—Viewing only	Usual diet	475	OC	M	M	H
TV ads—Experiment	Preferences	81	YCOC	M	M	M
TV ads—Viewing + other media	Adiposity	12,759	OCT	M	M	H
TV ads—Experiment	Preferences	70	OC	M	M	M
TV ads—Experiment	Beliefs and preferences	70	OC	M	M	M
TV ads—Experiment	Short-perm consumption	151	OC	H	H	M
TV ads—Experiment	Beliefs and preferences	151	OC	H	H	M
TV ads—Experiment	Short-term consumption	288	OC	H	H	H
TV ads—Viewing only	Adiposity	746	OCT	M	M	H
TV ads—Viewing only	Adiposity	391	T	L	L	H
TV ads—Viewing only	Adiposity	207	OC	L	L	H
TV ads—Viewing only	Adiposity	155	YCOCT	M	L	H
TV ads—Experiment	Preferences	1,647	T	M	M	H
TV ads—Experiment	Usual diet	1,647	T	M	H	H
TV ads—Viewing only	Adiposity	88	YCOC	M	L	H

continues

Reference Author(s)	Year	Relationship	Significance	Research Method
Guillaume et al.	1997	Health (TV)	Y	CS
Halford et al.	2004	Diet	Y	Exp
Harrison	2005	Precursors	Y	L-Pnl
Hernandez et al.	1999	Health (TV)	Y	CS
Heslop, Ryans	1980	Precursors	N	Exp
Hitchings, Moynihan	1998	Diet	Y	CS
Horn et al.	2001	Health (TV)	Y	L-Pnl
Horn et al.	2001	Health (TV)	Y	CS
Hoy et al.	1986	Precursors	Y	Exp
Isler et al.	1987	Precursors (TV)	Y	CS
Janz et al.	2002	Health (TV)	Y	CS
Jeffrey et al.	1982	Diet	Y	Exp
Jeffrey et al.	1982	Diet	Y	Exp
Kant, Graubard	2003	Diet (TV)	N	CS
Katzmarzyk et al.	1998	Health (TV)	N	CS
Kaur et al.	2003	Health (TV)	Y	L-Pnl
Kaur et al.	2003	Health (TV)	Y	CS
Klein-Platat et al.	2005	Health (TV)	Y	CS
Krassas et al.	2001	Health (TV)	Y	CS
Kunkel	1988	Precursors	Y	Exp
Levin et al.	2004	Health (TV)	N	CS
Lewis, Hill	1998	Precursors	Y	Exp

Cause Variable Category	Effect Variable Category	Sample		Measure Quality	Causality Evidence	Ecological Validity
		Size	Age			
TV ads— Viewing only	Adiposity and other	1,028	OC	M	L	H
TV ads— Experiment	Short-term consumption	42	OC	H	H	M
TV ads— Viewing only	Beliefs	134	OC	M	M	H
TV ads— Viewing only	Adiposity	461	OCT	L	L	H
TV ads— Experiment	Preferences	280	YCOC	M	H	M
TV ads— Viewing only	Usual diet	44	OC	M	L	L
TV ads— Viewing only	Adiposity	103	OC	L	L	H
TV ads— Viewing only	Adiposity	103	OC	L	L	H
TV ads— Experiment	Preferences	78	YC	M	M	L
TV ads— Viewing only	Requests	250	YCOC	M	L	H
TV ads— Viewing only	Adiposity	464	YCOC	M	L	H
TV ads— Experiment	Short-term consumption	47	YC	H	H	M
TV ads— Experiment	Short-term consumption	96	YCOC	H	H	M
TV ads— Viewing only	Usual diet	4,137	OCT	L	M	H
TV ads— Viewing only	Adiposity	784	OCT	L	L	H
TV ads— Viewing only	Adiposity	2,223	T	L	L	H
TV ads— Viewing only	Adiposity	2,223	T	L	L	H
TV ads— Viewing + other media	Adiposity	2,714	OC	L	L	H
TV ads— Viewing + other media	Adiposity	2,468	OCT	L	L	H
TV ads— Experiment	Beliefs, preferences, and requests	152	YCOC	M	M	M
TV ads— Viewing only	Adiposity	148	YC	M	L	L
TV ads— Experiment	Preferences	35	OC	M	H	L

continues

Reference Author(s)	Year	Relationship	Significance	Research Method
Lin et al.	2004	Health (TV)	N	CS
Locard et al.	1992	Health (TV)	N	CS
Macklin	1990	Precursors	N	Exp
Macklin	1994	Precursors	Y	Exp
Maffeis et al.	1998	Health (TV)	N	L-Pnl
Maffeis et al.	1998	Health (TV)	Y	CS
Manios et al.	2004	Health (TV)	Y	CS
Matheson et al.	2004	Diet (TV)	Y	CS
McMurray et al.	2000	Health (TV)	N	CS
Miller, Busch	1979	Precursors	Y	Exp
Morton	1990	Precursors	Y	CS
Muller et al.	1999	Diet (TV)	Y	CS
Muller et al.	1999	Health (TV)	Y	CS
Norton et al.	2000	Precursors	Y	CS
Obarzanek et al.	1994	Health (TV)	Y	CS
O'Loughlin et al.	2000	Health (TV)	N	L-Pnl
Palmer, McDowell	1981	Precursors	Y	CS
Pate, Ross	1987	Health (TV)	Y	CS
Peterson et al.	1984	Precursors	Y	Exp
Peterson et al.	1984	Diet	N	Exp
Pine, Nash	2003	Precursors	Y	CS
Proctor et al.	2003	Health (TV)	Y	L-Pnl

Cause Variable Category	Effect Variable Category	Sample Size	Age	Measure Quality	Causality Evidence	Ecological Validity
TV ads—Viewing only	Adiposity	1,651	OCT	M	M	H
TV ads—Viewing only	Adiposity	1,020	YC	L	L	H
Print ads	Beliefs, preferences, and requests	36	YC	M	M	L
TV ads—Experiment	Requests	40	YCOC	L	M	L
TV ads—Viewing only	Adiposity	112	OCT	L	L	H
TV ads—Viewing only	Adiposity	112	OCT	L	L	H
TV ads—Viewing + other media	Adiposity	198	OC	L	L	H
TV ads—Viewing only	Usual diet	214	OC	M	L	H
TV ads—Viewing + other media	Adiposity	2,389	OCT	L	L	H
TV ads—Experiment	Preferences	363	YCOC	M	H	L
TV ads—Viewing only	Requests	185	T	M	L	H
TV ads—Viewing only	Usual diet	1,497	YCOC	M	L	H
TV ads—Viewing only	Adiposity	1,497	YCOC	M	L	H
Price and promotion	Preferences	35	OCT	M	L	M
TV ads—Viewing + other media	Adiposity	2,379	OC	M	M	H
TV ads—Viewing only	Adiposity	2,634	OC	L	M	H
TV ads—Viewing only	Beliefs	64	YC	M	M	L
TV ads—Viewing only	Adiposity	2,372	OC	M	L	M
TV ads—Experiment	Beliefs and preferences	106	OC	M	M	M
TV ads—Experiment	Short-term consumption	106	OC	H	M	M
TV ads—Campaign	Preferences	75	YC	M	M	M
TV ads—Viewing only	Adiposity	106	YCOC	M	M	H

continues

Reference Author(s)	Year	Relationship	Significance	Research Method
Reid et al.	1980	Precursors (TV)	N	CS
Reilly et al.	2005	Health (TV)	Y	L-Pnl
Resnik, Stern	1977	Precursors	Y	Exp
Ritchey, Olson	1983	Precursors (TV)	N	CS
Ritchey, Olson	1983	Diet (TV)	Y	CS
Robinson	1999	Diet (TV)	N	Exp
Robinson	1999	Health (TV)	Y	Exp
Robinson et al.	1993	Health (TV)	N	CS
Robinson et al.	1993	Health (TV)	N	L-Pnl
Robinson, Killen	1995	Diet (TV)	Y	CS
Robinson, Killen	1995	Health (TV)	N	CS
Ross et al.	1981	Precursors	N	Exp
Ross et al.	1981	Precursors	Y	Exp
Shannon et al.	1991	Health (TV)	Y	L-Pnl
Shannon et al.	1991	Health (TV)	N	CS
Sherwood et al.	2003	Health (TV)	N	CS
Signorielli, Lears	1992	Precursors (TV)	Y	CS
Signorielli, Lears	1992	Diet (TV)	Y	CS
Signorielli, Staples	1997	Precursors (TV)	Y	CS
Stettler et al.	2004	Health (TV)	Y	CS
Stoneman, Brody	1981	Precursors	Y	Exp
Stoneman, Brody	1982	Precursors	Y	Exp

Cause Variable Category	Effect Variable Category	Sample Size	Age	Measure Quality	Causality Evidence	Ecological Validity
TV ads—Viewing only	Beliefs	138	OC	L	L	M
TV ads—Viewing only	Adiposity	5,493	YCOC	L	M	H
TV ads—Experiment	Preferences	45	OC	H	H	L
TV ads—Viewing only	Preferences	122	YC	M	L	H
TV ads—Viewing only	Usual diet	122	YC	L	M	M
TV ads—Viewing only	Usual diet	192	OC	M	H	H
TV ads—Viewing only	Adiposity	192	OC	M	H	H
TV ads—Viewing only	Adiposity	671	T	L	L	M
TV ads—Viewing only	Adiposity	279	T	L	M	M
TV ads—Viewing + other media	Usual diet	1,912	T	L	L	H
TV ads—Viewing + other media	Adiposity	1,912	T	L	L	H
TV ads—Experiment	Beliefs	100	YCOC	L	M	M
TV ads—Experiment	Beliefs	100	YCOC	L	M	L
TV ads—Viewing only	Adiposity	489	OC	M	L	H
TV ads—Viewing only	Adiposity	773	OC	M	L	H
TV ads—Viewing + other media	Adiposity	96	OC	L	L	H
TV ads—Viewing only	Beliefs	209	OC	M	M	H
TV ads—Viewing only	Usual diet	209	OC	M	M	H
TV ads—Viewing only	Beliefs and preferences	427	OC	M	M	H
TV ads—Viewing only	Adiposity	872	OC	M	M	H
TV ads—Experiment	Preferences	124	OC	M	H	L
TV ads—Experiment	Requests	36	YC	H	H	M

continues

| Reference | | | | Research |
Author(s)	Year	Relationship	Significance	Method
Storey et al.	2003	Health (TV)	Y	CS
Storey et al.	2003	Health (TV)	Y	CS
Sugimori et al.	2004	Health (TV)	Y	L-Pnl
Tanasescu et al.	2000	Health (TV)	Y	CS
Taras et al.	1989	Diet (TV)	Y	CS
Taras et al.	2000	Diet	Y	CS
Taras et al.	2000	Precursors	Y	CS
Toyran et al.	2002	Precursors	Y	CS
Toyran et al.	2002	Health (TV)	Y	CS
Tremblay, Willms	2003	Health (TV)	Y	CS
Trost et al.	2001	Health (TV)	N	CS
Tucker	1986	Health (TV)	N	CS
Utter et al.	2003	Diet (TV)	Y	CS
Utter et al.	2003	Health (TV)	Y	CS
Vandewater et al.	2004	Health (TV)	N	CS
Wake et al.	2003	Health (TV)	Y	CS
Waller et al.	2003	Health (TV)	N	CS
Wolf et al.	1993	Health (TV)	Y	CS
Wong et al.	1992	Health (TV)	Y	CS
Woodward et al.	1997	Diet (TV)	Y	CS
Yavas, Abdul-Gader	1993	Precursors	Y	CS
Zive et al.	1998	Diet (TV)	Y	CS

Cause Variable Category	Effect Variable Category	Sample		Measure Quality	Causality Evidence	Ecological Validity
		Size	Age			
TV ads— Viewing only	Adiposity	3,473	OCT	M	M	H
TV ads— Viewing only	Adiposity	8,772	OCT	M	M	H
TV ads— Viewing only	Adiposity	8,170	YCOC	L	L	H
TV ads— Viewing only	Adiposity	53	OC	L	L	H
TV ads— Viewing only	Usual diet	66	YCOC	L	L	H
TV ads— Campaign	Usual diet	237	YC	M	L	H
TV ads— Campaign	Requests	237	YC	L	L	H
TV ads— Viewing only	Requests	886	OC	L	L	H
TV ads— Viewing only	Adiposity	886	OC	L	L	H
TV ads— Viewing only	Adiposity	7,216	OC	L	L	H
TV ads— Viewing + other media	Adiposity	187	OC	L	L	H
TV ads— Viewing only	Adiposity	379	T	M	L	H
TV ads— Viewing + other media	Usual diet	4,480	T	M	M	M
TV ads— Viewing + other media	Adiposity	4,480	T	M	L	M
TV ads— Viewing only	Adiposity	2,831	ITYCOC	M	M	H
TV ads— Viewing only	Adiposity	2,862	OCT	L	L	H
TV ads— Viewing only	Adiposity	880	OC	L	L	H
TV ads— Viewing only	Adiposity	552	OCT	L	L	H
TV ads— Viewing only	Other	1,081	YCOCT	M	M	H
TV ads— Viewing only	Usual diet	2,082	T	L	L	H
TV ads— Viewing only	Requests	217	OC	M	L	H
TV ads— Viewing only	Usual diet	351	YC	M	L	H

REFERENCES

Andersen RE, Crespo CJ, Bartlett SJ, Cheskin LJ, Pratt M. 1998. Relationship of physical activity and television watching with body weight and level of fatness among children: Results from the Third National Health and Nutrition Examination Survey. *J Am Med Assoc* 279(12):938–942.

Anderson DR, Huston AC, Schmitt KL, Linebarger DL, Wright JC. 2001. Early childhood television viewing and adolescent behavior: The recontact study. *Mon Soc Res Child Dev* 66(1):I–VIII, 1–147.

Armstrong CA, Sallis JF, Alcaraz JE, Kolody B, McKenzie TL, Hovell MF. 1998. Children's television viewing, body fat, and physical fitness. *Am J Health Promot* 12(6):363–368.

Auty S, Lewis C. 2004. Exploring children's choice: The reminder effect of product placement. *Psychol Marketing* 21(9):697–713.

Bao Y, Shao AT. 2002. Nonconformity advertising to teens. *J Ad Res* 42(3):56–65.

Barry TE, Gunst RF. 1982. Children's advertising: The differential impact of appeal strategy. *Current Issues and Research in Advertising* 5:113–125.

Berkey CS, Rockett HR, Field AE, Gillman MW, Frazier AL, Camargo CA Jr, Colditz GA. 2000. Activity, dietary intake, and weight changes in a longitudinal study of preadolescent and adolescent boys and girls. *Pediatrics* 105(4):E56.

Berkey CS, Rockett HR, Gillman MW, Colditz GA. 2003. One-year changes in activity and in inactivity among 10- to 15-year-old boys and girls: Relationship to change in body mass index. *Pediatrics* 111(4 Pt 1):836–843.

Bogaert N, Steinbeck KS, Baur LA, Brock K, Bermingham MA. 2003. Food, activity and family—environmental vs. biochemical predictors of weight gain in children. *Eur J Clin Nutr* 57(10):1242–1249.

Bolton RN. 1983. Modeling the impact of television food advertising on children's diets. *Current Issues and Research in Advertising* 6(1):173–199.

Borzekowski DLG, Poussaint AF. 1998. *Latino American Preschoolers and the Media*. Philadelphia, PA: Annenberg Public Policy Center of the University of Pennsylvania.

Borzekowski DL, Robinson TN. 2001. The 30-second effect: An experiment revealing the impact of television commercials on food preferences of preschoolers. *J Am Diet Assoc* 101(1):42–46.

Boynton-Jarrett R, Thomas TN, Peterson KE, Wiecha J, Sobol AM, Gortmaker SL. 2003. Impact of television viewing patterns on fruit and vegetable consumption among adolescents. *Pediatrics* 112(6 Pt 1):1321–1326.

Brody GH, Stoneman Z, Lane TS, Sanders AK. 1981. Television food commercials aimed at children, family grocery shopping, and mother–children interactions. *Family Relations* 30:435–439.

Burke V, Beilin LJ, Simmer K, Oddy WH, Blake KV, Doherty D, Kendall GE, Newnham JP, Landau LI, Stanley FJ. 2005. Predictors of body mass index and associations with cardiovascular risk factors in Australian children: A prospective cohort study. *Int J Obes Relat Metab Disord* 29(1):15–23.

Cantor J. 1981. Modifying children's eating habits through television ads: Effects of humorous appeals in a field setting. *J Broadcasting* 23(1):37–47.

Carruth BR, Goldberg DL, Skinner JD. 1991. Do parents and peers mediate the influence of television advertising on food-related purchases? *J Adolesc Res* 6(2):253–271.

Christenson PG. 1982. Children's perceptions of TV commercials and products. The effects of PSAs. *Commun Res* 9(4):491–524.

Clancy-Hepburn K, Hickey AA, Nevill G. 1974. Children's behavior responses to TV food advertisements. *J Nutr Ed* 6(3):93–96.

Clarke TK. 1984. Situational factors affecting preschoolers' responses to advertising. *J Acad Marketing Sci* 12(4):25–40.

Coon KA, Goldberg J, Rogers BL, Tucker KL. 2001. Relationships between use of television during meals and children's food consumption patterns. *Pediatrics* 107(1):e7.

Crespo CJ, Smit E, Troiano RP, Bartlett SJ, Macera CA, Andersen RE. 2001. Television watching, energy intake, and obesity in US children: Results from the third National Health and Nutrition Examination Survey, 1988–1994. *Arch Pediatr Adolesc Med* 155(3):360–365.

Crooks DL. 2000. Food consumption, activity, and overweight among elementary school children in an Appalachian Kentucky community. *Am J Phys Anthropol* 112(2): 159–170.

Dawson BL, Jeffrey DB, Walsh JA. 1988. Television food commercials' effect on children's resistance to temptation. *J Appl Soc Psychol* 18(16):1353–1360.

Deheeger M, Rolland-Cachera MF, Fontvieille AM. 1997. Physical activity and body composition in 10 year old French children: Linkages with nutritional intake? *Int J Obes Relat Metab Disord* 21(5):372–379.

Dennison BA, Erb TA, Jenkins PL. 2002. Television viewing and television in bedroom associated with overweight risk among low-income preschool children. *Pediatrics* 109(6): 1028–1035.

Dietz WH Jr, Gortmaker SL. 1985. Do we fatten our children at the television set? Obesity and television viewing in children and adolescents. *Pediatrics* 75(5):807–812.

Donkin AJM, Neale RJ, Tilston C. 1993. Children's food purchase requests. *Appetite* 21(3): 291–294.

Donohue TR. 1975. Effect of commercials on black children. *J Advert Res* 15(6):41–47.

Dowda M, Ainsworth BE, Addy CL, Saunders R, Riner W. 2001. Environmental influences, physical activity, and weight status in 8- to 16-year-olds. *Arch Pediatr Adolesc Med* 155(6):711–717.

duRant RH, Baranowski T, Johnson M, Thompson WO. 1994. The relationship among television watching, physical activity, and body composition of young children. *Pediatrics* 94(4 Pt 1):449–455.

duRant RH, Thompson WO, Johnson M, Baranowski T. 1996. The relationship among television watching, physical activity, and body composition of 5- or 6-year-old children. *Pediatric Exerc Sci* 8:15–26.

Dwyer JT, Stone EJ, Yang M, Feldman H, Webber LS, Must A, Perry CL, Nader PR, Parcel GS. 1998. Predictors of overweight and overfatness in a multiethnic pediatric population. Child and Adolescent Trial for Cardiovascular Health Collaborative Research Group. *Am J Clin Nutr* 67(4):602–610.

Eisenmann JC, Bartee RT, Wang MQ. 2002. Physical activity, TV viewing, and weight in U.S. youth: 1999 Youth Risk Behavior Survey. *Obes Res* 10(5):379–385.

Faber RJ, Meyer TP, Miller MM. 1984. The effectiveness of health disclosures within children's television commercials. *J Broadcasting* 28(4):463–476.

Fontvieille AM, Kriska A, Ravussin E. 1993. Decreased physical activity in Pima Indian compared with Caucasian children. *Int J Obes Relat Metab Disord* 17(8):445–452.

Francis LA, Lee Y, Birch LL. 2003. Parental weight status and girls' television viewing, snacking, and body mass indexes. *Obes Res* 11(1):143–151.

French SA, Jeffery RW, Story M, Breitlow KK, Baxter JS, Hannan P, Snyder MP. 2001a. Pricing and promotion effects on low-fat vending snack purchases: The CHIPS Study. *Am J Public Health* 91(1):112–117.

French SA, Story M, Neumark-Sztainer D, Fulkerson JA, Hannan P. 2001b. Fast food restaurant use among adolescents: Associations with nutrient intake, food choices and behavioral and psychosocial variables. *Int J Obes Relat Metab Disord* 25(12):1823–1833.

Galst JP. 1980. Television food commercials and pro-nutritional public service announcements as determinants of young children's snack choices. *Child Dev* 51:935–938.

Galst JP, White MA. 1976. The unhealthy persuader: The reinforcing value of television and children's purchase-influencing attempts at the supermarket. *Child Dev* 47:1089–1096.

Giammattei J, Blix G, Marshak HH, Wollitzer AO, Pettitt DJ. 2003. Television watching and soft drink consumption: Associations with obesity in 11- to 13-year-old schoolchildren. *Arch Pediatr Adolesc Med* 157(9):882–886.

Goldberg ME. 1990. A quasi-experiment assessing the effectiveness of TV advertising directed to children. *J Marketing Res* 27(4):445–454.

Goldberg ME, Gorn GJ, Gibson W. 1978. TV messages for snack and breakfast foods: Do they influence children's preferences? *J Consum Res* 5:73–81.

Gordon-Larsen P, Adair LS, Popkin BM. 2002. Ethnic differences in physical activity and inactivity patterns and overweight status. *Obes Res* 10(3):141–149.

Gorn GJ, Florsheim R. 1985. The effects of commercials for adult products on children. *J Consumer Res* 11(4):962–967.

Gorn GJ, Goldberg ME. 1980. Children's responses to repetitive television commercials. *J Consum Res* 6:421–424.

Gorn GJ, Goldberg ME. 1982. Behavioral evidence of the effects of televised food messages on children. *J Consum Res* 9:200–205.

Gortmaker SL, Must A, Sobol AM, Peterson K, Colditz GA, Dietz WH. 1996. Television viewing as a cause of increasing obesity among children in the United States, 1986–1990. *Arch Pediatr Adolesc Med* 150(4):356–362.

Gracey D, Stanley N, Burke V, Corti B, Beilin LJ. 1996. Nutritional knowledge, beliefs, and behaviours in teenage school students. *Health Ed Res* 11(2):187–204.

Graf C, Koch B, Dordel S, Schindler-Marlow S, Icks A, Schuller A, Bjarnason-Wehrens B, Tokarski W, Predel HG. 2004. Physical activity, leisure habits and obesity in first-grade children. *Eur J Cardiovasc Prev Rehabil* 11(4):284–290.

Gray A, Smith C. 2003. Fitness, dietary intake, and body mass index in urban Native American youth. *J Am Diet Assoc* 103(9):1187–1191.

Greenberg BS, Brand JE. 1993. Television news and advertising in schools: The *Channel One* controversy. *J Commun* 43(1):143–151.

Grund A, Dilba B, Forberger K, Krause H, Siewers M, Rieckert H, Muller MJ. 2000. Relationships between physical activity, physical fitness, muscle strength and nutritional state in 5- to 11-year-old children. *Eur J Appl Physiol* 82(5-6):425–438.

Guillaume M, Lapidus L, Bjorntorp P, Lambert A. 1997. Physical activity, obesity, and cardiovascular risk factors in children. The Belgian Luxembourg Child Study II. *Obes Res* 5(6):549–556.

Halford JC, Gillespie J, Brown V, Pontin EE, Dovey TM. 2004. Effect of television advertisements for foods on food consumption in children. *Appetite* 42(2):221–225.

Harrison K. 2005. Is "fat free" good for me? A panel study of television viewing and children's nutritional knowledge and reasoning. *Health Commun* 17(2):117–132.

Hernandez B, Gortmaker SL, Colditz GA, Peterson KE, Laird NM, Parra-Cabrera S. 1999. Association of obesity with physical activity, television programs and other forms of video viewing among children in Mexico City. *Int J Obes Relat Metab Disord* 23(8): 845–854.

Heslop LA, Ryans AB. 1980. A second look at children and the advertising of premiums. *J Consumer Res* 6(4):414–420.

Hitchings E, Moynihan PJ. 1998. The relationship between television food advertisements recalled and actual foods consumed by children. *J Hum Nutr Diet* 11:511–517.

Horn OK, Paradis G, Potvin L, Macaulay AC, Desrosiers S. 2001. Correlates and predictors of adiposity among Mohawk children. *Prev Med* 33(4):274–281.

Hoy MG, Young CE, Mowen JC. 1986. Animated host-selling advertisements: Their impact on young children's recognition, attitudes, and behavior. *J Pub Policy Marketing* 5: 171–184.

Isler L, Popper ET, Ward S. 1987. children's purchase requests and parental responses: Results from a diary study. *J Advert Res* 27(5):28–39.

Janz KF, Levy SM, Burns TL, Torner JC, Willing MC, Warren JJ. 2002. Fatness, physical activity, and television viewing in children during the adiposity rebound period: The Iowa Bone Development Study. *Prev Med* 35(6):563–571.

Jeffrey DB, McLellarn RW, Fox DT. 1982. The development of children's eating habits: The role of television commercials. *Health Ed Q* 9(2 suppl 3):174–189.

Kant AK, Graubard BI. 2003. Predictors of reported consumption of low-nutrient-density foods in a 24-h recall by 8–16 year old US children and adolescents. *Appetite* 41(2): 175–180.

Katzmarzyk PT, Malina RM, Song TM, Bouchard C. 1998. Television viewing, physical activity, and health-related fitness of youth in the Quebec Family Study. *J Adolesc Health* 23(5):318–325.

Kaur H, Choi WS, Mayo MS, Harris KJ. 2003. Duration of television watching is associated with increased body mass index. *J Pediatr* 143(4):506–511.

Klein-Platat C, Oujaa M, Wagner A, Haan MC, Arveiler D, Schlienger JL, Simon C. 2005. Physical activity is inversely related to waist circumference in 12-y-old French adolescents. *Int J Obes Relat Metab Disord* 29(1):9–14.

Krassas GE, Tzotzas T, Tsametis C, Konstantinidis T. 2001. Determinants of body mass index in Greek children and adolescents. *J Pediatr Endocrinol Metab* 14(Suppl 5): 1327–1333.

Kunkel D. 1988. Children and host-selling television commercials. *Commun Res* 15(1): 71–92.

Levin S, Martin MW, Riner WF. 2004. TV viewing habits and body mass index among South Carolina Head Start children. *Ethn Dis* 14(3):336–339.

Lewis MK, Hill AJ. 1998. Food advertising on British children's television: A content analysis and experimental study with nine-year olds. *Int J Obes Relat Metab Disord* 22(3): 206–214.

Lin BH, Huang CL, French SA. 2004. Factors associated with women's and children's body mass indices by income status. *Int J Obes Relat Metab Disord* 28(4):536–542.

Locard E, Mamelle N, Billette A, Miginiac M, Munoz F, Rey S. 1992. Risk factors of obesity in a five year old population. Parental versus environmental factors. *Int J Obes Relat Metab Disord* 16(10):721–729.

Macklin MC. 1990. The influence of model age on children's reactions to advertising stimuli. *Psychol Market* 7(4):295–310.

Macklin MC. 1994. The effects of an advertising retrieval cue on young children's memory and brand evaluations. *Psychol Marketing* 11(3):291–311.

Maffeis C, Talamini G, Tato L. 1998. Influence of diet, physical activity and parents' obesity on children's adiposity: A four-year longitudinal study. *Int J Obes Relat Metab Disord* 22(8):758–764.

Manios Y, Yiannakouris N, Papoutsakis C, Moschonis G, Magkos F, Skenderi K, Zampelas A. 2004. Behavioral and physiological indices related to BMI in a cohort of primary schoolchildren in Greece. *Am J Hum Biol* 16(6):639–647.

Matheson DM, Killen JD, Wang Y, Varady A, Robinson TN. 2004. Children's food consumption during television viewing. *Am J Clin Nutr* 79(6):1088–1094.

McMurray RG, Harrell JS, Deng S, Bradley CB, Cox LM, Bangdiwala SI. 2000. The influence of physical activity, socioeconomic status, and ethnicity on the weight status of adolescents. *Obes Res* 8(2):130–139.

Miller JH, Busch P. 1979. Host selling vs. premium TV commercials: An experimental evaluation of their influence on children. *J Market Res* 16(3):323–332.

Morton HN. 1990. A survey of the television viewing habits, food behaviours, and perception of food advertisements among south Australian year 8 high school students. *J Home Econ Assoc Australia* 22(2):34–36.

Muller MJ, Koertzinger I, Mast M, Langnase K, Grund A. 1999. Physical activity and diet in 5 to 7 years old children. *Public Health Nutr* 2(3A):443–444.

Norton PA, Falciglia GA, Ricketts C. 2000. Motivational determinants of food preferences in adolescents and pre-adolescents. *Ecology Food Nutr* 39(3):169–182.

Obarzanek E, Schreiber GB, Crawford PB, Goldman SR, Barrier PM, Frederick MM, Lakatos E. 1994. Energy intake and physical activity in relation to indexes of body fat: The National Heart, Lung, and Blood Institute Growth and Health Study. *Am J Clin Nutr* 60(1):15–22.

O'Loughlin J, Gray-Donald K, Paradis G, Meshefedjian G. 2000. One- and two-year predictors of excess weight gain among elementary schoolchildren in multiethnic, low-income, inner-city neighborhoods. *Am J Epidemiol* 152(8):739–746.

Palmer EL, McDowell CN. 1981. Children's understanding of nutritional information presented in breakfast cereal commercials. *J Broadcasting* 25(3):295–301.

Pate RR, Ross JG. 1987. Factors associated with health-related fitness. The National Children and Youth Fitness Study II. *J Physical Ed Recreat Dance* 58:93–95.

Peterson PE, Jeffrey DB, Bridgwater CA, Dawson B. 1984. How pronutrition television programming affects children's dietary habits. *Dev Psychol* 20(1):55–63.

Pine KJ, Nash A. 2003. Barbie or Betty? Preschool children's preference for branded products and evidence for gender-linked differences. *Dev Behav Pediatr* 24(4):219–224.

Proctor MH, Moore LL, Gao D, Cupples LA, Bradlee ML, Hood MY, Ellison RC. 2003. Television viewing and change in body fat from preschool to early adolescence: The Framingham Children's Study. *Int J Obes Relat Metab Disord* 27(7):827–833.

Reid LN, Bearden WO, Teel JE. 1980. Family income, TV viewing and children's cereal ratings. *Journalism Q* 57(2):327–330.

Reilly JJ, Armstrong J, Dorosty AR, Emmett PM, Ness A, Rogers I, Steer C, Sherriff A. 2005. Early life risk factors for obesity in childhood: Cohort study. *Br Med J* 330(7504): 1357–1364.

Resnik A, Stern BL. 1977. Children's television advertising and brand choice: A laboratory experiment. *J Advert* 6:11–17.

Ritchey N, Olson C. 1983. Relationships between family variables and children's preference for and consumption of sweet foods. *Ecology Food Nutr* 13:257–266.

Robinson TN. 1999. Reducing children's television viewing to prevent obesity. A randomized controlled trial. *J Am Med Assoc* 282(16):1561–1567.

Robinson TN, Killen JD. 1995. Ethnic and gender differences in the relationships between television viewing and obesity, physical activity, and dietary fat intake. *J Health Educ* 26(2):S91–S98.

Robinson TN, Hammer LD, Killen JD, Kraemer HC, Wilson DM, Hayward C, Taylor CB. 1993. Does television viewing increase obesity and reduce physical activity? Cross-sectional and longitudinal analyses among adolescent girls. *Pediatrics* 91(2):273–280.

Ross RP, Campbell T, Huston-Stein A, Wright JC. 1981. Nutritional misinformation of children: A developmental and experimental analysis of the effects of televised food commercials. *J Appl Dev Psychol* 1:329–347.

Shannon B, Peacock J, Brown MJ. 1991. Body fatness, television viewing and calorie-intake of a sample of Pennsylvania sixth grade children. *J Nutr Educ* 23(6):262–268.

Sherwood NE, Story M, Neumark-Sztainer D, Adkins S, Davis M. 2003. Development and implementation of a visual card-sorting technique for assessing food and activity preferences and patterns in African American girls. *J Am Diet Assoc* 103(11):1473–1479.

Signorielli N, Lears M. 1992. Television and children's conceptions of nutrition: Unhealthy messages. *Health Commun* 4(4):245–257.

Signorielli N, Staples J. 1997. Television and children's conceptions of nutrition. *Health Commun* 9(4):289–301.

Stettler N, Signer TM, Suter PM. 2004. Electronic games and environmental factors associated with childhood obesity in Switzerland. *Obes Res* 12(6):896–903.

Stoneman Z, Brody GH. 1981. Peers as mediators of television food advertisements aimed at children. *Dev Psychol* 17(6):853–858.

Stoneman Z, Brody GH. 1982. The indirect impact of child-oriented advertisements on mother–child interactions. *J Appl Dev Psychol* 2:369–376.

Storey ML, Forshee RA, Weaver AR, Sansalone WR. 2003. Demographic and lifestyle factors associated with body mass index among children and adolescents. *Int J Food Sci Nutr* 54(6):491–503.

Sugimori H, Yoshida K, Izuno T, Miyakawa M, Suka M, Sekine M, Yamagami T, Kagamimori S. 2004. Analysis of factors that influence body mass index from ages 3 to 6 years: A study based on the Toyama cohort study. *Pediatr Int* 46(3):302–310.

Tanasescu M, Ferris AM, Himmelgreen DA, Rodriguez N, Perez-Escamilla R. 2000. Bio-behavioral factors are associated with obesity in Puerto Rican children. *J Nutr* 130(7): 1734–1742.

Taras HL, Sallis JF, Patterson TL, Nader PR, Nelson JA. 1989. Television's influence on children's diet and physical activity. *Dev Behav Pediatr* 10(4):176–180.

Taras H, Zive M, Nader P, Berry CC, Hoy T, Boyd C. 2000. Television advertising and classes of food products consumed in a paediatric population. *Int J Ad* 19:487–493.

Toyran M, Ozmert E, Yurdakok K. 2002. Television viewing and its effect on physical health of schoolage children. *Turk J Pediatr* 44(3):194–203.

Tremblay MS, Willms JD. 2003. Is the Canadian childhood obesity epidemic related to physical inactivity? *Int J Obes Relat Metab Disord* 27(9):1100–1105.

Trost SG, Kerr LM, Ward DS, Pate RR. 2001. Physical activity and determinants of physical activity in obese and non-obese children. *Int J Obes Relat Metab Disord* 25(6):822–829.

Tucker LA. 1986. The relationship of television viewing to physical fitness and obesity. *Adolescence* 21(84):797–806.

Utter J, Neumark-Sztainer D, Jeffery R, Story M. 2003. Couch potatoes or French fries: Are sedentary behaviors associated with body mass index, physical activity, and dietary behaviors among adolescents? *J Am Diet Assoc* 103(10):1298–1305.

Vandewater EA, Shim MS, Caplovitz AG. 2004. Linking obesity and activity level with children's television and video game use. *J Adolesc* 27(1):71–85.

Wake M, Hesketh K, Waters E. 2003. Television, computer use and body mass index in Australian primary school children. *J Paediatr Child Health* 39(2):130–134.

Waller CE, Du S, Popkin BM. 2003. Patterns of overweight, inactivity, and snacking in Chinese children. *Obes Res* 11(8):957–961.

Wolf AM, Gortmaker SL, Cheung L, Gray HM, Herzog DB, Colditz GA. 1993. Activity, inactivity, and obesity: Racial, ethnic, and age differences among schoolgirls. *Am J Public Health* 83(11):1625–1627.

Wong ND, Hei TK, Qaqundah PY, Davidson DM, Bassin SL, Gold KV. 1992. Television viewing and pediatric hypercholesterolemia. *Pediatrics* 90(1):75–79.

Woodward DR, Cumming FJ, Ball PJ, Williams HM, Hornsby H, Boon JA. 1997. Does television affect teenagers' food choices? *J Human Nutr Diet* 10:229–235.

Yavas U, Abdul-Gader A. 1993. Impact of TV commercials on Saudi children's purchase behaviour. *Marketing Intelligence Planning* 11(2):37–43.

Zive MM, Frank-Spohrer GC, Sallis JF, McKenzie TL, Elder JP, Berry CC, Broyles SL, Nader PR. 1998. Determinants of dietary intake in a sample of white and Mexican-American children. *J Am Diet Assoc* 98(11):1282–1289.

G

Children and Youth Marketing
and Advertising Regulations
and Guidelines in Selected Countries

TABLE G-1 Statutory Regulations and Voluntary Guidelines for Television Advertising to Children in Selected Countries

Region/Country	Statutory Regulations	Voluntary Guidelines	Specific Restrictions or Guidelines for Television Advertising to Children
Africa			
South Africa	*Regulatory Authorities*	*Self-Regulatory Organizations* Advertising Standards Authority of South Africa	Advertisements addressed to or likely to influence children should not contain any statement or visual presentation which might result in harming them, mentally, morally, physically, or emotionally. A child is defined as younger than 18 years of age.
Asia			
China	*Regulatory Authorities* State Administration of Industry and Commerce	*Self-Regulatory Organizations*	Advertisements must not impair the physical and mental health of minors. Product placement is discouraged wherever possible. A child is defined as younger than 15 years of age.
Japan		National Association of Commercial Broadcasters in Japan	A child is defined as younger than 18 years of age.
Australasia and Pacific			
Australia	*Regulatory Authorities* Australian Broadcasting Authority	*Self-Regulatory Organizations* Commercial Television Australia Advertising Standards Bureau oversees the Advertising Standards Board and the	Prohibits advertising during programs aimed at younger children, restricts the amount of advertising during programming for older children, and limits advertisements featuring

continues

TABLE G-1 Continued

Region/Country	Statutory Regulations	Voluntary Guidelines	Specific Restrictions or Guidelines for Television Advertising to Children
			children's television personalities. A child is defined as 14 years of age and younger.
		Advertising Claims Board	
New Zealand		Advertising Standards Authority New Zealand Television Broadcasters' Council	No advertisements are allowed to be broadcast on preschool television or Sunday mornings. There is limited advertising in school-age children's television. Prohibits products from being advertised within a television program that come directly from a program or its licensed characters. Repetition of advertisements is limited per hour and per channel.
Philippines		AdBoard	
Europe		*Self-Regulatory Organizations*	
EU[a]	*Regulatory Authorities* EU Television Without Frontiers Directive	European Advertising Standards Alliance (EASA) International Chamber of Commerce (ICC)	Prohibits advertisements to children that (1) exploit their inexperience or credulity; (2) understate the degree of skill or age level required to use or enjoy the product; and (3) contain any statement or visual presentation that could have the effect of harming mentally, morally, or physically. The ICC's Commission on Marketing and Advertising adheres to the Framework for Responsible Food and Beverage Communications. Minors are defined under national laws.
Belgium	EU Television Without Frontiers Directive	Jury for Ethical Practices in Advertising	Prohibits advertising before and after children's television programs.

	The Ministry of Economic Affairs; Ministry of Public Health; High Audiovisual Council; Flemish Media Commissariat	The World Federation of Advertisers oversees the Responsible Advertising and Children Programme	See EU. A child is defined as younger than 12 years of age.
Czech Republic	EU Television Without Frontiers Directive	Rada Pro Reklamu	Advertising of various content is banned to children that shows them in dangerous situations. See EU.
Denmark	EU Television Without Frontiers Directive The Market Court; The Consumer Ombudsman; The Consumer Council; The Radio and Television Advertisements Board; The National Food Institute	Reklame Forum	Prohibits figures and puppets that appear in children's programs from appearing in advertisements. See EU. A child is defined as younger than 18 years of age.
Finland	Consumer Protection Act Consumer Ombudsmen	Board of Business Practice	Advertisements are prohibited that attempt to persuade a child to buy a product through a direct offer. Advertisements are prohibited in which sales pitches are delivered by familiar cartoon characters or children. A child is defined as younger than 12 years of age.
France	EU Television Without Frontiers Directive	Bureau de Vérification de la Publicité	Provides several recommendations to ensure that advertising does not exploit the inexperience or innocence of children. See EU.

continues

TABLE G-1 Continued

Region/Country	Statutory Regulations	Voluntary Guidelines	Specific Restrictions or Guidelines for Television Advertising to Children
Greece	EU Television Without Frontiers Directive	Hellenic Association of Advertising Communications and Greek Advertisers' Association	Enforces restrictions on advertising to children during specific times. See EU.
Hungary	EU Television Without Frontiers Directive Országos Rádió és Televízió Testület (National Radio and Television Commission)	Hungarian Advertising Association created the Hungarian Code of Advertising Ethics	Provides guidelines pertaining to advertising made for or featuring children. See EU.
Ireland	EU Television Without Frontiers Directive Broadcasting Commission of Ireland	Advertising Standards Authority of Ireland Radio Telefis Eireann (RTE)	RTE prohibits broadcast sponsorship of any children's programs. See EU.
Italy	EU Television Without Frontiers Directive	Istituto di Autodisciplina Publicitaria (IAP) (Institute for Self-Regulation in Advertising)	Enforces advertising guidelines developed for programs featuring children including during cartoons and using cartoon characters before and after the television programs in which they appear.
Netherlands	EU Directive on Comparative Advertising	The Advertising Foundation	Bans advertising of alcohol and sweets on television to children. A child is defined as younger than 12 years of age.
Norway	Norwegian Mass Authority The Consumer Ombudsmen		Instituted a ban on advertising to children younger than 12 years of age in 1992.

Country	Regulatory body / instrument	Description
Sweden	EU Television Without Frontiers Directive The Consumer Ombudsmen Council on Market Ethics	Prohibits broadcast advertising before and after children's programs through the Norwegian Marketing Control Act. Instituted a ban on advertising to children younger than 12 years of age in 1991. Prohibits advertising during children's programs and on using television characters or presenters in advertisements.
United Kingdom	EU Television Without Frontiers Directive Office of Communications (Ofcom) Advertising Standards Authority	Prohibits children's television personalities from advertising before a specific time and includes language prohibiting merchandising within two hours of a television program. Created advertising-free children's television channels. A child is defined as younger than 16 years of age.
Latin America Argentina	*Regulatory Authorities* Federal regulations for advertising *Self-Regulatory Organizations* Camara Argentina de Anunciantes (Argentine Chamber of Advertisers) Association of Advertising Agencies in Argentina, Unified Code of Ethics of the Mercosur	Advertising directed at children and adolescents must adhere to established guidelines.
Brazil	Consumer Defense Code Association of Advertising Agencies in Brazil, Unified Code of Ethics of the Mercosur Self-regulating Advertising Council (CONAR)	Advertising directed at children and adolescents must adhere to established guidelines.

continues

TABLE G-1 Continued

Region/Country	Statutory Regulations	Voluntary Guidelines	Specific Restrictions or Guidelines for Television Advertising to Children
Chile	Antitrust and Unfair Advertising Competition Commission	CONAR	Alcohol advertising must not contain messages or be broadcast in media or at times especially addressed to minors and must not encourage them to consume alcoholic beverages.
Mexico	Attorney General for Consumer Protection Ministry of the Interior Ministry of Health	Consejo Nacional de la Publicidad (National Council for Advertising)	Guidelines provide direction on how to avoid taking advantage of children's credulity or lack of experience. Regulations for children's television advertising have not yet been developed.
Paraguay	Federal regulations connected to the subject	Council for Self-Regulatory Advertising Associations of Advertising Agencies in Paraguay, Unified Code of Ethics of the Mercosur	Prohibits publicity of tobacco and alcoholic beverages that use minors as well as characters or people that are representative of children or adolescents. Advertising directed at children and adolescents are advised to follow guidelines.
Peru		Asociación Nacional de Anunciantes (ANDA)	
Middle East	*Regulatory Authorities*	*Self-Regulatory Organizations*	
Israel	Ministry of Communications		Regulates content and hours of television and radio broadcasting according to the 2001 Law of Classification, Labeling, and Prohibition of Harmful Broadcasts and the 1991 consumer protection law that regulates advertising content directed to minors.

	Regulatory Authorities	Self-Regulatory Organizations	
Kuwait	None		Regulations for children's television advertising have not yet been developed.
Saudi Arabia	None		Regulations for children's television advertising have not yet been developed.
North America			
Canada	Canadian Broadcasting Corporation (CBC) Broadcast Code for Advertising to Children Canadian Radio-Television and Telecommunications Commission Office de la Protection du Consommateur (Quebec)	Advertising Standards Canada	The province of Quebec instituted a ban on advertising to children under the age of 13 years in 1980. Restricts the use of puppets and subliminal messages to encourage children to purchase products. CBC prohibits advertising of any kind in programs directed to children under the ages of 12 years. A child is defined as younger than 12 years of age in Canada and younger than 13 years of age in Quebec.
United States	Federal Trade Commission (FTC) Federal Communications Commission (FCC)	Children's Advertising Review Unit (CARU)	The Children's Television Act restricts advertising during programs targeted at children under the age of 12 years to 10.5 minutes per hour on weekends, and 12 minutes per hour during the week. A child is defined as younger than 12 years of age.

NOTE: EU = European Union.

aAll EU countries follow the EU Television Without Frontiers Directive. However, certain EU countries also have their own self-regulatory agencies and additional restrictions or guidelines regarding television advertising to children. Some of the countries with regulations specific to children and television advertising have been listed separately from the EU.

SOURCES: BCI (2001); Friedman and Dickler (2003); Hawkes (2004); Personal communication. K. Tessmann Diaz. Arochi, Marroquin and Lindner, S.C., Mexico, August 12, 2005, for guidelines on Mexico. Personal communication. Elizabeth Levy. The National Council for the Child, Jerusalem, Israel, November 27, 2005, for guidelines on Israel.

TABLE G-2 Statutory or Voluntary Regulations for Marketing Approaches Used for Food and Beverage Promotion to Children

Selected Region or Country	Television Advertising	In-School Marketing	Sponsorship	Product Placement[a]	Internet Marketing[b]	Sales Promotions
Africa						
South Africa	X		X			
Asia						
China	X		X	X		
India	X		X			X
Japan	X	X			X	
Russian Federation						
Thailand	X					
Australasia and Pacific						
Australia	X	X	X		X	X
New Zealand	X		X			
Philippines	X			X		
Latin America						
Argentina	X					
Brazil	X	X				
Chile	X					
Mexico	X				X	
Europe						
Austria	X			X	X	
Belgium	X	X		X		X
Czech Republic	X			X		
Denmark	X	X		X	X	
Finland	X	X	X	X	X	X
France	X	X			X	X
Germany	X	X		X		X
Greece	X	X		X		X

	Television advertising	In-school marketing	Sponsorship	Product placement	Internet marketing	Sales promotions
Ireland	X	X	X	X		X
Italy	X			X	X	X
Netherlands	X	X	X	X		X
Norway	X		X	X	X	
Poland	X					
Portugal	X	X				X
Spain	X				X	X
Sweden	X			X	X	X
Switzerland	X			X		
United Kingdom	X		X	X		X
Middle East						
Saudi Arabia		X				
North America						
Canada	X	X			X	
Quebec	X	X				
United States	X	X		X	X	X

NOTE: The following definitions were used for the purpose of this table and may differ from terms used throughout the report: *television advertising* is the use of television as a medium to promote a product or service; *in-school marketing* is a technique used to spread advertising messages targeted at children while they are in the school environment; *sponsorship* is the provision of funds and other resources to an event or activity in return for access to the exploitable commercial potential associated with that activity; *product placement* is the use of any message, logo, object, or prop that appears in a visual or graphic in exchange for payment; *Internet marketing* is a promotional activity on the Internet to connect consumers to a marketer's products; and *sales promotions* are marketing tools used to create an incentive to buy a product or service at the point of sale.

aStatutory restrictions on product placement in television programs only; product placement in films is not subject to statutory regulations.

bRegulations on Internet marketing with clauses specific to children.

SOURCE: Hawkes (2004).

REFERENCES

BCI (Broadcasting Commission of Ireland). 2001. *Children's Advertising Code*. Dublin, Ireland: BCI.

Friedman AE, Dickler H. 2003. *International Advertising Clearance*. Amsterdam, Netherlands: Global Advertising Lawyers Alliance.

Hawkes C. 2004. *Marketing Food to Children: The Global Regulatory Environment*. Geneva: World Health Organization.

ENDNOTES FROM CHAPTER 6

1. Similarly, the court rejected the claim that McDonald's had failed to warn consumers about the unhealthy attributes of its food on the grounds that the plaintiffs had not shown that such products "were dangerous in any way other than that which was open and obvious to a reasonable consumer." *Id.* at 541. The federal court also found that the plaintiffs had failed to "draw an adequate causal connection between their consumption of McDonald's food and their alleged injuries." *Pelman* v. *McDonald's Corporation*, 2003 WL 22052778, at *11 (2003). Plaintiffs failed to answer "pertinent" questions that would help establish causation, including: What else did the plaintiffs eat? How much did they exercise? Is there a family history of the diseases which are alleged to have been caused by McDonald's products? Without this additional information, McDonald's does not have sufficient information to determine if its foods are the cause of plaintiffs' obesity, or if instead McDonald's foods are only a contributing factor. *Id.* at *11. The district court was recently reversed on the ground that the plaintiffs ought to be able to pursue discovery on the issue of whether their obesity (and related medical conditions) were caused by McDonald's deceptive practices. *Pelman* v. *McDonald's Corporation*, No. 03-9010, slip op. at 6 (2d Cir. Jan. 25, 2005).

2. The FTC "will find deception if there is a representation, omission or practice that is likely to mislead the consumer acting reasonably in the circumstances, to the consumer's detriment." Federal Trade Commission Policy Statement on Deception, *appended to* Cliffdale Associates, Inc., 103 F.T.C. 110, 174 (1984). An "unfair" act or practice is one that "causes or is likely to cause substantial injury to consumers which is not reasonably avoidable by consumers themselves and not outweighed by countervailing benefits to consumers or to competition." 15 U.S.C. § 45(n), 2002.

3. The statute defines the term "false advertisement" to mean "an advertisement, other than labeling, which is misleading in a material respect; and in determining whether any advertisement is misleading, there shall be taken into account (among other things) not only representations made or suggested by statement, word, design, device, sound, or any combination thereof, but also the extent to which the advertisement fails to reveal facts material in the light of such representations or material with respect to consequences which may result from the use of the commodity to which the advertisement relates under the conditions prescribed in said advertisement, or under such conditions as are customary or usual." 15 U.S.C. § 55(a)(1), 2002.

4. See, e.g., 16 C.F.R. § 410.1, 2005, rule on deceptive advertising as to sizes of viewable pictures on television sets; 16 C.F.R. § 239.1-5, 2005, rule on deceptive advertising of guarantees.

5. In assessing products liability claims involving children, for example, courts often distinguish between what can be expected of a "reasonable child" and a "reasonable adult." See, e.g., *Swix* v. *Daisy Manufacturing Company*, 2004 (holding, in a products liability action, that the "reasonable child"—and not "reasonable adult"— standard should apply when typical user of the product is a child); *Bunch* v. *Hoffinger Industries, Inc.*,

2004 (upholding a trial court's application of the "reasonable child" standard in a products liability case. In explaining its decision, the court stated "a distinction must be made between an adult's ability to recognize and appreciate certain risks and a minor's corresponding ability. Certain conditions considered harmless to adults may not be so to the general class of children who, by reason of their immaturity, might be incapable of appreciating the risk involved.")

6. Codified as amended in scattered sections of 15 U.S.C. (2002).

7. The *Central Hudson* test has been applied in very inconsistent ways by the Court itself. Compare, e.g., *Posadas de Puerto Rico Associates v. Tourism Company* (1986), with *Rubin v. Coors Brewing Company* (1995). More than a majority of the Justices have indicated their dissatisfaction with the test. See *44 Liquormart, Inc. v. Rhode Island*, (1996). Yet the Court has continued to apply the test, with increasing severity, despite its discomforts. See, e.g., *Greater New Orleans Broadcasting Association v. United States*, 1999; *Lorillard Tobacco Company v. Reilly*, 2001; *Thompson v. Western States Medical Center*, 2002.

8. *Peel v. Attorney Registration and Disciplinary Commission*, 1990; In R.M.J., 455 U.S. 191, 203 (1982) ("Truthful advertising related to lawful activities is entitled to the protections of the First Amendment. But when the particular content or method of the advertising suggests that it is inherently misleading or when experience has proved that in fact such advertising is subject to abuse, the States may impose appropriate restrictions. Misleading advertising may be prohibited entirely.)

9. In a pre-*Central Hudson* case, the Supreme Court suggested that certain marketing or advertising practices aimed at children can be regulated by the FTC, even when no fraud or deception has occurred, because they target "children, too young to be capable of exercising an intelligent judgment of the transaction" and such practices "exploit consumers . . . who are unable to protect themselves" (*FTC v. R. F. Keppel & Brothers, Inc.*, 1934).

10. See *Central Hudson Gas & Electric Company v. Public Service Commission*, 1980; *Rubin v. Coors Brewing Company* (1995); *United States v. Edge Broadcasting Company*, 1993.

11. *Lorillard Tobacco Company v. Reilly*, 2001, at 556 (quoting Fla. Bar v. Went For It, Inc., 515 U.S. 618, 632 (1995) (quoting Bd. of Trustees of State Univ. of N.Y. v. Fox, 492 U.S. 469, 477 (1989).

12. "A commercial advertisement is constitutionally protected not so much because it pertains to the seller's business as because it furthers the societal interest in the 'free flow of commercial information.'" (Quoting *Virginia State Board of Pharmacy v. Virginia Citizens Consumer Council, Inc.*, 1976.)

13. "It is only when the decision to censor a school-sponsored [speech] . . . has no valid educational purpose that the First Amendment . . . require[s] judicial intervention to protect students' constitutional rights." (Quotations omitted.) (*Hazelwood School District v. Kuhlmeier*, 1988).

14. *Red Lion Broadcasting Company v. FCC*, at 376, 383, 389 (1969) (holding a broadcast licensee can, consistent with the First Amendment, be required to serve "as a proxy or fiduciary with obligations to present those views and voices which are representative of his community and which would otherwise, by necessity, be barred from the airwaves"); see also *Columbia Broadcasting System, Inc. v. Democratic National Committee*, 1973. In most areas of First Amendment jurisprudence, the rights of speakers are paramount. In the context of the broadcast media, however, the Court has said, "[T]he people as a whole retain their interest in free speech by radio and their collective right to have the medium function consistently with the ends and purposes of the First Amendment. It is the right of the viewers and listeners, not the right of the broadcasters, which is paramount." *Red Lion Broadcasting Company v. FCC* (1969).

15. Codified as amended in scattered sections of 47 U.S.C. (2002).
16. 47 U.S.C. § 303a(b) (2002). The Act applies to all television broadcasters including cable operators, home shopping stations, and educational, and noncommercial broadcasters. Policies and Rules Concerning Children's Television Programming (Memorandum Opinion and Order), 6 FCC Record 5093, paragraphs 4, 16, 44 (1991). The FCC exempts cable operators in circumstances where a "cable system's passive retransmission of a broadcast signal and its passive role with respect to access channel programming." *Id.* at para. 6. The FCC also exempts noncommercial broadcasters from the "record compilation, filing and submission requirements." *Id.* at para 45. Since March 2004, the Act has also applied to direct broadcast satellite (DBS). Implementation of Section 25 of the Cable Television Consumer Protection and Competition Act of 1992; Direct Broadcast Satellite Public Interest Obligations, 19 FCC Record 5647, paragraph 48 (2004).
17. Policies and Rules Concerning Children's Television Programming (Report and Order), 6 FCC Record. 2111, paragraph 3 (1991).
18. 6 FCC Record 5093, paragraph 39.
19. 6 FCC Record 2111, paragraph 44. The FTC also has promulgated rules regulating program-length commercials. These rules mandate certain disclosure requirements for program-length commercials.
20. Congress enacted the Children's Online Privacy Protection Act (COPPA) in 1998, and the FTC rules implementing the Act went into effect in April 2000. Children's Online Privacy Protection Rule, 16 C.F.R. § 312.1 et seq. (2005) (implementing COPPA).
21. The FCC also regulates some uses of Internet-related advertising. Under rules promulgated by the FCC, during television programming directed at children 12 years old and under, Internet website addresses can be displayed only if the website offers a substantial amount of *bona fide* program-related or other noncommercial content, the website is not primarily intended for commercial purposes (including either e-commerce or advertising), the website's home page and other menu pages are clearly labeled to distinguish noncommercial from commercial sections, and the page of the website to which viewers are directed by the website address is not used for e-commerce, advertising, or other commercial purposes. 47 C.F.R. § 73.670(b) (2004). In addition, website addresses cannot be displayed during a program or the commercials that air during that program if the website uses characters from the program to sell products or services.

H

Workshop Program

Marketing Strategies That Foster Healthy Food and Beverage
Choices in Children and Youth

Workshop sponsored by the
Institute of Medicine
Committee on Food Marketing and the Diets of Children and Youth

January 27, 2005
8:30 am–5:00 pm

Keck Center of The National Academies
500 Fifth Street, NW, Keck 100
Washington, DC 20001

Program

8:30 am   **Welcome, Introductions, and Overview of Open Session**
J. Michael McGinnis, Committee Chair

8:45 am   **Panel 1: Industry Perspectives**
Ellen Taaffe, M.S., Vice President, Health and Wellness
Marketing, PepsiCo Inc., Chicago, IL

9:00 am Lance Friedmann, M.B.A., Senior Vice President, Global
         Health and Wellness, Kraft Foods, Inc., Northfield, IL

9:15 am Marlena Peleo-Lazar, Chief Creative Officer and Vice
         President, McDonald's Corporation, Oak Brook, IL

9:30 am Ken Powell, M.B.A., Executive Vice President, General Mills,
         Inc., Minneapolis, MN

9:45 am **Committee Discussion with Panelists**

10:30 am **Break**

10:40 am **Panel 2: Youth-Focused Media and Marketing Perspectives**
         Marva Smalls, M.P.A., Executive Vice President, Public Affairs
         and Chief of Staff, Nickelodeon, TV Land, and Spike TV,
         New York, NY

11:00 am Bob McKinnon, Yellow Brick Road, New York, NY

11:20 am Morris Reid, Blue Fusion and Founding Partner and Managing
         Director, The Westin Rinehart Group, Washington, DC

11:40 am **Committee Discussion with Panelists**

12:30 pm **Lunch**

1:30 pm **Panel 3: Research Perspectives**
         Leann Birch, Ph.D., Distinguished Professor, Department of
         Human Development and Family Studies, The Pennsylvania
         State University, University Park, PA

1:50 pm Elizabeth Moore, Ph.D., Associate Professor of Marketing,
         University of Notre Dame, IN

2:10 pm Victoria Rideout, M.A., Vice President and Director, Program
         for the Study of Entertainment Media and Health, Henry J.
         Kaiser Family Foundation, Menlo Park, CA

2:30 pm **Committee Discussion with Panelists**

3:30 pm **Break**

3:45 pm   **Open Forum**
          Elizabeth Lascoutx, The Children's Advertising Review Unit
          William Cochran, Geisinger Clinic and American Academy of
             Pediatrics (AAP) Representative
          David McCarron, Shaping America's Youth
          David Gipp, United Tribes Technical College
          Warlene Gary, National PTA
          Keith Scarborough, Association of National Advertisers
          Susan Laramee, American Dietetic Association
          David Katz, Partnership for Essential Nutrition
          Margo Wootan, Center for Science in the Public Interest
          Elizabeth Pivonka, Produce for Better Health Foundation
          Richard Martin, Grocery Manufacturers of America
          Patti Miller, Children Now
          Bill MacLeod, Collier Shannon Scott, PLLC
          Wendy Miller, Beaumont Healthy Kids Program, William
             Beaumont Hospital
          Karen Tucker, American Association of Family and Consumer
             Sciences
          Diana Zuckerman, National Research Center for Women and
             Families

5:00 pm   **Adjourn**

I

Biographical Sketches of Committee Members and Staff

J. Michael McGinnis, M.D., M.P.P. *(Chair)*, is a Senior Scholar at the Institute of Medicine (IOM), The National Academies. He was previously Senior Vice President and Counselor to the President at the Robert Wood Johnson Foundation. He holds degrees in political science, medicine, and public policy from University of California, Berkeley, University of California, Los Angeles (UCLA), and Harvard University. For nearly three decades, he has been a participant in national prevention policy, including a continuous appointment—Assistant Surgeon General and Deputy Assistant Secretary for Health—throughout the Carter, Reagan, Bush, and Clinton Administrations, from 1977 to 1995, with responsibility for coordinating health-promotion and disease-prevention activities. From 1978 to 1995, he was Chairman of the Nutrition Policy Board at the U.S. Department of Health and Human Services (DHHS). Internationally, Dr. McGinnis held leadership positions in 1974–1975 to eradicate smallpox in India, and in 1995–1996 for the post-war reconstruction of the health sector in Bosnia. His academic work has included appointments as Scholar-in-Residence at the National Academy of Sciences and to the faculties of George Washington, Princeton, and Duke Universities. He has published numerous papers on health policy, public health, preventive medicine, nutrition, and tobacco, and served on various journal, scientific, and community boards. He is a member of the Institute of Medicine and a Fellow in the American College of Epidemiology and the American College of Preventive Medicine, and has received various public service awards. Recent IOM committee work includes the IOM Committee on Establishing a National Cord Blood

Stem Cell Bank Program, and the IOM Roundtable on Environmental Health Sciences, Research, and Medicine. Earlier National Academies' service includes the Food and Nutrition Board and the Committee on Agricultural Biotechnology, Health, and the Environment.

Daniel R. Anderson, Ph.D., is a Professor in the Department of Psychology at the University of Massachusetts. He received his Ph.D. in psychology from Brown University. Dr. Anderson's research focuses on children and television, particularly the cognitive and educational aspects. His published work concerns attention, comprehension, viewing behavior, and the long-term impact of television on children's development. Dr. Anderson's current research interests include toddler understanding of television, the effects of adult background television on infant and toddler behavior, and brain activation during television viewing. He is currently on national advisory boards for PBS Ready to Learn, Children's Digital Media Center (CDMC), and the Children's Advertising Review Unit of the Council of Better Business Bureaus. Dr. Anderson has been involved in the development of many television programs, including *Allegra's Window, Gullah Gullah Island, Bear in the Big Blue House, Blue's Clues,* and *Dora the Explorer.* He was also an advisor to *Captain Kangaroo, The Wubbulous World of Dr. Seuss, Sesame Street,* and *Fimbles* (BBC).

J. Howard Beales III, Ph.D., is an Associate Professor of Strategic Management and Public Policy at George Washington University in Washington, DC. From 2001 to early August 2004, Dr. Beales served as Director of the Bureau of Consumer Protection at the Federal Trade Commission (FTC), where he was responsible for the development and implementation of the National Do Not Call Registry. Dr. Beales received his Ph.D. in economics from the University of Chicago and his B.A. in economics from Georgetown University. Dr. Beales began his career at the FTC in 1977 as an economist specializing in consumer protection. In 1981, he was appointed Assistant to the Director of the Bureau of Consumer Protection, the first economist to hold that position, and served as Associate Director for Policy and Evaluation in the Bureau from 1983 to 1987. He developed policy in a number of key areas, including the Commission's Deception and Advertising Substantiation Policy Statements. Dr. Beales left the FTC in 1987 for a 1-year appointment as Branch Chief in the Office of Management and Budget's Office of Information and Regulatory Affairs, where he managed the review of regulations proposed by the Departments of Labor, Health and Human Services (DHHS), Housing and Urban Development, and Treasury. His areas of expertise include consumer research, contract law, economics of commercial free speech, applied microeconomics, marketing and advertising, public policy toward business, and safety and health regulations.

David V. B. Britt, M.P.A., is the retired President and Chief Executive Officer of the Sesame Workshop. Mr. Britt's professional experience includes executive positions with the U.S. Agency for International Development, Equal Employment Opportunity Commission, and the Overseas Private Investment Corporation. He has presented to various congressional committees on media and informal education, federal support of educational media, advertising limits, and mandatory educational programming requirements for commercial television. Since his retirement, Mr. Britt has been engaged in consulting and leadership development for nonprofit organizations. He is currently a Director of the Education Trust and Board Chair of Kids Voting USA. Mr. Britt is a member of the Council on Foreign Relations. He is also a member of the Board of Advisors for the Initiative on Social Enterprise at the Harvard Business School, as well as the Hauser Center at the Kennedy School of Government at Harvard University. He is a former member of the Board on Children, Youth, and Families (BCYF). He received a B.A. from Wesleyan University and an M.P.A. from the John F. Kennedy School of Government at Harvard University.

Sandra L. Calvert, Ph.D., is a Professor of Psychology at Georgetown University and the Director of the Children's Digital Media Center (CDMC). She received her Ph.D. in developmental and child psychology from the University of Kansas. Dr. Calvert's interdisciplinary work, spanning the fields of psychology, communications, public policy, and education, seeks to improve the well-being of children and adolescents by bridging the gap between knowledge generation and knowledge application. She has examined social policy issues revolving around the Children's Television Act, in which broadcasters are legally required to provide educational and informational television programs for children. She is currently examining the role that interactivity and identity play in children's learning from entertainment media at the CDMC, a National Science Foundation-based research consortium at Georgetown University, the University of California, Riverside, the University of California, Los Angeles, Northwestern University, and the University of Texas at Austin. She has received additional support for the CDMC from the Stuart Family Foundation. Dr. Calvert is a fellow of the American Psychological Association and a member of the Society for Research in Child Development and the International Communication Association. Dr. Calvert previously served on the National Academy of Sciences Committee which assessed Tools and Strategies for Protecting Children from Pornography and Other Objectionable Content on the Internet. In 2005, she received the Applied or Public Research Award from the International Communication Association. Professor Calvert has consulted for Nickelodeon Online, Sesame Workshop, and *Blue's Clues* to influence the development of children's television programs, computer and Internet software, and online educational games.

Keith T. Darcy, M.B.A., is the Executive Director of the Ethics Officer Association in Waltham, MA. Previously, he served as Chairman and Chief Executive Officer of Darcy Partners, Inc. (DPI). He has combined a 30-year career in the financial services industry with his profession as an educator and his long-term involvement in business ethics, corporate governance, and organizational leadership. DPI consults with boards and senior executives in the areas of leadership, ethics, governance, and reputation risk, as well as the alignment of corporate culture, brand loyalty, and organizational performance. Mr. Darcy currently serves on the boards of directors of E*Trade Bank and New York National Bank, is Chairman of the Board of the Better Business Bureaus Foundation, and chairs its Audit Committee. Additionally he is Director Emeritus of the Ethics Officer Association. Mr. Darcy teaches *Ethics & Leadership* in the Executive Programs at the Wharton School at the University of Pennsylvania. He is also Executive-in-Residence at the University of Maryland University College; a Teaching Fellow at the R. H. Smith School of Business, University of Maryland; and Executive-in-Residence at Manhattanville College, Purchase, NY. Mr. Darcy is an Executive Fellow and Vice Chairman of the Center for Business Ethics at Bentley College in Waltham, MA. In addition, he moderates programs for the Aspen Institute in Aspen, Colorado. He previously served as Associate Dean and Distinguished Professor of Business at Georgetown University's McDonough School of Business. Mr. Darcy holds a B.S. from Fordham University's College of Business and an M.B.A. from the Hagan Graduate School of Business at Iona College, and has completed additional post-graduate study at New York Theological Seminary.

Aimée Dorr, Ph.D., is the Dean of the UCLA Graduate School of Education and Information Studies. She received her Ph.D. in developmental psychology from Stanford University. Her research interests include the role of electronic media in formal and informal education and socialization; processes by which young people make sense of, utilize, and are affected by electronic media; and media literacy. Dr. Dorr's professional memberships include the American Educational Research Association, American Library Association, American Psychological Association, International Communication Association, National Society for the Study of Education, and Society for Research in Child Development among others. She is the Co-chair of Educational Outreach for UCLA. Dr. Dorr has been a consultant for numerous television and other media-related projects, most recently *La*

Opinión, a Los Angeles Spanish-language daily newspaper for the Latino Parents Awareness Campaign, and a Spanish-language guide to K–12 standards and college preparation. She is currently consulting for KCEd, an initiative using public television and the Internet to educate and train child caregivers, and she serves as a member of the Board of Educational Advisers for the Children's Advertising Review Unit of the Better Business Bureaus.

Lloyd J. Kolbe, Ph.D., has held appointments in academic, private-sector, and federal agencies, and is currently Professor of Applied Health Science at Indiana University. He received his Ph.D. from the University of Toledo. Dr. Kolbe has served as President of the American School Health Association, Vice President of the International Union for Health Promotion and Education, Visiting Professor at Beijing Medical University, Lead for Health Promotion within the U.S.–Russian Joint Commission on Economic and Technological Cooperation, Chairman of the World Health Organization Expert Committee on School Health Programs, member of the U.S. Senior Biomedical Research Service, and founding Director of the Division of Adolescent and School Health at the U.S. Centers for Disease Control and Prevention. For his efforts to improve child and adolescent health, Dr. Kolbe has received awards given by the U.S. Public Health Service, the DHHS, and the International Union for Health Promotion and Education. Dr. Kolbe has authored more than 120 publications and he currently serves as Vice Chair of the BCYF's Committee on Adolescent Health and Development, a standing IOM committee.

Dale L. Kunkel, Ph.D., is a Professor of Communication at the University of Arizona in Tucson. He is the former Director of the University of California (UC) Santa Barbara Washington Program at the UC Washington Center in Washington, DC. He studies children and media issues from several diverse perspectives, including television effects research as well as assessments of media industry content and practices. Dr. Kunkel received his Ph.D. from the Annenberg School of Communication at the University of Southern California. He was awarded a Congressional Science Fellowship from the Society for Research in Child Development. During that fellowship he served as an advisor to Congress on children and media issues. Dr. Kunkel is considered an expert on children's media policy and has delivered invited testimony at hearings before the U.S. Senate, the U.S. House of Representatives, and the Federal Communications Commission. He is a former Chair of the American Psychological Association's Committee on Children, Youth, and Families, and was senior author on the scientific report of the APA Task Force on Advertising and Children in 2003. He served as a Principal Investigator on the National Television Violence Study (1994–98), and more recently directed projects examining the V-chip program ratings and sexual socialization messages supported by the Henry J. Kaiser Family Foundation.

Paul Kurnit, M.A., is Founder and President of Kurnit Communications and KidShop, two marketing consulting firms in Chappaqua, New York, and a Clinical Professor of Marketing at Pace University's Lubin School of Business. He earned an M.A. in communication (theory and media) from Queens College in New York City and a B.A. in communication (rhetoric and public address) from the University of Wisconsin. Mr. Kurnit has broad experience in marketing and communications, advertising, entertainment, brand strategy, new product development, and teaching with special expertise in youth and family marketing and cultural trends. He previously served as President of Griffin Bacal, a DDB Worldwide advertising agency, where he had oversight for advertising, promotion, and public relations for a wide range of clients including Hasbro, PepsiCo, General Mills, Pillsbury, and Nestlé as well as assignments from Disney, McDonald's, General Mills, Good Humor, Veryfine, Mead Johnson, and others. At Griffin Bacal, he created specialty business units to focus on a diverse range of marketing services including youth trend tracking (Trend Walk™), youth consulting (Kid Think Inc.™), and online research (LiveWire: Today's Families Online™). He also served as Executive Vice President of Sunbow Entertainment, producers of hundreds of half hours of children's television programming including, the Peabody Award receiving *The Great Space Coaster*, two after-school specials for CBS and ABC, and two network television series for Fox and CBS. Mr. Kurnit is a member of the Advertising Council Creative Review Committee and serves on the advisory boards of the Children's Advertising Review Unit (CARU) and the board of the Advertising Educational Foundation. Mr. Kurnit has contributed his expertise to a number of social marketing initiatives to address youth cheating, teen smoking, bias and diversity, marijuana use, child abuse, gender, and nutrition.

Robert C. Post, Ph.D., J.D., is the David Boies Professor of Law at Yale Law School in New Haven. He received his A.B. from Harvard College, his Ph.D. in the history of American civilization from Harvard University, and his J.D. from Yale Law School. Dr. Post served as a Law Clerk to Justice William J. Brennan on the U.S. Supreme Court and to David Bazelon on the U.S. Court of Appeals for the District of Columbia Circuit. He was an associate at the law firm of Williams & Connolly. For many years he was the Alexander F. and May T. Morrison Professor of Law at the University of California, Berkeley. Dr. Post's expertise includes constitutional law (with particular emphasis on the First Amendment), legal history, and jurisprudence. He has authored or co-authored more than 60 articles and edited several books. Dr. Post is a Councilor of the American Academy of Arts and Sciences.

Richard Scheines, Ph.D., is a Professor of Philosophy at Carnegie Mellon University in Pittsburgh, and holds courtesy appointments in the Center for Automated Learning and Discovery and the Human–Computer Interaction Institute. He received his B.A. in history from Hobart College and joined the Carnegie Mellon faculty after receiving his Ph.D. in history and philosophy of science from the University of Pittsburgh in 1987. Dr. Scheines' research focuses on the connections between causal structure and data, especially social science and behavioral science data. He has collaborated for more than two decades with statisticians and computer scientists on a project to characterize what can and cannot be learned about causal claims from statistical data in a variety of empirical settings, and to develop and implement algorithms for causal discovery. His research interests emphasize the problem of inferring the causal relations among latent variables, such as intelligence, which cannot be measured directly. He has applied this work to several policy areas, including estimating the effects of low-level exposure to lead on the cognitive capacities of children, and determining the effects of welfare reform on single mothers and their ability to effectively parent. Dr. Scheines currently receives support from the McDonnell Foundation for developing online courseware in causal and statistical reasoning. He has co-authored dozens of articles and three books on causal inference and causal discovery, and designed an online course in causal and statistical reasoning.

Frances H. Seligson, Ph.D., R.D., is a Nutrition Consultant and Adjunct Associate Professor in the Department of Nutrition at The Pennsylvania State University. She is retired as the Associate Director of Nutrition at Hershey Foods Corporation. During her tenure at Hershey Foods, she held the positions of Senior Manager of Nutrition and Food Safety, Manager of Nutrition and Food Safety, and Manager of Nutrition Affairs. She has also worked for The Procter & Gamble Company and was Assistant Professor of Nutrition at the University of North Carolina at Chapel Hill. Dr. Seligson received her undergraduate degree in dietetics from Drexel University in Philadelphia, completed a dietetic internship at the Massachusetts General Hospital in Boston, and earned a Ph.D. in nutrition from the University of California, Berkeley. She has published extensively in the areas of nutrition and food consumption. Her professional memberships include the American Society for Nutritional Sciences and the American Dietetic Association, and she has served on the IOM Committee on Use of Dietary Reference Intakes in Nutrition Labeling. Dr. Seligson is currently a consultant on scientific issues to Hershey Foods and has represented Hershey Foods on

International Life Sciences Institute technical committees on dietary lipids, carbohydrates, energy, and lifestyle and weight management. She also has consulted for the International Food Information Council Committee on Dietary Sugars and previously was involved with its childhood obesity prevention initiative.

Mary Story, Ph.D., R.D., is a Professor in the Division of Epidemiology and Associate Dean for Student and Academic Affairs in the School of Public Health at the University of Minnesota in Minneapolis. She is an Adjunct Professor in the Department of Pediatrics, School of Medicine at the University of Minnesota. Dr. Story received a Ph.D. in human nutrition science from Florida State University. Her M.S. is in food science. Dr. Story's research focuses on understanding factors related to eating behaviors of youth, and community-, school-, and family-based interventions for obesity prevention, healthful eating, and physical activity among children, adolescents, and families. Several projects have focused on working with low-income communities and communities of color. Her research also focuses on environmental interventions to promote healthful food choices. Dr. Story has received awards for her work with child and adolescent nutrition and obesity prevention from the American Public Health Association, American Dietetic Association, Association of State and Territorial Public Health Nutrition Directors, Minnesota Department of Health and Department of Pediatrics at the University of Minnesota. She is active in national professional associations and is the immediate past chair of the Food and Nutrition Section of the American Public Health Association. Dr. Story is currently on the editorial board for the *Journal of Adolescent Health* and the *Journal of the American Dietetic Association.*

Ellen A. Wartella, Ph.D., is the Executive Vice Chancellor and Provost of the University of California, Riverside. She is a Distinguished Professor of Psychology. Dr. Wartella received her Ph.D. in mass communications from the University of Minnesota. She studies the role of media in child development. Dr. Wartella was a co-principal investigator on the National TV Violence Study and is currently a co-principal investigator of the Children's Digital Media Center. She is also serving on the Kraft Food Global Health and Wellness Advisory Council, the Decade of Behavior National Advisory Committee, the Board of Trustees of Sesame Workshop, and the National Educational Advisory Board for CARU. Dr. Wartella is a member of the American Psychological Association and the Society for Research in Child Development and is the past President of the International Communication Association; she has recently been awarded the International Communication Association's Steven Chaffee Career Productivity Award. Dr. Wartella is a member of the Board on Children, Youth, and Families.

Jerome D. Williams, Ph.D., is the F. J. Heyne Centennial Professor in Communication in the Department of Advertising at the University of Texas at Austin (UT). He also holds a joint appointment in the Center for African and African American Studies. Prior to joining the UT faculty, he was a faculty member in the Marketing Department in Howard University's School of Business, where he was also Director of the Center for Marketplace Diversity. Prior to his appointment at Howard, he was a member of the Pennsylvania State University Marketing Department faculty for 14 years. During that period, he had a number of visiting appointments nationally and internationally. He has also worked for General Electric Company in Energy Systems Information and for the U.S. Department of Energy's Solar Energy Research Institute. Dr. Williams' research interests cover several areas in the business-to-business and consumer marketing domains, with emphasis on ethnic minority marketing. He has conducted research on long-term business relationships, industrial marketing communications and promotion, and consumer behavior involving marketing communications strategies. Dr. Williams has testified in a number of court cases as an expert witness on consumer response to advertising strategies. Dr. Williams received his Ph.D. in business administration and marketing from the University of Colorado.

FNB Liaison

Nancy F. Krebs, M.D., R.D., is an Associate Professor of Pediatrics and Section Head of Nutrition in the Department of Pediatrics at the University of Colorado School of Medicine. Dr. Krebs received her M.S. from the University of Maryland and her M.D. from the University of Colorado School of Medicine. Her expertise and research interests are in pediatrics and general nutrition, breast-feeding, nutrition support, and growth problems. She is a member of the American Academy of Pediatrics, American Society for Clinical Nutrition (ASCN), American Society for Nutritional Sciences, and American Dietetic Association. She has received numerous awards for excellence in teaching and was a recipient of the ASCN's Physician Nutrition Specialist Award.

IOM Staff

Rosemary Chalk is Director of the Board on Children, Youth, and Families within the Division of Behavioral and Social Sciences and Education and the Institute of Medicine within the National Academies. She has more than 17 years of experience directing studies on vaccines and immunization finance, educational finance, family violence, child abuse and neglect, and research ethics. From 2000 to 2003, Ms. Chalk was a part-time Study Director at the IOM. She also directed the child abuse/family violence research area at Child Trends, a nonprofit research center in Washington, DC, where she conducted studies on the development of child well-being indicators for the child welfare system. As part of her work at Child Trends and the National Academies, Ms. Chalk has directed a range of projects sponsored by the William T. Grant Foundation, Doris Duke Charitable Foundation, the Carnegie Corporation of New York, The David and Lucile Packard Foundation, and various agencies within the DHHS, among others. Earlier in her career, Ms. Chalk was a consultant and writer for a broad array of science and society research projects. She has authored publications on issues related to child and family policy, science and social responsibility, research ethics, and child abuse and neglect. She was the first Program Head of the Committee on Scientific Freedom and Responsibility of the American Association for the Advancement of Science from 1976 to 1986 and is a former Section Officer for the same organization. She served as a Science Policy Analyst for the Congressional Research Service at the Library of Congress from 1972 to 1975. She has a B.A. in foreign affairs from the University of Cincinnati.

Jennifer Appleton Gootman, M.A., is a Senior Program Officer in the Food and Nutrition Board (FNB) at the IOM. She recently completed an Ian Axford Fellowship in Public Policy, working and living in New Zealand with the purpose of publishing a report on New Zealand's national youth development strategy and related child and youth policies. Prior to the fellowship, she directed and disseminated two studies—*Community Programs to Promote Youth Development* and *Working Families and Growing Kids*—for the IOM and National Research Council's BCYF. She was previously a Social Science Analyst for the Office of Planning and Evaluation in the DHHS. Her work there focused on child and family policy for low-income families, including welfare reform, child care, child health, youth development, and teen pregnancy prevention issues. She has directed a number of community youth programs in Los Angeles and New York City, involving young people in leadership development, job preparedness, and community service. She received her B.A. in education and fine arts from the University of Southern California and her M.A. in public policy from the New School for Social Research.

Vivica I. Kraak, M.S., R.D., is a Senior Program Officer in the FNB at the IOM. In addition to staffing the congressionally mandated IOM study and subsequent report, *Preventing Childhood Obesity: Health in the Balance*, she is also the Co-study Director for the IOM study on Progress in Preventing Childhood Obesity. Prior to joining the IOM in 2002, she worked as a Clinical Dietitian at Columbia–Presbyterian Medical Center and as a Public Health Nutritionist specializing in HIV disease in New York City. From 1994 to 2000, she was a Research Nutritionist in the Division of Nutritional Sciences at Cornell University where she collaborated on several domestic and international food policy and community nutrition research initiatives. She has co-authored a variety of publications related to food security and community food systems, nutrition and HIV/AIDS, international food aid and food security, viewpoints about genetically engineered foods, use of dietary supplements, and the influence of commercialism on the food and nutrition-related decisions and behaviors of children and youth. She received her B.S. in nutritional sciences from Cornell University and completed a coordinated M.S. in nutrition and dietetic internship at Case Western Reserve University and the University Hospitals of Cleveland. She is a member of the American Public Health Association and the American Dietetic Association.

Linda D. Meyers, Ph.D., is Director of the FNB at the IOM, and has also served as the Deputy Director and a Senior Program Officer in FNB. Prior to joining the IOM in 2001, she worked for 15 years in the Office of Disease Prevention and Health Promotion in the DHHS where she was a Senior Nutrition Advisor, Deputy Director, and Acting Director. Dr. Meyers has received a number of awards for her contributions to public health, including the Secretary's Distinguished Service Award for *Healthy People 2010* and the Surgeon General's Medallion. Dr. Meyers has a B.A. in health and physical education from Goshen College in Indiana, an M.S. in food and nutrition from Colorado State University, and a Ph.D. in nutritional sciences from Cornell University.

Leslie J. Sim is a Research Associate in the FNB at the IOM and also provides Web support for all of the FNB activities. In 2003, she received recognition within FNB as a recipient of an IOM inspirational staff award. Ms. Sim has previously worked both as a Teaching Assistant and Laboratory Assistant for an undergraduate food science laboratory class. She is also working on a military nutrition study to determine if modifications are needed in the military ration composition to prevent possible adverse health and performance consequences of consuming such rations while in short-term high-stress situations. Previously, she has worked on other military nutrition reports including *Caffeine for the Sustainment of Mental Task Performance*; *High-Energy, Nutrient-Dense Emergency Relief Food Product*; *Weight Management: State of the Science and Opportunities for Military Programs*; *Monitoring Metabolic Status: Predicting Decrements in Physiological and Cognitive Performance*; and most recently *Nutritional*

Needs for Short-Term, High-Stress Operations. Ms. Sim also provided research support for the IOM reports, *Infant Formula: Evaluating the Safety of New Ingredients* and *Dietary Reference Intakes: Applications in Dietary Planning.* She received a B.S. in biology with an emphasis on food science from Virginia Tech.

Shannon L. Wisham is a Research Associate in the FNB at the IOM where she staffed the congressionally mandated IOM study and subsequent report, *Preventing Childhood Obesity: Health in the Balance.* She has also worked on several National Research Council reports, including *Partnerships for Reducing Landslide Risk, Fair Weather: Effective Partnerships in Weather and Climate Services,* and *Resolving Conflicts Arising from the Privatization of Environmental Data.* She has been with the National Academies since 2001. She holds a B.A. in environmental science from LaSalle University in Philadelphia. Previously, she worked as a Researcher for Booz-Allen & Hamilton in the Environmental Protection Agency's Region 3 Comprehensive Environmental Response, Compensation, and Liability Act/Superfund Records Center.

Index

Research
dietary assessment methods, 50–51
ecological perspective, 26–28
goals, 23–24
on healthful diet promotion, 304
international efforts, 32–33, 300–302
on labeling to communicate nutritional
content, 378
on marketing other than television, 302,
304
on marketing products other than food
and beverage, 234–235
marketing research by food and
beverage industry, 135, 142–143,
190–191, 233, 376–377
on marketing to youth, 6, 23, 33–34, 380
measurement issues, 303, 304, 309
methodology, 24–28
proprietary, 7, 15, 34, 143, 377, 387
recommendations for, 15, 303–306, 309,
386–387
shortcomings of, 7, 30, 302–303, 374–375
for social marketing, 334, 339
See also Data sources; Systematic
evidence review
Restaurants
advertising spending, 164
beverage consumption patterns in, 68
brand loyalty, 104
calorie intake from, 71–72, 113, 375
consumption patterns and trends in,
113–115, 151
diet quality in, 114
neighborhood sociodemographic
characteristics and, 114–115
nutrition labeling requirements for, 323–
324
portion sizes, 71, 102
promotion of healthful diets in, *10*, 204–
205, 210–211, 374
proximity to schools, 114
recommendations for health promoting
practices, 11, 382
regional variation in eating behaviors, 82
sales, 113–114, 151
See also Fast food and quick serve
restaurants
Retail outlets
children's influence on food choices,
103, 155
consumer behavior, 150, 151
consumer use of food labels, 324

food sales, 144
health promotion efforts, 205, 378
in-store product requests, 102–104
marketing strategies, 150
neighborhood characteristics, 115–116
product offerings, 146
recommendations for product displays,
11–12, 383
supermarket revenues, 150
trade promotion in, 137–138
trends, 151
Riboflavin intake
current sources, 56
regional variation, 81
trends, 54–55
Rice, 61
Rickets, 44

S

Sales promotion, 137
Salty taste, 94
Saturated fats in youth diet
associated health risks, 1–2, 43
current concerns, 2, 18
dietary recommendations and guidelines,
57, 58
economic status and, 80
family meal contents, 109
healthy and balanced diet, 45
patterns, 19, 49, 57, 58, 82
sources, 56
School Breakfast Program, 14, 78–79, 112,
121, 122, 326, 328, 386
School Meals Initiative, 322
Schools, 112–113
after-school programs, 14, 111, 386
calorie intake in, 71–72, 112
contracts for food and beverage sales,
188, 329–330
food choices in, 112–113
food programs, 14, 41, 64, 79, 111,
112, 121, 122, 327–328, 386
industry self-regulation of marketing in,
200, 203, 206–207
industry-sponsored educational
materials, 190, 326
marketing practices and trends, 187–
190, 377
media literacy training in, 326–327
nutrition education interventions, 322,
323, 325–326